Biological
Responses in Cancer

Volume 4

Biological Responses in Cancer

Series Editor
ENRICO MIHICH
Grace Cancer Drug Center
Roswell Park Memorial Institute
Buffalo, New York

Biological Responses in Cancer

Volume 4

Edited by
Enrico Mihich

Grace Cancer Drug Center
Roswell Park Memorial Institute
Buffalo, New York

PLENUM PRESS • NEW YORK AND LONDON

The Library of Congress cataloged the first volume in this series as follows:

Main entry under title:

Biological responses in cancer.

Includes bibliographical references and index.
1. Cancer—Immunological aspects. 2. Immune response. I. Mihich, Enrico.
[DNLM: 1. Neoplasms—Physiopathology. 2. Cell transformation, Neoplastic. 3.
Neoplasm invasiveness. 4. Neoplasm metastasis. QZ 202 B6157]
RC268.3.B56   1982   616.99′4079   82-18041

ISBN 978-1-4684-1238-3   ISBN 978-1-4684-1236-9 (eBook)
DOI 10.1007/978-1-4684-1236-9

© 1985 Plenum Press, New York
Softcover reprint of the hardcover 1st edition 1985

A Division of Plenum Publishing Corporation
233 Spring Street, New York, N.Y. 10013

CONTRIBUTORS

MOZEENA BANO, Laboratory of Pathophysiology, National Cancer Institute, National Institutes of Health, Bethesda, Maryland 20205

MAITREYI BHATTACHARJEE, Laboratory of Pathophysiology, National Cancer Institute, National Institutes of Health, Bethesda, Maryland 20205

YOON SANG CHO-CHUNG, Laboratory of Pathophysiology, National Cancer Institute, National Institutes of Health, Bethesda, Maryland 20205

PIETRO M. GULLINO, Laboratory of Pathophysiology, National Cancer Institute, National Institutes of Health, Bethesda, Maryland 20205

GLORIA H. HEPPNER, Michigan Cancer Foundation, Detroit, Michigan 48201

FREESIA L. HUANG, Laboratory of Pathophysiology, National Cancer Institute, National Institutes of Health, Bethesda, Maryland 20205

C. LAL KAPOOR, Laboratory of Pathophysiology, National Cancer Institute, National Institutes of Health, Bethesda, Maryland 20205

WILLIAM R. KIDWELL, Laboratory of Pathophysiology, National Cancer Institute, National Institutes of Health, Bethesda, Maryland 20205

UNTAE KIM, Department of Pathology, Roswell Park Memorial Institute, Buffalo, New York 14263

LANCE A. LIOTTA, Laboratory of Pathology, National Cancer Institute, National Institutes of Health, Bethesda, Maryland 20205

GARTH L. NICOLSON, Department of Tumor Biology, The University of Texas–M. D. Anderson Hospital and Tumor Institute, Houston, Texas 77030

YOUCEF M. RUSTUM, Department of Experimental Therapeutics and Grace Cancer Drug Center, Roswell Park Memorial Institute, Buffalo, New York 14263

HARRY K. SLOCUM, Department of Experimental Therapeutics and Grace Cancer Drug Center, Roswell Park Memorial Institute, Buffalo, New York 14263

SUSAN J. TAYLOR, Laboratory of Pathophysiology, National Cancer Institute, National Institutes of Health, Bethesda, Maryland 20205

UNNUR P. THORGEIRSSON, Laboratory of Pathology, National Cancer Institute, National Institutes of Health, Bethesda, Maryland 20205

TAINA TURPEENNIEMI-HUJANEN, Laboratory of Pathology, National Cancer Institute, National Institutes of Health, Bethesda, Maryland 20205

BARBARA K. VONDERHAAR, Laboratory of Pathophysiology, National Cancer Institute, National Institutes of Health, Bethesda, Maryland 20205

PREFACE

The series of volumes entitled *Biological Responses in Cancer* provides information on approaches through which the interaction between neoplastic and normal cells may be modified. Topics discussed in various volumes include immunological and host defense systems, control mechanisms of cell and population growth, cell differentiation, and cell transformation. This volume is specifically concerned with various aspects of cell interactions and regulation within heterogeneous tumor cell populations, and their role in tumor progression and metastasis. Knowledge in this area is likely to provide new leads toward the exploitation of novel cellular sites and mechanisms in the development of new types of therapies of cancer. Several topics are discussed within these general areas of consideration. The possibly unique characteristics and mechanisms of tumor vascularization and the potential sites of interference with angiogenesis that might have therapeutic implications are critically evaluated. Tumor cell–normal tissue interactions involved in different phases of the growth and metastatic processes are discussed in two chapters dealing with mechanisms of tumor invasion and with the role of collagen in mammary tumor growth; here again potential leads are identified that may be exploited toward the development of new therapeutic approaches. The evolution of phenotypic diversity as a phenomenon complicating the biology of tumor metastasis and consequently affecting the opportunities offered by chemotherapy is also critically considered. Various aspects of tumor cell population heterogeneity are dealt with in three chapters using the mammary gland and tumor models as a focus for discussion: diversity in relation to hormone responsiveness, diversity in relation to differentiation and the onset of preneoplasia, and aspects of the genomic regulation of mammary carcinoma growth are considered as examples providing new leads for possible therapeutic intervention. The final chapter deals with the overall problem of tumor cell heterogeneity and its therapeutic implications.

Overall, the concept discussed in this volume is that fundamental biological aspects of cell regulation and cell population interactions are critical in attempts to develop novel types of therapies. The limitations of currently available therapies are also evident in light of the phenomena discussed. The large number of questions that need to be answered for an understanding and therapeutic exploitation of several of the phenomena discussed are outlined. It is hoped that this volume will contribute to progress in the areas discussed and will stimulate therapeutically oriented research through productive interactions among readers with diversified expertise.

ACKNOWLEDGMENT. The editor wishes to express appreciation for the excellent support provided by Ms. Jessie Crowe in editorial matters related to the preparation of this volume.

Buffalo, New York   Enrico Mihich

CONTENTS

CHAPTER 3

MAMMARY TUMOR GROWTH ARREST BY COLLAGEN
SYNTHESIS INHIBITORS

WILLIAM R. KIDWELL, MOZEENA BANO, AND SUSAN J. TAYLOR

CHAPTER 7

ROLE OF CYCLIC AMP IN MODIFYING THE GROWTH OF MAMMARY
CARCINOMAS: GENOMIC REGULATION

YOON SANG CHO-CHUNG, FREESIA L. HUANG, AND C. LAL KAPOOR

CHAPTER 8

CELLULAR HETEROGENEITY OF HUMAN TUMORS: IMPLICATIONS FOR
UNDERSTANDING AND TREATING CANCER

HARRY K. SLOCUM, GLORIA H. HEPPNER, AND YOUCEF M. RUSTUM

CHAPTER 1

ANGIOGENESIS, TUMOR VASCULARIZATION, AND POTENTIAL INTERFERENCE WITH TUMOR GROWTH

PIETRO M. GULLINO

1. INTRODUCTION

The objective of this chapter is to evaluate the role that neovascularization may have in tumor growth and to assess the present knowledge of tumor angiogenesis. New formation of a vascular network has been recognized to be indispensable for tumor growth since the transplantability of neoplastic tissues was first discovered. Increased knowledge of the angiogenic process is sought for two main purposes: (1) to define the possible relationship between acquisition of angiogenic capacity by a cell population and risk of its neoplastic transformation and (2) to investigate possibilities for effectively influencing angiogenesis and consequently tumor growth. Both questions will be discussed here after the pertinent characteristics of the tumor vascular network have been outlined.

2. THE VASCULAR NETWORK AS A COMPONENT OF THE NEOPLASTIC TISSUE

2.1. Vascular and Interstitial Compartments in Tumors

The angioarchitecture of tumors was initially studied with the hope of improving the biological characterization of neoplastic tissues. It became

---

PIETRO M. GULLINO • Laboratory of Pathophysiology, National Cancer Institute, National Institutes of Health, Bethesda, Maryland 20205.

rapidly apparent that the approach was rewarding only in the area of diagnosis. Visualization of the vascular network, particularly in metastatic growth, often shows changes in the normal angioarchitecture of the host tissue that have diagnostic value.

From the time when tumors were induced in tar-painted mice, the alteration of the vascular network in the dermis and hypodermis had been observed to represent an early event of the carcinogenesis process (Kreyberg, 1927). Direct observation of tumor explants within a transparent chamber has repeatedly shown that lack of vessel proliferation results in failure of tumor growth. Indeed, production of capillaries was particularly intense around rapidly growing tumors and appearance of vascular buds required only 2–3 days, while around slower growing implants 8 days or more were required for capillary budding. (Ide et al., 1939; Algire et al., 1945, 1947; Algire and Legallais, 1947).

The initial formation of capillaries around a tumor implant consists of a dense and highly unpatterned brush that becomes incorporated into the invading neoplastic population. Later the architecture of the capillary bed is dictated by the growth patterns of the cell population, i.e., a lobular arrangement may have a basketwork type of capillary pattern and poorly differentiated areas have no consistent architecture (Warren, 1979; Shubik, 1982).

An important point to be emphasized is the behavior of the arterial system in the organ invaded by the tumor. In general, the arteries of the infiltrated tissue persist and become part of the tumor vascular system. Documentation of this event can be clearly obtained in tumors implanted into a kidney. Vinylate casts of the arterial vessels show that the main branches supplying the kidney become the main vessels supplying the invading tumor. The original arteries are "stretched" to supply a tumor mass severalfold larger than the kidney itself (Gullino and Grantham, 1964).

This observation is important because of a common misconception that blood to the neoplastic cell population is supplied by a unitary and homogeneous network. The neoplastic cells invade the normal host tissue by commandeering the supply of blood via new formation of capillary-type vessels and incorporation of host vessels. The arteries, in particular, are preserved for a long time with most of their structures intact. Results of treatments that are supposed to change the supply of blood to a tumor will, therefore, depend a good deal on the degree of preservation of the host network. Because this is a parameter impossible to evaluate, and quite variable from one tumor to another, the data on drug action on tumor blood supply are poorly reproducible, as the literature shows.

Since the host supplies the newly formed vessels to the growing tumor, is the size of the vascular compartment controlled by the host or by the neoplastic cell population? There is evidence that the latter is the case. In a series of carcinogen-induced hepatocarcinomas transplanted in rats, the size of the vascular space varied from $4.5 \pm 0.6\%$ to $12.4 \pm 0.3\%$ of tissue weight, but remained constant for each tumor type regardless of the transplantation site. Moreover, two different neoplastic cell populations isolated from the same tumor produced two tumor types upon transplantation, one with a vascular space of 8.0 ± 0.8% and the other of 12.4 ± 0.3% of tissue weight. This difference persisted over many transplant generations, suggesting that a permanent change in the neoplastic cell population corresponded to a permanent change in the vascular space of the growing tumor (Gullino and Grantham, 1964).

These conclusions are based on data obtained in tumors of a few grams and by relying on the diffusion of markers within the tumor vascular network. Morphometric analysis, on the other hand, confirmed the relative stability of the average vascular space of growing tumors (Hilmas and Gillette, 1975) but also showed that a continuous change in the capillarylike portion of the tumor network occurs as the tumor grows. These vessels tend to become larger and shorter. Consequently, even if the total vascular volume does not change substantially, the surface and therefore the functional efficiency of the network is reduced as time passes (Vogel, 1965).

The possibility of reaching the cell population of a tumor via the vascular network is also profoundly influenced by the interstitial compartment, i.e., the area between the capillary wall and the cell outer membrane. Three characteristics of the tumor interstitial compartment are usually not fully appreciated: the size, the anisotropy, and the lack of an anatomically stable lymphatic network. In rat hepatocarcinomas the interstitial water space was evaluated by marker diffusion and was found to constitute 40–50% of the tumor water, i.e., an amount about three times larger than that of the liver (Gullino et al., 1965). In rat sarcomas, the extracellular volume was estimated at 0.35–0.50 ml/g tissue as compared with 0.13 ml/g in the muscles that originated the sarcoma (Appelgren et al., 1973). In human gliomas, the intracellular space was 20–40% as compared to 6–7% in normal brain tissue as evaluated by electron microscopy (Bakay, 1970).

The reasons for this enlarged interstitial compartment of tumors are not clear. One possibility can be related to the lack of anatomically well defined lymphatic vessels within the compartment. We calculated that 5–10% of the fluid passing through the tumor vessels does not return to the general circulation via the venous route; instead, it oozes out at the tumor surface through the interstitial compartment (Butler et al., 1975). The hydrostatic pressure generated within the interstitial compartment of the tumor, as measured with a micropore chamber attached to a manometer, was found to be consistently higher than the pressure in the subcutaneous tissue into which the tumor was transplanted (Butler et al., 1975). Values up to 30 mm H_2O were measured, indicating that interstitial fluid pressures may reach levels sufficient to collapse capillaries.

The effects of this hypertension on tissue necrosis are difficult to assess, but are probably relevant. The increase in pressure may be the consequence of fluid drainage across a compartment lacking preformed lymphatic channels. Indeed, the presence of convective currents within the interstitial compartment of tumors was revealed by the spread of pyronine dyes along irregular directions at a rate greater than that predictable by diffusion alone (Reinhold, 1971). The entity of these currents and their possible importance in transferring molecules within the tumor extracellular space depend on the blood supply and the anisotropy of its distribution.

2.2. Blood Flow and Regional Supply in Tumors

Conventionally, the term *blood flow to a tumor* refers to the total volume of blood entering or leaving the whole tumor and also to the volume flow distributed within a tumor. The two concepts must be kept separated.

Measurement of total volume of blood requires a tumor isolated from the vascular network of the invaded tissues. This was obtained in preparations in which neoplastic cells implanted into a rat ovary (30 mg) produced tumors 3–6 g in size and growing within a paraffin sack. Since only the ovarian artery and vein supplied the tumor, blood flow of the whole tumor was evaluated by cannulating the ovarian vein and measuring the tumor efferent blood. Isolation from the surrounding tissues was guaranteed by the paraffin sack. The absence of the original ovarian network was insured by the extensive tumor growth (100- to 200-fold larger than the host organ). Indeed, vinylate casts of the vascular system revealed the destruction of the ovarian network and its substitution with a newly formed tumor-induced network.

With this approach, we observed that rat hepatocarcinomas 3–10 g in size had a blood supply 10- to 20-fold smaller than that in normal rat liver, and decreasing per unit weight as the tumor volume increased (Gullino and Grantham, 1961a,b). In chemically induced primary mammary carcinoma, the efferent blood was found to be 0.03–0.13 ml/min per g in tumors grown isolated from the surrounding tissues and weighing 2.0–3.5 g (Gullino and Grantham, 1962). Comparable values were later obtained by Vaupel (1975) using a similar approach. By plethysmography, which can be considered a method measuring arterial inflow (Appelgren, 1982), values of 0.22–0.58 ml/min per g of tissue have been obtained for 20-methycholanthrene-induced carcinomas (Kjartansson *et al.*, 1976).

Indirect methods using tracers of different nature have been extensively utilized to measure blood supply, particularly in humans. The blood flow of primary human hepatocarcinomas was found to be 12 ± 6 ml/min per 100 g tissue as contrasted with 29 ± 10 ml/min per 100 g in normal liver (Plengvanit *et al.*, 1972). Using ^{133}Xe clearing techniques in human tumors, Mäntylä *et al.* (1976) measured a blood flow of 38 ± 14 ml/min per 100 g in lymphomas, 11 ± 5 ml/min per 100 g in anaplastic carcinomas, and 14 ± 9 ml/min per 100 g in differentiated malignant tumors.

The large number of blood flow determinations done with a variety of methods points to one general conclusion, i.e., the overall blood supply to growing tumors in humans, as well as in experimental animals, is usually smaller than that to the normal tissue of origin. It is a common misconception that a fast growing tumor should be "well vascularized" because it requires a "good" blood supply. In our experience, the blood supply to a 30-mg rat ovary is sufficient to sustain the growth of a 5123 hepatocarcinoma up to 6 g (200-fold) over a period of 25 days with little necrosis and without any enlargement or hypertrophy of the ovarian artery, the only afferent vessel.

The limited overall supply of blood is only one aspect of the inefficiency of tumor blood flow; the anisotropy of blood distribution within the tumor vascular network is another important aspect.

Microcirculation in tumors has been analyzed primarily by the transparent chamber technique. The tumor is grown between two transparent plates as a thin sheet of cells supported by a band of host connective tissue, often rich in inflammatory-type vessels. In the anesthesized animal the vessels are examined with a microscope adapted for *in vivo* observation and video techniques. Capillaries and precapillary vessels within the tumor are compared with adjacent vessels of regions not invaded by neoplastic cells. Some consistent events are observed regardless of tumor type: a redundant development of enlarged, venous-type vessels occurs at the periphery of the tumor implant; the newly developing vessels sprout mostly from veins; the structure and functions of single arteries appear to be only slightly affected by the spreading tumor; large fluctuations of red blood cell velocity within the capillaries consistently occur; regurgitation and intermittent circulation, i.e., stasis followed by resumption of flow, sometimes in a direction opposite to the previous one, are often observed. The total numbers of nonflowing capillaries varied greatly during the observation period and tissue pressure appeared to be the dominant cause of flow arrest (Ide *et al.*, 1939; Eddy and Casarett, 1973; Intaglietta *et al.*, 1977; Endrich *et al.*, 1979). The presence of arteriovenous shunting was observed in several tumor types (Göthlin, 1977; Reinhold, 1979). In areas of stabilized tumor microcirculation, Endrich *et al.* (1979) measured perfusion rates of 0–101 ml/min per 100 g with a high average of 15–18 ml/min per 100 g; toward the center of the tumor the perfusion rate dropped to an average of 2–4 ml/min per 100 g.

These and similar results show that it is unrealistic to assign a single value to the blood perfusion rate of a tumor. Inhomogeneity of blood perfusion is, therefore, both local and temporal.

The diffusion coefficients of circulating molecules appear to be higher in tumors, particularly for macromolecules. This was predicted from the frequently incomplete structure of the newly formed tumor capillaries. Nugent and Jain (1984), for instance, observed that tissue diffusion coefficients for intravascular transport of a 19,400-MW fluorescein–isothiocyanate–dextran conjugate were 2.3 and 7.5 for granulation tissue and tumor capillaries, respectively, and the diffusion coefficients were 0.061 and 1.9 for a 62,000-MW conjugate. These values, however, must be considered only a rough indication of the vascular–extravascular exchange because the fluid distribution in the extracellular compartment is highly heterogeneous. For instance, the extravasation velocity of "pyranin," a water-soluble nontoxic and nonbinding dye, was found to range from 25 μm/sec to values lower than 1 μm/sec (Reinhold, 1979).

The differences of the intravascular pressure in various parts of the microcirculatory circuit, the high pressure of the interstitial fluid mentioned earlier, and the permeability characteristics of the vessel walls contribute to making the extravascular fluid distribution in tumors highly unpredictable and anisotropic. Consequently, the microcirculatory network of a tumor is a system in which every section is continuously subjected to fluctuations of blood flow which, in turn, produce highly variable perfusion rates of the extravascular compartment. This situation is responsible for a highly heterogeneous environment around the neoplastic cell population. For instance, we were surprised to find differences in temperature of up to 2°C between two regions of the same tumor just millimeters apart (Gullino et al., 1982). To the well recognized heterogeneity of the cell populations, one must add the heterogeneity of the environment existing in vivo within each tumor. However inefficiently, the neoplastic cell population is able to induce the host to produce a vascular network sufficient to sustain tumor growth. The understanding of the mechanism of this induction may offer an approach to alter or block tumor growth.

3. ACQUISITION OF ANGIOGENIC CAPACITY AND RISK OF NEOPLASTIC TRANSFORMATION

The ability to induce neovascularization has been studied for a variety of tissues, cells, or extracts thereof. The methodology is usually based on implanting the angiogenesis effectors into an appropriate location where neoformation of vessels can be easily detected, such as the cornea of the rabbit or the chorioallantoic membrane of the chicken (Gullino, 1981). The tests in vivo require special care in both execution and interpretation because of the frequency of interfering events, such as inflammation, that make the results unreliable. Using these approaches, results from the literature indicate that, in general, normal adult tissues are rarely angiogenic while neoplastic tissues are frequently angiogenic (Folkman and Cotran, 1976; Gullino, 1981).

To study the acquisition of angiogenic capacity we selected two models, the subcutaneous fibroblasts and the mammary epithelium of the adult mouse and rat. These cells are angiogenic in less than 5% of implants under physiological conditions, but induce angiogenesis in more than 70% of implants when neoplastically transformed. We first tested whether angiogenic capacity was acquired during carcinogenesis. BALB/c fibroblasts, removed from the subcutaneous region, are not angiogenic in the rabbit cornea assay. When cultivated in vitro in a standard medium (DMEM + 10% calf serum), the fibroblasts remained not angiogenic for the first three culture passages. At passage 4, about 50% of the implants induced an angiogenic response and at passage 7 practically all implants were angiogenic in the rabbit cornea assay (Ziche and Gullino, 1982). When the fibroblasts of passage 7 were reinjected into the subcutaneous tissue of the donor or into a syngeneic mouse, a tumor was never observed. Production of a sarcoma occurred at culture passages 18–20, not before. Thus, in this model, angiogenic capacity was acquired during neoplastic transformation, but long before the fibroblasts were neoplastic, i.e., had the capacity to form a sarcoma in vivo (Ziche and Gullino, 1982).

Comparable findings were obtained in another model of carcinogenesis in vivo. It is known that plastic coverslips implanted in the subcutaneous tissue of CBA mice produce a sarcoma (Brand, 1975). When the plastic coverslip is 25 × 15 × 0.2 mm in size, the first sarcomas usually appear after 6–7 months and by 16 months almost every mouse has a tumor. We implanted coverslips in the subcutaneous tissue of CBA adult mice, but removed them after 2–4 weeks, i.e., long before any tumor was present or was expected to occur. At this time a layer of cells adhered to the plastic and was tested for angiogenic activity. While normal subcutaneous tissue is not angiogenic, the cells attached to the plastic, i.e., the cells that several months later would have produced a sarcoma, already showed an angiogenic response in 43% of corneal implants (Ziche and Gullino, 1981).

When the size of the plastic coverslip is small, i.e., 7 × 11 × 0.2 mm, sarcomas are still produced, but the first tumors appear about 15 months after the implant and about 70% of the animals die of old age before a sarcoma is evident (Brand, 1975). In the same CBA mouse, we implanted a large coverslip (25 × 15 × 0.2 mm) in the right lumbar region and a small coverslip (7 × 11 × 0.2 mm) in the left lumbar region. After 2–4 weeks, the coverslips were removed simultaneously and the angiogenic capacity of the cells attached to the plastic coverslip was tested. In the same rabbit, one cornea received cells from the large coverslip and the contralateral cornea received cells from the small coverslip. The angiogenic response of the cells from the large coverslip was four- to fivefold more frequent than that of the cornea implanted with the cells from the small coverslip. Thus, the cell population at higher risk of neoplastic transformation had acquired angiogenic capacity more rapidly than that at lower risk. This suggests that acquisition of angiogenic capacity by a cell population normally lacking it indicates a progression toward neoplastic transformation.

The validity of this hypothesis was tested in human mammary epithelium. Gaffney (1982) succeeded in cultivating an epithelial line from human milk that could be passaged in culture. At culture passage 6 there were enough cells available to us for a test of angiogenic activity: 4 out of 6 implants were found to be positive. The transplantation of these cells into athymic nude mice failed to produce a tumor. At culture passage 23 the cell population was tested again: 8 out of 13 implants were positive for angiogenesis, but transplantation into athymic nudes failed again to produce a tumor. Only at culture-passage 103 was the cell population able to form a tumor in athymic nudes, and at this time almost every implant induced angiogenesis in the cornea test. We concluded that for human mammary epithelium as well, the acquisition of angiogenic capacity preceded the neoplastic transformation as expressed by formation of a tumor in vivo.

The confirmation of this finding was pursued with two types of experiments in vivo.

The human mammary gland removed for a carcinoma is in the majority of cases particularly rich in hyperplastic ductal or lobular epithelium in areas distant from the tumor (Wellings and Rice, 1978). These lesions are often considered "preneoplastic," i.e., at higher risk than normal parenchyma of becoming neoplastic, although direct proof is lacking. We compared the angiogenic capacity of these hyperplastic lesions with that of the normal mammary tissue and found that, while the latter is only exceptionally angiogenic, 28% of the hyperplastic lesions were strongly angiogenic (S. Brem et al., 1978).

A situation similar to that in the human breast occurs in the mouse mammary gland. Females of the C3H A^{vy} strain show numerous hyperplastic lesions very early in life and by age 15 months almost all have breast cancer. This hyperplastic epithelium implanted in the mammary fat pad very often survives and colonizes the whole fat pad. From nodules of hyperplastic epithelium Medina (1973) developed two lines that are morphologically identical but have different behaviors. Both lines colonize the mammary fat pad and remain as a normal mammary tissue for the lifespan of the host. However, one line (D1) generates carcinomas in about 5% of implants, and the other line (D2) produces carcinomas in about 45% of implants.

We tested the angiogenic capacity of the D1 and D2 lines before any neoplastic transformation was evident and found that the D2 line induced an angiogenic response twice as frequently as the D1 line. Thus, the angiogenic response could indicate that D2 was at higher risk of neoplastic transformation than D1, despite the identical morphological appearance of the two lines and a histological picture of simple hyperplasia (Gimbrone and Gullino, 1976).

Strum (1983) has recently confirmed our observation that mammary hyperplastic lesions at high risk of neoplastic transformation have an angiogenic response much more frequent than normal parenchyma. An accurate evaluation in humans by Jensen et al. (1982) revealed a higher angiogenic capacity even in histologically normal lobules from a carcinoma-bearing breast as compared to a noncancerous breast.

An elevated angiogenic activity before a tumor is fully established has been demonstrated to occur in vivo (Cohen et al., 1980) during chemical carcinogenesis. Fisher 344 rats fed 0.2% N-[4-(5-nitro-2-furyl)-2-thiazolyl]formamide in the diet have tumors of the bladder epithelium within about 20 weeks of feeding. After 6 weeks of feeding small foci of nodular or papillary hyperplasia are already present in the bladder epithelium. Corresponding to these foci, a high-density plexus of narrow capillaries with multiple, short terminal branches is visible in the subepithelial plexus. Return to a normal diet after 6 weeks of feeding the carcinogen resulted in the return to normal of the epithelium within 4 weeks, and in the simultaneous disappearance of the capillary proliferation beneath the hyperplastic epithelium. Thus, angiogenic activity was present when the epithelium was in a "pre-neoplastic" state, and a reversal of the carcinogenic process was followed by a reversal of the vascular proliferation.

In the previous sections, it has been emphasized that formation and growth of a tumor are strongly dependent upon the new formation of a vascular network. Normal adult tissues in most cases do not have the capacity to induce neovascularization, but neoplastic tissues show angiogenic activity to a high frequency. Our experiments with fibroblasts and mammary epithelium suggest that angiogenic capacity is a property acquired in the course of neoplastic transformation and that it is present before unrestrained growth becomes the predominant characteristic of the tissue. Detection of angiogenic capacity in a tissue normally deprived of it could, therefore, be an important marker of progression toward neoplastic transformation, i.e., formation of a growing tumor in vivo. The experiments reported in this section support this hypothesis. However, the methodology presently available to evaluate the angiogenic capacity of a tissue is insufficient to permit routine clinical application for screening purposes. A better knowledge of the mechanism of angiogenesis is necessary to devise a test that may have value in detecting high-risk cell populations with accuracy.

4. MECHANISM OF ANGIOGENESIS

A blood vessel in its simplest structure consists of a continuous tube of endothelium limited by a basement membrane. Endothelial cells are able to produce a basement membrane (Howard et al., 1976); therefore, it is generally assumed that the endothelium is the protagonist in angiogenesis. From this premise, the formation of a capillary requires at least two events, mobilization and proliferation of endothelial cells. The study of the mechanism of angiogenesis has evolved through two stages. In the first, attention was focused on the angiogenic capacity of tissues or cells or fractions thereof; in the second stage the prevalent purpose was to find and characterize substances with chemotactic and/or growth-stimulating activity on the endothelium.

4.1. Angiogenesis by Tissues or Cells

In vivo transplantation techniques were used to evaluate the ability of normal tissues, adult or embryonic, to induce neovascularization. The rabbit cornea or chicken chorioallantoic membrane assay was predominantly utilized (Gullino, 1981). Most normal tissues are not angiogenic, but several exceptions were found: the testes of the 1-day-old mouse (Huseby et al., 1975), the corpus luteum (Jakob et al., 1977; Gospodarowicz and Thakral, 1978), the salivary gland (Hoffman et al., 1976), and the epithelium of the epidermis under particular circumstances (Nishioka and Ryan, 1972; Wolf and Harrison, 1973). On the contrary, most neoplastic tissues are strongly angiogenic (Folkman, 1974; Folkman and Cotran, 1976). In our experience, however, 10–20% of implants from a primary tumor strongly angiogenic in the rabbit cornea assay (Gimbrone et al., 1974) usually failed to induce neovascularization despite the presence in the negative implants of neoplastic tissue histologically similar to the tissue of the positive implants. Azizkhan et al. (1981) reported similar findings. These observations have a counterpart in normal tissue, as shown by an experiment reported by Federman et al. (1980). Retina from one eye of a New Zealand White rabbit was implanted into a corneal pocket of the contralateral eye. Fragments from the vascular retina induced new formation of limbal vessels that anastomosed with the vessels of the implant in 15 of 29 experiments. However, when fragments of the peripheral avascular retina were implanted under the same conditions, angiogenesis was not observed. Since the implant is autologous, one assumes that the events triggering angiogenesis should not represent an "immunological" type of response.

On the other hand, implants of mouse or rabbit lymph nodes or spleen were found to induce an angiogenic response in the chick chorioallantoic membrane assay (Auerbach et al., 1976). Autologous macrophages obtained from the peritoneal cavity and implanted in the cornea of the guinea pig showed angiogenic activity in only 8% of implants, but when they were activated in vivo by thioglycollate or paraffin oil, the angiogenic response increased to 75% of implants (Polverini et al., 1977). Similar observations were reported for murine spleen cells treated with the T-cell mitogen phytohemagglutinin and transferred to the chorioallantoic membrane of chicken eggs (Pliskin et al., 1980).

Angiogenic capacity has been attributed to a variety of other cell populations, i.e., neutrophils (Fromer and Klintworth, 1975a,b, 1976) (although angiogenesis in wound repair proceeds in neutropenic animals as effectively as in normal animals) (Stein and Levenson, 1966; Simpson and Ross, 1972); embryonic yolk sac cells (Auerbach and Sidky, 1978); mast cells (Kessler et al., 1976); cells from regenerating deer antler (Auerbach et al., 1976); vitreous body and retina (Glaser et al., 1980a; Chen and Chen, 1980); and hypothalamus (Maciag et al., 1979).

From all these observations, one conclusion seems justified: Angiogenesis can be triggered by a variety of effectors that could act through a common mechanism. The existence of an angiogenesis factor produced by a variety of tissues under the appropriate conditions was postulated (Folkman et al., 1971).

4.2. Angiogenesis Factors

The search for an angiogenesis factor(s) concentrated first on the neoplastic tissue, known to be strongly angiogenic. Several fractions of different degrees of characterization were reported to be angiogenic in vivo and to have an effect on endothelium *in vitro* (Tuan *et al.*, 1973; Phillips and Kumar, 1979; McAuslan and Hoffman, 1979; Fenselau *et al.*, 1981; Kumar *et al.*, 1983). Neoplastic tissue, however, was not the sole source of angiogenesis factors. Bovine parotid gland (Hoffman *et al.*, 1976); retina of human, bovine, and feline origin (Glaser *et al.*, 1980a); wound fluid (Greenburg and Hunt, 1978); and synovial fluid of patients with rheumatoid arthritis or ankylosing spondylitis (Brown *et al.*, 1980) were all found to contain angiogenesis factors apparently identical to that derived from tumors (Weiss *et al.*, 1983).

The work on tissue fractionation in search of factors able to induce neovascularization produced two observations important for the interpretation of the mechanism of angiogenesis: (1) Material of very small molecular weight (<500 MW) can trigger angiogenesis *in vivo* (Weiss *et al.*, 1979) and (2) several factors can be mitogenic or chemotactic or both on endothelial cells *in vitro* (Gospodarowicz *et al.*, 1977; Castellot *et al.*, 1980; Glaser *et al.*, 1980a–c; Banda *et al.*, 1982; Maciag *et al.*, 1982). Obviously, a chemotactic or mitogenic effect on endothelium in culture is not equivalent to an angiogenic event *in vivo*. However, the need to quantitate the effect of an angiogenesis factor expanded the experimental procedures from the utilization of *in vivo* assays useful primarily for detecting inducers of neovascularization (such as the rabbit cornea or the chick chorioallantoic membrane assays) into the *in vitro* measurements of migration and growth of endothelial cells capable of yielding quantitative data. Comparison of the results obtained with the *in vivo* and *in vitro* assays appears to be the most promising approach to increase our knowledge of the mechanism of angiogenesis.

We first addressed the question of whether the angiogenic activity displayed by neoplastic tissues *in vivo* was a property of the cell population or an event dependent on substances present in the fluid surrounding the cells, i.e., was the putative angiogenesis factor(s) excreted? A chamber with walls composed of millipore filters of average pore size less than 0.5 μm was implanted in rats in a pouch of subcutaneous tissue and about 200 mg of Walker carcinoma fragments were seeded around the chamber. Within a few days, a tumor developed and incorporated the chamber. The neoplastic cells grew against the filter, but did not penetrate into the chamber cavity, whereas the fluid surrounding the cells did penetrate and was sampled, lyophilized, and tested for angiogenic capacity in the rabbit cornea assay (Gimbrone *et al.*, 1974). The acellular fluid was angiogenic, but often produced an inflammatory response; the ethanol extract, however, was strongly angiogenic, but not inflammatory. We concluded that *in vivo* the putative angiogenesis factor(s) was present in the interstitial fluid of growing tumors (Ziche *et al.*, 1982).

We also observed that the tumor interstitial fluid was very rich in prostaglandins (PG) of E and $F_{2\alpha}$ species. The angiogenic capacity of several prostaglandins was then tested, and PGE_1 was found to be the most effective inducer of neovascularization in the rabbit cornea at a dosage unable to mobilize inflammatory-type cells (Ziche *et al.*, 1982). This observation confirmed a similar report by Ben Ezra (1979). The hypothesis that PGE_1 could be involved in the angiogenesis process was sustained by the effect of in-domethacin, which blocks production of prostaglandin. Corneal vasculari-zation induced by neoplastic cells could be prevented by intense indometh-acin treatment of the test rabbit (Ziche et al., 1982).

PGE$_1$ incorporated into slow-release Elvax pellets prepared according to the method of Langer and Folkman (1976) offered the opportunity to obtain a consistent and direct invasion of the cornea by capillaries originating from the limbal vessels. The capillary buds appeared 70–80 hr after pellet im-plantation. With this experimental model, we tested the composition of the corneal tissue during angiogenesis. In the same rabbit, one cornea was im-planted with PGE$_1$ and the contralateral cornea with PGI$_2$ or PGE$_2$ at a dose of 1 μg for each pellet, i.e., a dose angiogenic for PGE$_1$ but not angiogenic for PGI$_2$ or PGE$_2$. About 80 hr after implantation, the fragment of cornea underlying the pellet was removed. (The time of 80 hr was selected on the assumption that determinations should be done before the capillary invasion of the cornea altered any change which might occur at a time when the cornea was ready for vascular penetration.) We found that copper ion con-centration was enhanced within the cornea treated with PGE$_1$, as compared with the contralateral cornea of the same rabbit treated with PGE$_2$ or PGI$_2$, not angiogenic. The hypothesis that copper ions were involved in the an-giogenesis process was sustained by the finding that in copper-deficient rabbits angiogenesis was prevented or severely impaired (Ziche et al., 1982).

If copper ions are required in angiogenesis, ceruloplasmin, the copper-carrier protein of plasma, may also be involved in the process. We found that ceruloplasmin was angiogenic, but only when copper was bound to the molecule; apoceruloplasmin was not angiogenic. Indeed, the whole molecule is not necessary to induce neovascularization of the cornea. An 11,000-MW fraction obtained from trypsinized ceruloplasmin and containing about 50% of the total copper of the intact molecule was equally able to induce angio-genesis and equally unable to do so when copper was removed from the peptides (Raju et al., 1982).

These observations prompted us to test whether a molecule, normally not angiogenic, could be transformed into an angiogenesis effector when complexed with copper. Heparin and the tripeptide Glycyl-L-histidyl-L-lysine were found to be angiogenic when complexed with copper, whereas they failed to induce neovascularization of the cornea when copper was not bound to the molecule (Raju et al., 1982). These findings are indirectly corroborated by previous observations of enhanced phagokinesis in cultured aortal endothelial cells stimulated by ceruloplasmin or copper ions (Mc-Auslan and Reilly, 1980).

The cornea assay is very effective in revealing an angiogenic response but is much less reliable when quantitation of the process is necessary. Mobilization of endothelium in vitro permits precise quantitation, but ob-viously it mimics only one of the first events in angiogenesis, i.e., cell mo-bilization occurring in an environment that permits experimental manipu-lations but does not reproduce the in vivo conditions. Since a better approach is not presently available, Boyden chamber (Boyden, 1962) and gelatin–agarose (Alessandri et al., 1983) assays were utilized to compare angiogenic activity in vivo with the capacity to mobilize endothelial cells in vitro by angiogenesis effectors. Bovine capillary endothelium was used in all of these experiments.

The fragments of corneas underlying an Elvax pellet that incorporated an angiogenesis effector consistently mobilized endothelial cells in larger numbers and for a longer distance than fragments of the contralateral cornea from the same rabbit tested with a nonangiogenic material (Alessandri et al., 1983). This increment in mobilization occurred regardless of the effector used to treat the cornea, i.e., PGE_1, ceruloplasmin or fragments thereof, or heparin + copper. The mobilization was selective for capillary endothelium; it did not affect fibroblasts from human skin or from rabbit cornea. Endothelium from fetal bovine aorta was also not mobilized, suggesting the existence of differences between the endothelium of large vessels and that of capillaries. Presently these differences are not well defined and even less well understood. Zetter (1980) and Keegan et al. (1982) also reported that tumor-derived factors could stimulate the migration of capillary endothelium but not the migration of aortic endothelium.

The angiogenesis effectors that induced, in the cornea, the capacity to mobilize capillary endothelium in vitro were also tested alone, i.e., without the intermediary action of the cornea. None of them was able to mobilize capillary endothelium except the heparin + copper complex. In both the Boyden chamber and gelatin–agarose assays, endothelial cell mobilization by the heparin + copper complex was two- to threefold above the level observed with heparin alone. Heparin without copper exhibited a chemokinetic effect not much different from that of the culture medium alone, but no chemotactic action (Alessandri et al., 1983, 1984).

At this time, the heparin + copper complex appears to be the only angiogenesis effector chemically well defined and capable of inducing neovascularization of the rabbit cornea in vivo, as well as promoting strong migration of bovine capillary endothelium in vitro (Alessandri et al., 1984).

4.3. Antiangiogenesis

The reasons why tissues such as cartilage are not vascularized remain obscure. It has been observed that fragments of hyaline cartilage explanted onto the chick chorioallantoic membrane are not invaded by the proliferating mesenchyme (Eisenstein et al., 1973), but that cartilage extracted with 1.0 M guanidine HCl is rapidly invaded (Sorgente et al., 1975). The accepted interpretation of this finding is that guanidine HCl extracts a structural component of the cartilage that prevents vascularized mesenchyme from colonizing the hyaline cartilage. Indeed, a fragment of cartilage implanted in the rabbit cornea between the limbal vessels and a fragment of V_2 carcinoma prevented formation of new vessels and vascular colonization of the tumor in the area surrounding the cartilage. The same event was observed when the tumor was implanted in the chorioallantoic membrane close to a hyaline cartilage fragment (H. Brem and Folkman, 1975). The hypothesis that this finding was due to "leakage" of an antiangiogenesis factor from the cartilage was corroborated by two observations: (1) isolation of a cartilage fraction that inhibited tumor neovascularization (Langer et al., 1976; Lee and Langer, 1983) or growth of capillary endothelium (Sorgente and Dorey, 1980) and (2) growth depression or arrest of V_2 carcinoma or B16 melanoma when a partially purified extract of cartilage was infused into the area bearing the tumor (Langer et al., 1980).

The work on the identification and characterization of the antiangiogenesis activity of cartilage revealed that chondrocytes in culture synthesized substances with antiprotease activity (Kuettner et al., 1974) and that a trypsin inhibitor could be isolated from cartilage (Sorgente et al., 1976). In particular, the guanidine HCl extract of cartilage contains a potent inhibitor of the collagenolytic activity as released, for instance, by endothelial cells in culture (Kuettner and Pauli, 1978). The elimination of this inhibitor of collagenolysis could be responsible for the invasion of the hyaline cartilage as observed after guanidine HCl extraction (Sorgente et al., 1975).

Lytic enzymes must play a major role during angiogenesis because any movement of an endothelial cell within a tissue requires a "digestion" of the components constituting the cell environment. In fact, endothelial cells cultured in serum-free media produce more collagenolytic activity during the growth and cell movement phase of the culture than after they have reached the monolayer phase (Kuettner and Pauli, 1978). Consequently, the observation that heparin stimulates the collagenolytic activity of human mammary carcinomas in vitro (Sadove and Kuettner, 1977) becomes important for the interpretation of the mechanism of angiogenesis.

As reported in Section 4.2, the heparin + copper complex is an angiogenesis effector in vivo and is also able to mobilize capillary endothelium in vitro (Alessandri et al., 1983, 1984). Taylor and Folkman (1982) have found that protamine is a specific inhibitor of angiogenesis and that this property is related to the ability of protamine to bind heparin, thus blocking migration of capillary endothelium. Later on, Folkman's group also observed that heparin fragments administered with high doses of cortisone inhibited angiogenesis and caused regression of some large tumor masses (Folkman et al., 1983). More recently, a tumor-derived growth factor that stimulates the proliferation of capillary endothelium was found to have a strong affinity for heparin (Shing et al., 1984).

From all these observations, it appears that heparin or fragments thereof may have an important role in angiogenesis, particularly in the initial phase of the process, when mobilization of the endothelium occurs. Blocking of this mobilization may contribute substantially to antiangiogenesis, which may in turn profoundly alter tumor growth, metastatic spread, wound healing, and chronic alterations of tissues where neovascularization is a determinant component of the lesions.

5. CONCLUDING REMARKS

The possibility of modifying the biological characteristics of tumor growth by influencing angiogenesis has been postulated since tumor transplantability was discovered. Lack of tumor growth was very soon correlated with lack of neovascularization of the transplant. The determinant importance of angiogenesis was further supported by the observation that in avascular tissues neoplastic cells were unable to form solid tumors of clinical importance for the host unless neovascularization occurred. This finding constituted the basis for the hypothesis that an "angiogenesis factor" was produced by neoplastic cells and was responsible for neovascularization. Despite the fact that a chemically well defined angiogenesis factor was never found, the hypothesis stimulated a deeper analysis of the angiogenetic mechanism. It became clear that the strong angiogenic capacity of tumors was a property that appeared during neoplastic transformation and long before the apparent unrestrained growth became the predominant symptom of the neoplastic disease. Two conclusions of practical significance were drawn from these findings: (1) Adult tissues normally lacking angiogenic capacity are at higher risk of becoming neoplastically transformed when angiogenic capacity is acquired, and (2) fluids in contact with neoplastic tissues—such as urine, aqueous humor, or cerebrospinal fluid—acquire angiogenic capacity. In the first case, angiogenesis could be a marker of neoplastic progression (S. Brem et al., 1977, 1978); in the second case angiogenic capacity can indicate tumor regrowth after surgery, for instance in the bladder (Chodak et al., 1981), eye (Tapper et al., 1979), or nervous system (López-Pousa et al., 1981).

The need to understand the mechanism of the angiogenic response is, therefore, related to the possibility of an immediate clinical application in diagnosis, prognosis, and treatment of neoplastic lesions. At this time, angiogenesis appears as the end point in a sequence of events, driven by effectors such as PGE_1, copper ions, ceruloplasmin, heparin, and probably fibronectin. The most interesting part of the latest findings is that fragments of molecules normally present in the interstitial compartment are able to either trigger angiogenesis in vivo or mobilize the endothelial cells in vitro or both. Whether these molecular fragments act singly or in a coordinated fashion is not yet clear. One working hypothesis can already be formulated: The lytic action on molecules normally present in the extracellular compartment is probably sufficient to create the conditions for mobilization of capillary endothelium, i.e., the first step of neovascularization. It is not necessary to postulate the production of angiogenesis factors to explain the triggering of neovascularization. Mobilization of capillary endothelium can be triggered by fragments of molecules such as ceruloplasmin (Alessandri et al., 1983), heparin (Alessandri et al., 1984), and fibronectin (work in progress in our laboratory). These fragments may be produced by lytic enzymes liberated by neoplastic cells or by tissue destruction, as in wounds, or may be present during tissue remodeling, as in chronic artropathies. Mol-

ecules normally present in the interstitial compartment can become "angiogenesis factors" when fragmented by lytic enzymes. The most pressing
question now is whether or not a few of these fragments must be arranged
in some specific combination to become the driving force for neovascularization to be established.

REFERENCES

Alessandri, G., Raju, K., and Gullino, P. M., 1983, Mobilization of capillary endothelium in
    vitro induced by effectors of angiogenesis in vivo, Cancer Res. 43:1790–1797.
Alessandri, G., Raju, K., and Gullino, P. M., 1984, Angiogenesis in vivo and selective mobili-
    zation of capillary endothelium in vitro by heparin + copper complex, Microcirculation,
    Endothelium Lymphatics 1:329–346.
Algire, G. H., and Legallais, F. Y., 1947, Growth rate of transplanted tumors in relation to latent
    period and host vascular reaction, Cancer Res. 7:724.
Algire, G. H., Chalkley, H. W., Legallais, F. Y., and Park, H. D., 1945, Vascular reactions of
    normal and malignant tissues in vivo. I. Vascular reactions of mice to wounds and to normal
    and neoplastic transplants, J. Natl. Cancer Inst. 6:73–85.
Algire, G. H., Legallais, F. Y., and Park, H. D., 1947, Vascular reactions of normal and malignant
    tissues in vivo. II. The vascular reaction of normal and neoplastic tissues of mice to bacterial
    polysaccharide from Serratia marcesens (Bacillus prodigiosus) culture filtrates, J. Natl.
    Cancer Inst. 8:53–62.
Appelgren, L. K., 1982, Methods of recording tumor blood flow, in: Tumor Blood Circulation
    (H.-I. Peterson, ed.), CRC Press, Boca Raton, Florida, pp. 87–101.
Appelgren, L., Peterson, H.-I., and Rosengren, B., 1973, Vascular and extravascular spaces in
    two transplantable tumors of the rat, Bibl. Anat. 12:504–510.
Auerbach, R., and Sidky, Y. A., 1978, Studies on the maturation of immune responsiveness in
    the mouse. III. Ontogeny of immunocompetence as measured by the ability of embryonic
    yolk sac cells to evoke angiogenesis in allogeneic hosts, in: Animal Models of Comparative
    and Developmental Aspects of Immunity and Disease (M. E. Gershwin and E. L. Cooper,
    eds.), Pergamon Press, New York, pp. 166–174.
Auerbach, R., Kubai, L., and Sidky, Y., 1976, Angiogenesis induction by tumors, embryonic
    tissues, and lymphocytes, Cancer Res. 36:3435–3440.
Azizkhan, R. G., Azizkhan, J. C., Klagsbrun, M., Darling, R. C., III, Rochman, E., and Folkman,
    J., 1981, An avascular subpopulation of chondrosarcoma exhibits limited growth in vivo
    and is unable to stimulate capillary endothelial cells in vitro, Surg. Forum 32:424–426.
Bakay, L., 1970, The extracellular space in brain tumors. I. Morphological considerations, Brain
    93:695–698.
Banda, M. J., Knighton, D. R., Hunt, T. K., and Werb, Z., 1982, Isolation of a nonmitogenic
    angiogenesis factor from wound fluid, Proc. Natl. Acad. Sci. USA 79:7773–7777.
Ben Ezra, D., 1979, Neovasculogenesis: Triggering factors and possible mechanisms, Surv.
    Ophthalmol. 24:167–176.
Boyden, S., 1962, The chemotactic effect of mixtures of antibody and antigen on polymor-
    phonuclear leucocytes, J. Exp. Med. 115:453–466.
Brand, K. G., 1975, Foreign body induced sarcomas, in: Cancer: A Comprehensive Treatise,
    Volume 1 (F. F. Becker, ed.), Plenum Press, New York, pp. 485–511.
Brem, H., and Folkman, J., 1975, Inhibition of tumor angiogenesis mediated by cartilage, J. Exp.
    Med. 141:427–439.
Brem, S., Gullino, P. M., and Medina, D., 1977, Angiogenesis: A marker for neoplastic trans-
    formation of mammary papillary hyperplasia, Science 195:880–882.
Brem, S., Jensen, H. M., and Gullino, P. M., 1978, Angiogenesis as a marker of preneoplastic
    lesions of the human breast, Cancer 41:239–244.

Brown, R. A., Weiss, J. B., Tomlinson, I. W., Phillips, P., and Kumar, S., 1980, Angiogenic factor from synovial fluid resembling that from tumours, Lancet 1:682–685.

Butler, T. P., Grantham, F. H., and Gullino, P. M., 1975, Bulk transfer of fluid in the interstitial compartment of mammary tumors, Cancer Res. 35:3084–3088.

Castellot, J. J., Jr., Karnowsky, M. J., and Spiegelman, B. M., 1980, Potent stimulation of vascular endothelial cell growth by differentiated 3T3 adipocytes, Proc. Natl. Acad. Sci. USA 77:6007–6011.

Chen, C.-H., and Chen, S. C., 1980, Angiogenic activity of vitreous and retinal extract, Invest. Ophthalmol. Vis. Sci. 19:596–602.

Chodak, G. W., Scheiner, C. J., and Zetter, B. R., 1981, Urine from patients with transitional-cell carcinoma stimulates migration of capillary endothelial cells, N. Engl. J. Med. 305:869–874.

Cohen, S. M., Tatematsu, M., Shinohara, Y., Nakanishi, K., and Ito, N., 1980, Neovascularization in rats during urinary bladder carcinogenesis induced by N-[4-(5-nitro-2-furyl)-2-thiazolyl]formamide, J. Natl. Cancer Inst. 65:145–148.

Eddy, H. A., and Casarett, G. W., 1973, Development of the vascular system in the hamster malignant neurilemmoma, Microvasc. Res. 6:63–82.

Eisenstein, R., Sorgente, N., Soble, L. W., Miller, A., and Kuettner, K. E., 1973, The resistance of certain tissues to invasion: Penetrability of explanted tissues by vascularized mesenchyme, Am. J. Pathol. 73:765–774.

Endrich, B., Reinhold, H. S., Gross, J. F., and Intaglietta, M., 1979, Tissue perfusion in homogeneity during early tumor growth in vitro, J. Natl. Cancer Inst. 62:387–395.

Federman, J. L., Brown, G. C., Felberg, N. T., and Felton, S. M., 1980, Experimental ocular angiogenesis, Am. J. Ophthalmol. 89:1231–1237.

Fenselau, A., Watt, S., and Mello, R. J., 1981, Tumor angiogenic factor: Purification from the Walker 256 rat tumor, J. Biol. Chem. 256:9605–9611.

Folkman, J., 1974, Tumor angiogenesis, Adv. Cancer Res. 19:331–358.

Folkman, J., and Cotran, R., 1976, Relation of vascular proliferation to tumor growth, Int. Rev. Exp. Pathol. 16:207–248.

Folkman, J., Merler, E., Abernathy, C., and Williams, G., 1971, Isolation of a tumor factor responsible for angiogenesis, J. Exp. Med. 133:275–288.

Folkman, J., Langer, R., Linhardt, R. J., Haudenschild, C., and Taylor, S., 1983, Angiogenesis inhibition and tumor regression caused by heparin or a heparin fragment in the presence of cortisone, Science 221:719–725.

Fromer, C. H., and Klintworth, G. K., 1975a, An evaluation of the role of leukocytes in the pathogenesis of experimentally induced corneal vascularization. I. Comparison of experimental models of corneal vascularization, Am. J. Pathol. 79:537–550.

Fromer, C. H., and Klintworth, G. K., 1975b, An evaluation of the role of leukocytes in the pathogenesis of experimentally induced corneal vascularization. II. Studies on the effect of leukocytic elimination on corneal vascularization, Am. J. Pathol. 81:531–544.

Fromer, C. H., and Klintworth, G. K., 1976, An evaluation of the role of leukocytes in the pathogenesis of experimentally induced corneal vascularization. III. Studies related to the vasoproliferative capability of polymorphonuclear leukocytes and lymphocytes, Am. J. Pathol. 82:159–167.

Gaffney, E. V., 1982, A cell line (HBL 100) established from human breast milk, Cell Tissue Res. 227:563–568.

Gimbrone, M. A., Jr., and Gullino, P. M., 1976, Angiogenic capacity of preneoplastic lesions of the murine mammary gland as a marker of neoplastic transformation, Cancer Res. 36:2611–2620.

Gimbrone, M. A., Jr., Cotran, R. S., Leapman, S. B., and Folkman, J., 1974, Tumor growth and neovascularization: An experimental model using the rabbit cornea, J. Natl. Cancer Inst. 52:413–427.

Glaser, B. M., D'Amore, P. A., Michels, R. G., Patz, A., and Fenselau, A., 1980a, Demonstration of vasoproliferative activity from mammalian retina, J. Cell Biol. 84:298–304.

Glaser, B. M., D'Amore, P. A., Seppa, H., Seppa, S., and Schiffmann, E., 1980b, Adult tissues contain chemoattractants for vascular endothelial cells, Nature 288:483–484.

Glaser, B. M., D'Amore, P. A., Lutty, G. A., Fenselau, A. H., Michels, R. G., and Patz, A., 1980c, Chemical mediators of intraocular neovascularization, *Trans. Ophthalmol. Soc. UK* **100**:369–373.

Gospodarowicz, D., and Thakral, K. K., 1978, Production of a corpus luteum angiogenic factor responsible for proliferation of capillaries and neovascularization of the corpus luteum, *Proc. Natl. Acad. Sci. USA* **75**:847–851.

Gospodarowicz, D., Mescher, A. L., and Birdwell, C. R., 1977, Stimulation of corneal endothelial cell proliferation in vitro by fibroblasts and epidermal growth factors, *Exp. Eye Res.* **25**:75–89.

Göthlin, J., 1977, Arteriovenous shunting in carcinomas evaluated by a dye dilution technique, *Scand. J. Urol. Nephrol.* **11**:159–163.

Greenburg, G. B., and Hunt, T. K., 1978, The proliferative response in vitro of vascular endothelial and smooth muscle cells exposed to wound fluids and macrophages, *J. Cell Physiol.* **97**:353–360.

Gullino, P. M., 1981, Angiogenesis factor(s), in: *Tissue Growth Factors* (R. Baserga, ed.), Springer-Verlag, New York, pp. 427–449.

Gullino, P. M., and Grantham, F. H., 1961a, Studies on the exchange of fluid between host and humor. I. A method for growing "tissue isolated" tumors in laboratory animals, *J. Natl. Cancer Inst.* **27**:679–693.

Gullino, P. M., and Grantham, F. H., 1961b, Studies on the exchange of fluids between host and tumor. II. The blood flow of hepatomas and other tumors in rats and mice, *J. Natl. Cancer Inst.* **27**:1465–1491.

Gullino, P. M., and Grantham, F. H., 1962, Studies on the exchange of fluids between host and tumor. III. Regulation of blood flow in hepatomas and other rat tumors, *J. Natl. Cancer Inst.* **28**:211–229.

Gullino, P. M., and Grantham, F. H., 1964, The vascular space of growing tumors, *Cancer Res.* **24**:1727–1732.

Gullino, P. M., Grantham, F. H., and Smith, S. H., 1965, The interstitial water space of tumors, *Cancer Res.* **25**:727–731.

Gullino, P. M., Jain, R. K., and Grantham, F. H., 1982, Temperature gradients and blood perfusion in a mammary carcinoma, *J. Natl. Cancer Inst.* **68**:519–533.

Hilmas, D. E., and Gillette, E. L., 1975, Tumor microvasculature following fractionated x-irradiation, *Radiology* **116**:165–169.

Hoffman, H., McAuslan, B., Robertson, D., and Burnett, E., 1976, An endothelial growth-stimulating factor from salivary glands, *Exp. Cell Res.* **102**:269–275.

Howard, B. V., Macarak, E. J., Gunson, D., and Kefalides, N. A., 1976, Characterization of the collagen synthesized by endothelial cells in culture, *Proc. Natl. Acad. Sci. USA* **73**:2361–2364.

Huseby, R. A., Currie, C., Lagerborg, V. A., and Garb, S., 1975, Angiogenesis about and within grafts of normal testicular tissue: A comparison with transplanted neoplastic tissue, *Microvasc. Res.* **10**:396–413.

Ide, A. G., Baker, N. H., and Warren, S. C., 1939, Vascularization of the Brown–Pearce rabbit epithelioma transplant as seen in the transparent ear chamber, *Am. J. Roentgenol.* **42**:891–899.

Intaglietta, M., Myers, R. R., Gross, J. F., and Reinhold, H. S., 1977, Dynamics of microvascular flow in implanted mouse mammary tumors, *Bibl. Anat.* **15**:273–276.

Jakob, W., Jentzsch, K. D., Mauersberger, B., and Oehme, P., 1977, Demonstration of angiogenesis-activity in the corpus luteum of cattle, *Exp. Pathol. (Jena)* **13**:231–236.

Jensen, H. M., Chen, I., DeVault, M. R., and Lewis, A. E., 1982, Angiogenesis induced by "normal" human breast tissue: A probable marker for precancer, *Science* **218**:293–295.

Keegan, A., Hill, C., Kumar, S., Phillips, P., Schor, A., and Weiss, J., 1982, Purified tumor angiogenesis factor enhances proliferation of capillary, but not aortic, endothelial cells in vitro, *J. Cell Sci.* **55**:261–276.

Kessler, D. A., Langer, R. S., Pless, N. A., and Folkman, J., 1976, Mast cells and tumor angiogenesis, *Int. J. Cancer* **18**:703–709.

Kjartansson, I., Appelgren, L., Ivarsson, L., Peterson, H.-I., and Sivertsson, R., 1976, Total blood flow in a 20-methylcholanthrene induced rat sarcoma determined by plethysmography: Effect of aging and a single dose of x-ray irradiation, *Act. Chir. Scand. (Suppl.)* **471**:45–57.

Kreyberg, L., 1927, On local alterations of the blood-vessels of tar-painted white mice, Br. J. Exp. Pathol. 8:465–470.

Kuettner, K. E., and Pauli, B. U., 1978, Resistance of cartilage to normal and neoplastic invasion, Calcif. Tissue Abstr. Spec. Suppl. 251–278.

Kuettner, K. E., Croxen, R. L., Eisenstein, R., and Sorgente, N., 1974, Proteinase inhibitor activity in connective tissues, Experientia 30:595–597.

Kumar, S., West, D., and Daniel, M., 1983, Human lung tumor cell line adapted to grow in serum-free medium secretes angiogenesis factor, Int. J. Cancer 32:461–464.

Langer, R., and Folkman, J., 1976, Polymers for the sustained release of proteins and other macromolecules, Nature 263:797–800.

Langer, R., Brem, H., Falterman, K., Klein, M., and Folkman, J., 1976, Isolation of a cartilage factor that inhibits tumor neovascularization, Science 193:70–72.

Langer, R., Conn, H., Vacanti, J., Haudenschild, C., and Folkman, J., 1980, Control of tumor growth in animals by infusion of an angiogenesis inhibitor, Proc. Natl. Acad. Sci. USA 77:4331–4335.

Lee, A., and Langer, R., 1983, Shark cartilage contains inhibitors of tumor angiogenesis, Science 221:1185–1187.

López-Pousa, S., Ferrier, I., Vich, J. M., and Domenech-Mateu, J., 1981, Angiogenic activity in the CSF in human malignancies, Experientia 37:413–415.

McAuslan, B. R., and Hoffman, H., 1979, Endothelium stimulating factor from Walker carcinoma cells: Relation to tumor angiogenesis factor, Exp. Cell Res. 119:181–190.

McAuslan, B. R., and Reilly, W., 1980, Endothelial cell phagokinesis in response to specific metal ions, Exp. Cell Res. 130:147–157.

Maciag, T., Cerundolo, J., Ilsley, S., Kelley, P. R., and Forand, R., 1979, An endothelial cell growth factor from bovine hypothalamus: Identification and partial characterization, Proc. Natl. Acad. Sci. USA 76:5674–5678.

Maciag, T., Hoover, G. A., van der Spek, J., Stemerman, M. B., and Weinstein, R., 1982, Growth and differentiation of human umbilical-vein endothelial cells in culture, in: Growth of Cells in Hormonally Defined Medium, Book A (G. Sato, A. B. Pardee, and D. A. Sirbajku, eds.), Cold Spring Harbor Laboratory, Cold Spring Harbor, New York, pp. 525–538.

Mäntylä, M., Kuikka, J., and Rekonen, A., 1976, Regional blood flow in human tumours with special reference to the effect of radiotherapy, Br. J. Radiol. 49:335–338.

Medina, D., 1973, Preneoplastic lesions in mouse mammary tumorigenesis, in: Methods in Cancer Research, Volume 7 (C. H. Busch, ed.), Academic Press, New York, pp. 3–53.

Nishioka, K., and Ryan, T. J., 1972, The influence of the epidermis and other tissues on blood vessel growth in the hamster cheek pouch, J. Invest. Dermatol. 58:33–45.

Nugent, L. J., and Jain, R. K., 1984, Intravascular diffusion in normal and neoplastic tissues, Cancer Res. 44:238–244.

Phillips, P., and Kumar, S., 1979, Tumor angiogenesis factor (TAF) and its neutralisation by a xenogenic antiserum, Int. J. Cancer 23:82–88.

Plengvanit, U., Suwanik, R., Chearanai, O., Intrasupt, S., Sutayavanich, S., Kalayasiri, C., and Viranuvatti, V., 1972, Regional hepatic blood flow studied by intrahepatic injection of ^{133}xenon in animals and patients with carcinoma of the liver, with particular reference to the effect of hepatic artery ligation, Aust. NZ J. Med. 2:44–48.

Pliskin, M. E., Ginsberg, S. M., and Carp, N., 1980, Induction of neovascularization by nitrogen-activated spleen cells and their supernatants, Transplantation 29:255–258.

Polverini, P. J., Cotran, R. S., Gimbrone, M. A., Jr., and Unanue, E. R., 1977, Activated macrophages induce vascular proliferation, Nature 269:804–806.

Raju, K., Alessandri, G., Ziche, M., and Gullino, P. M., 1982, Ceruloplasmin, copper ions and angiogenesis, J. Natl. Cancer Inst. 69:1183–1188.

Reinhold, H. S., 1971, Improved microcirculation in irradiated tumors, Eur. J. Cancer 7:273–280.

Reinhold, H. S., 1979, In vivo observations of tumor blood flow, in: Tumor Blood Circulation (H.-I. Peterson, ed.), CRC Press, Boca Raton, Florida, pp. 115–128.

Sadove, A. M., and Kuettner, K. E., 1977, Inhibition of mammary carcinoma invasiveness with cartilage-derived inhibitor, Surg. Forum 28:499–501.

Shing, Y., Folkman, J., Sullivan, R., Butterfield, C., Murray, J., and Klagsbrun, M., 1984, Heparin affinity: Purification of a tumor-derived capillary endothelial cell growth factor, *Science* **223**:1296–1299.

Shubik, P., 1982, Vascularization of tumors: A review, *J. Cancer Res. Clin. Oncol.* **103**:211–226.

Simpson, D. M., and Ross, R., 1972, The neutrophilic leukocyte in wound repair: A study with antineutrophil serum, *J. Clin. Invest.* **51**:2009–2023.

Sorgente, N., and Dorey, C. K., 1980, Inhibition of endothelial cell growth by a factor isolated from cartilage, *Exp. Cell Res.* **128**:63–71.

Sorgente, N., Kuettner, K. E., Soble, L. W., and Eisenstein, R., 1975, The resistance of certain tissues to invasion. II. Evidence for extractable factors in cartilage which inhibit invasion by vascularized mesenchyme, *Lab. Invest.* **32**:217–222.

Sorgente, N., Kuettner, K. E., and Eisenstein, R., 1976, The isolation, purification, and partial characterization of proteinase inhibitors from bovine cartilage and cornea, in: *Protides of the Biological Fluids*, Volume 23 (H. Peeters, ed.), Pergamon Press, New York, pp. 227–230.

Stein, J. M., and Levenson, S. M., 1966, Effect of the inflammatory reaction on subsequent wound healing, *Surg. Forum* **17**:484–485.

Strum, J. M., 1983, Angiogenic responses elicited from chorioallantoic membrane vessels by neoplastic, preneoplastic, and normal mammary tissues from GR mice, *Am. J. Pathol.* **111**:282–287.

Tapper, D., Langer, R., Bellows, A. R., and Folkman, J., 1979, Angiogenesis capacity as a diagnostic marker for human eye tumors, *Surgery* **86**:36–40.

Taylor, S., and Folkman, J., 1982, Protamine is an inhibitor of angiogenesis, *Nature* **297**:307–312.

Tuan, D., Smith, S., Folkman, J., and Merler, E., 1973, Isolation of the nonhistone proteins of rat Walker carcinoma 256: Their association with tumor angiogenesis, *Biochemistry* **12**:3159–3165.

Vaupel, P., 1975, Interrelationship between mean arterial blood pressure, blood flow, and vascular resistance in solid tumor tissue of DS-carcinosarcoma, *Experientia* **31**:587–589.

Vogel, A. W., 1965, Intratumoral vascular changes with increased size of a mammary adenocarcinoma: New method and results, *J. Natl. Cancer Inst.* **34**:571–578.

Warren, B. A., 1979, The vascular morphology of tumors, in: *Tumor Blood Circulation* (H.-I. Peterson, ed.), CRC Press, Boca Raton, Florida, pp. 1–47.

Weiss, J. B., Brown, R. A., Kumar, S., and Phillips, P. 1979, An angiogenic factor isolated from tumours: A potent low-molecular-weight compound, *Br. J. Cancer* **40**:493–496.

Weiss, J. B., Hill, C. R., McLaughlin, B., and Elstow, S., 1983, Potentiating effect of heparin in the activation of procollagenase by a low M_r angiogenesis factor, *FEBS Lett.* **163**:62–65.

Wellings, S. R., and Rice, J. D., 1978, Preneoplastic lesions in the human breast, in: *Early Diagnosis of Breast Cancer: Methods and Results* (E. Grundmann and L. Beck, eds.), G. Fischer Verlag, New York, pp. 91–106.

Wolf, J. E., Jr., and Harrison, R. G., 1973, Demonstration and characterization of an epidermal angiogenic factor, *J. Invest. Dermatol.* **61**:130–141.

Zetter, B. R., 1980, Migration of capillary endothelial cells is stimulated by tumour-derived factor, *Nature* **285**:41–43.

Ziche, M., and Gullino, P. M., 1981, Angiogenesis and prediction of sarcoma formation by plastic, *Cancer Res.* **41**:5060–5063.

Ziche, M., and Gullino, P. M., 1982, Angiogenesis and neoplastic progression in vitro, *J. Natl. Cancer Inst.* **69**:483–487.

Ziche, M., Jones, J., and Gullino, P. M., 1982, Role of prostaglandin E_1 and copper in angiogenesis, *J. Natl. Cancer Inst.* **69**:475–482.

CHAPTER 2

MECHANISMS OF TUMOR INVASION AND THEIR POTENTIAL THERAPEUTIC MODIFICATIONS

UNNUR P. THORGEIRSSON,
TAINA TURPEENNIEMI-HUJANEN, and
LANCE A. LIOTTA

1. INTRODUCTION

Invasion and metastases are the major causes of morbidity and mortality for patients with malignant solid tumors. Many patients already have metastases at the time of primary tumor diagnosis. Individual patients' tumors vary widely in aggressiveness. One patient's tumor may grow to a larger size and fail to metastasize. Another patient's tumor of similar histologic appearance may metastasize at a very early stage. Consequently, there is a great clinical need to develop new methods to (1) prevent local tumor invasion, (2) identify and treat clinically occult micrometastases, and (3) predict the aggressiveness of a patient's individual tumor. The purpose of this chapter is to summarize basic science developments in oncology that provide strategies for developing such methods.

Cell surface components provide targets for labeled antibodies used in experimental models of in vivo metastases localization. Therefore, in the first section of this chapter, we will consider current research on cell membrane components altered in neoplastic cells. Invasion may be a process distinct from proliferation. We will examine the experimental evidence for this hypothesis and its implications for antiinvasion therapy. The role of the

UNNUR P. THORGEIRSSON, TAINA TURPEENNIEMI-HUJANEN, and LANCE A. LIOTTA • Laboratory of Pathology, National Cancer Institute, National Institutes of Health, Bethesda, Maryland 20205.

extracellular matrix in invasion and metastasis will be discussed. The matrix has been found to be consistently altered during the transition from benign to invasive neoplasms. Tumor cells may interact with or modify the matrix via special receptors or proteolytic enzymes. The important proteases will be considered along with the evidence for their role in metastasis. Inhibition of these enzymes may provide a therapeutic strategy for arresting the metastatic process.

2. CELLULAR PROPERTIES RELATING TO INVASION

2.1. Cell Membrane Alterations

Many cancer-associated phenotypic abnormalities may be related to alterations of the cell surface membrane. Alterations of the cell surface molecules may produce altered antigenic determinants such as reduced levels of glycosyltransferase (Grimes, 1970), which results in a lack of the terminal sugar residue glycolipids (Tal, 1965). Augmentation of the Forssman-like antigens in some transformed cells can also be explained by a similar mechanism (Robertson and Black, 1969). Many types of experimentally induced tumors and a variety of human cancers have altered cell membrane glycolipid composition (Hakomori and Kannagi, 1983). Tumor cells are thought to release cell surface glycoconjugates and glycosyltransferase into plasma. These factors may induce an immunosuppressive state by inhibiting lymphocyte proliferation. Augmented levels of normal surface glycoproteins have been observed in some transformed cells. The p53 protein is expressed at high levels in a variety of transformed cell lines (Linzer and Levine, 1979). It is hypothesized that this protein may play a central role in the cell cycle and in growth control (N. Reich and Levine, 1982). Studies of surface glycoproteins in lymphoproliferative malignancies have revealed changes that suggest an arrested maturation stage. Examples of neoplasms include T-cell leukemia (Anderson *et al.*, 1977), Burkitt's lymphoma (Nilsson *et al.*, 1977), and erythroleukemia (Gahmberg *et al.*, 1979).

Cell surface sialic acid and the degree of sialation may correlate with metastatic potential in certain model systems (Yogeeswaran and Salk, 1981). The altered sialation may affect antigenicity and alter receptor function, and it could relate to intracellular transport of glycoproteins. A sialogalactoprotein (GP-580) has been identified on the cell surface of lung metastases from human and rat mammary adenocarcinoma, and expression of this protein on the rat cells correlated with their spontaneous metastatic potential (Steck *et al.*, 1984). Changes in sialic acid content may also relate to fetal determinants. Elevated levels in fetal livers were observed to fall sharply after birth but began to rise after administration of a carcinogen and reached maximum level in poorly differentiated hepatomas.

Antigens augmented on tumors compared to normal tissues may be exploited for monoclonal antibody localization or treatment of metastases

(Koprowski *et al.*, 1981; Sears *et al.*, 1982). Monoclonal antibodies against cell surface antigens of melanoma cells were found to be cytotoxic both *in vitro* and *in vivo* (Koprowski *et al.*, 1978; Bernstein *et al.*, 1980). A melanoma cell surface antigen was identified that is a core glycoprotein for chondroitin sulfate proteoglycan (Bumol and Reisfeld, 1982). Monoclonal antibodies and antibody–toxin conjugates against this proteoglycan suppress growth of melanoma in athymic nude mice (Bumol *et al.*, 1983). Tissue-specific antibodies for breast epithelium have been developed by Ceriani's group using human milk fat globule membrane. The antigen was derived from the apical portion of breast epithelial cells during milk secretion (Ceriani *et al.*, 1977). The breast-specific antigens have been found in neoplastic breast epithelial cells although to a lesser extent than in their normal counterparts. Studies using nude mice implanted with human breast carcinoma demonstrated high plasma levels of milk fat globule membrane antigens, which dropped sharply upon removal of the tumor (Sasaki *et al.*, 1981). High levels of the mammary epithelial antigens were detected in plasma of breast cancer patients while normal controls and patients with other types of disseminated cancer did not have detectable antigen levels (Ceriani *et al.*, 1982). This avenue of research indicates that tumor-specific antibodies are not required for metastasis immunolocalization.

The discovery of α-fetoprotein (AFP) and carcinoembryonic antigen (CEA) in the 1960s demonstrated that fetal and tumor tissues sometimes share cell surface antigens. This similarity between tumor cells and embryonic cells has supported the concept that neoplasia may, in part, involve activation of genes that were repressed during cellular differentiation. The association of AFP with normal pregnancy and tumor growth was first made by Abelev in 1963 (Abelev *et al.*, 1963; Abelev, 1974). AFP production has been demonstrated in normal hepatocellular proliferation, regeneration of liver following partial hepatectomy or liver injury, fetal development, tumors of the liver and gastrointestinal tract, and germinal tumors containing yolk sac elements. AFP is a serum protein with a molecular weight (MW) of 70,000 (Watanabe, 1974). Its biological function in the fetus is not known. AFP may act as an estrogen-binding protein to protect the fetus from the effects of maternal estrogen, or it may inhibit immune response and thus protect the fetus from maternal immune attack, or it may function as fetal albumin.

CEA is a generic name for antigens from extracts of fetal colon and tumors of the gastrointestinal tract (Gold and Freedman, 1965). It is a glycoprotein with an MW of 200,000 (Krupey *et al.*, 1968) and is often significantly elevated in tumors of the gastrointestinal tract. Since it may also be mildly elevated in smokers and individuals with inflammatory bowel disease, it cannot be used as an absolute screening test for malignancy. Nevertheless, CEA levels may be of great clinical importance in monitoring the effects of cancer therapy.

Additional classes of oncodevelopmental antigens elevated in tumor tissues or plasma of cancer patients which may prove to be important are: beta-oncofetal antigen (Fritze and Mach, 1975), pancreatic oncofetal antigen

(Banwo et al., 1974), fetal sulfoglycoprotein (Häkkinen, 1974), fetal gut antigen (Smith and O'Neill, 1971), carcinofetal ferritin (Alpert et al., 1973), melanoma fetal antigens (Avis et al., 1973), and tissue polypeptide antigen (Björklund, 1976). These antigens may all be considered as candidates for immunolocalization studies.

2.2. Tumor Invasion—Active or Passive Process?

The relative contribution of active versus passive factors in tumor cell invasion has recently been studied both qualitatively and quantitatively. Local tumor growth can lead to pressure atrophy of surrounding host tissues. However, it has previously been unclear whether tumor "growth pressure" or tumor cell proliferation is absolutely necessary for tumor cell invasion of host connective tissue barriers (Sträuli, 1980). This question is difficult to address in the complex in vivo environment, where tumor cell proliferation cannot be separated from active tumor cell migration. These factors, however, can be separated in an in vitro invasion model. Mareel et al. (1979) have shown that nonproliferating tumor cells can invade organ fragments as judged by histology.

Thorgeirsson et al. (1984) have used the amnion invasion assay to study quantitatively whether basic cellular functions such as DNA synthesis, cell proliferation, and protein synthesis are necessary for tumor cell invasion. Human amnion, which contains a continuous basement membrane (BM) and a uniform nonvascular collagenous stroma (Van Herendael et al., 1978), is used in this assay. Tumor cells are inoculated on the BM surface of the amnion, which has been denuded of its epithelial layer, and the cells that invade through the full thickness of the amnion are collected on a Millipore filter (Thorgeirsson et al., 1982).

The tumor cells (M5076) used in this study were derived from a murine reticulum cell sarcoma (Talmadge et al., 1981; Hart et al., 1981). Previously, we demonstrated that the M5076 tumor cells were able to invade the amnion in vitro and that their invasiveness was stimulated by the chemoattractant FMLP (Thorgeirsson et al., 1982). FMLP is a synthetic tripeptide that is chemotactic for inflammatory cells and some tumor cells (Showell et al., 1976; Wass et al., 1981).

Attempts were made to identify basic cellular activities that are relevant to the invasive process. Tumor cell proliferation has been closely associated with invasion although the relationship between these two processes has not been studied systematically. Therefore, the amnion system was used to measure invasiveness of M5076 cells under pharmacologic conditions under which protein synthesis, DNA synthesis, or cell proliferation was inhibited.

The results indicated that at least M5076 tumor cells do not require DNA synthesis and proliferation in order to invade normal host connective tissues. Therefore, it is likely that cell proliferation and invasion are under separate genetic control. This may be of clinical significance since most chemotherapeutic agents used today are directed against proliferating tumor cells. Tumor cells that are not proliferating but are in the process of active invasion may be resistant to chemotherapy. Further studies of the genetic control and biochemical mechanisms of tumor invasion may lead to pharmacologic strategies designed specifically to inhibit invading tumor cells.

2.3. Anchorage Independence, Locomotion, and Chemotaxis

Transformed cells lose anchorage-dependent growth, which is a fundamental requirement for *in vitro* propagation of most normal nonhematopoietic cells (Todaro *et al.*, 1964). The cell adhesive and cytoskeletal changes associated with anchorage-independent growth have been studied in retrovirus-induced tumors. The transforming RSV oncogene-coded protein, pp60[src] and its tyrosine protein kinase activity have been associated with both the inner face of the plasma membrane and the cytoskeleton. This protein is enriched at the intercellular junctions (Willingham *et al.*, 1979) and is localized together with vinculin in the substrate adhesion plaques of the transformed cells (Rohrschneider, 1980). This suggests that pp60[src] kinase phosphorylates vinculin at the focal adhesion sites (Rohrschneider *et al.*, 1982). Thus, tumorigenic properties of the RSV-transformed cells correlate with the membrane association of the pp60[src] protein (Krueger *et al.*, 1982), which may alter the cytoskeletal architecture (Leavitt *et al.*, 1982).

Tumor cells are motile but it is still unproven that they have increased random locomotive ability compared to normal cells (Easty and Easty, 1976; Gershman *et al.*, 1978). Tumor cell motility studies are usually performed on monolayer cultures. Therefore, extrapolation of the *in vitro* observations to the complex *in vivo* situation should be made with reservations. The cytoskeletal apparatus is the major locomotive engine of the cell. Its three main components are microfilaments, microtubules, and intermediate filaments. Visualization of the cytoskeletal structures has been possible through the use of antibodies to their major proteins, i.e., actin, tubulin, and vimentin. Reports on structural cytoskeletal changes in malignancy are controversial and conflicting. Disorganization of the microfilament system was demonstrated in cells transformed by oncogenic viruses (Wang and Goldberg, 1976). Raz and co-workers observed increased metastatic potential in tumor cells that showed disarray of their actin organization (Raz and Geiger, 1982). Such a complex cell function as locomotion might require a highly organized rather than disorganized cytoskeleton. An increase in actin-containing structures of malignant cells was shown in one study (Gabbiani, 1979), while others have concluded that an increase in contractile proteins like actin is not a prerequisite for malignant behavior. *In vitro* studies by Mareel and coworkers, showing that microtubule inhibitors prevent invasion of malignant cells into embryonic chick tissues, suggest that directional cellular migration mediated through the cytoskeleton plays a crucial role in tumor invasion (Mareel and de Brabander, 1978).

Chemotactic factors may stimulate directional migration of tumor cells during local invasion and vascular dissemination by a mechanism similar

to polymorphonuclear leukocyte chemotaxis. A chemotactic factor was isolated from solid tumor tissue by Hayashi and co-workers in 1970 (H. Hayashi
et al., 1970). Subsequent work has indicated that secretion of this factor is
controlled by a neutral protease possibly released by destroyed host cells
(Koono et al., 1974). The second chemotactic factor was obtained from human or animal serum by proteolysis of the fifth complement component (C5).
This factor is chemically related to or possibly derived from the C5 chemotactic factor for leukocytes (Romualdez and Ward, 1975). Additional chemotactic factors for tumor cells include a bone-derived factor that was identified in the culture fluid of resorbed bone (Orr et al., 1980) and a synthetic
tripeptide, N-formyl-methionyl-leucyl-phenylalanine (Varani and Ward, 1982;
Thorgeirsson et al., 1982). Cellular changes have been observed that are
associated with the chemotactic response. These include increase in size
(Wass et al., 1980) and increased adherence to foreign surfaces (Varani et
al., 1981). Furthermore, a positive correlation was found between chemotactic responsiveness and metastatic capacity in fibrosarcoma cells (Varani
et al., 1979). Inhibition of chemotaxis could be an important pharmacologic
approach to the control of invasion and prevention of extravasation.

2.4. Heterogeneity

It is now generally accepted that tumors are composed of heterogeneous
populations of cells. Highly malignant subpopulations are thought to arise
spontaneously when tumor cells are subjected to various host selection pressures during progressive tumor growth. Foulds's tumor evolution hypothesis
(1956) suggested that tumor cells undergo irreversible changes to gain autonomy from their host regulatory processes (Foulds, 1956). Nowell extended
this concept to propose that tumor progression resulting in the emergence
of cell populations with different malignant potential is due to acquired
genetic alterations (Nowell, 1976). At present, it is generally accepted that
most spontaneously arising tumors have a clonal origin and will acquire
genetic instability with growth that results in heterogeneous cell populations
(Fialkow, 1976; Iannaccone et al., 1978; Calabresi et al., 1979; Baylin, 1982).
Cell populations can be distinguished based on their heterogeneity in karyotypes, growth characteristics, antigenicities, immunogenicities, and sensitivities to chemotherapeutic drugs and radiation.

Heterogeneity in metastatic capacity within the same tumor was first
demonstrated by Fidler and Kripke (1977). Subsequent studies using a wide
range of tumors of different histologic origin have confirmed their findings,
which suggest that only certain subpopulations of tumor cells possess the
properties required to complete successfully all the steps in the metastatic
process. It has also been determined that tumor cell clones develop into
heterogeneous cell populations during prolonged cultivation in vitro (Fidler
and Nicolson, 1981) and that biological diversity can rapidly develop in vivo
within individual metastases (Talmadge et al., 1979). Such instability is not
expressed if several clones are mixed and cocultivated, suggesting that they

exert regulatory restraints on each other (Poste *et al.*, 1981). Mutations of malignant cell lines produce clones with variable metastatic capacities and even nonmetastatic clones (Boon and Kellerman, 1977; Fisher and Cifone, 1981; Kerbel *et al.*, 1982).

The mechanism by which phenotypic instability is generated is not clear. Goldberg (1974) proposed that tumor cells may undergo somatic cell hybridization *in vivo*. Hybridization could lead to either emergence of more malignant cells or genotypic stability. Schirrmacher (1980) suggested that genetic programs exist in tumor cells that can be activated by environmental signals and could eventually lead to phenotypic diversity. Poste and co-workers (Poste *et al.*, 1984) believe that the clonal evolution during tumor progression may occur in three phases: (1) initial generation of clones with diverse but stable metastatic phenotype, (2) evolution of unstable metastatic clones that are stabilized by interactions with other clones, and (3) emergence of unstable metastatic clones that are unresponsive to the stabilizing effects of other clones (Poste *et al.*, 1984). Tumor progression may be influenced by different modifications in the microenvironment, such as changes in cell nutrients, hormones, and other factors, which could contribute to the generation of phenotypic diversity (Nicolson and Poste, 1983). Pharmacologic approaches to the control of heterogeneity must await further biochemical studies of the mechanisms involved.

2.5. Host Defenses

The metastatic process is relatively inefficient, and only a minute fraction of disseminated tumor cells survive to form metastases (Fidler, 1970; Liotta *et al.*, 1974; Butler and Gullino, 1975; Weiss, 1980; Weiss *et al.*, 1982; Schirrmacher and Waller, 1982). Mechanical as well as immune factors play a role. There is substantial experimental evidence to show that the immune system plays a role in elimination of tumor cells in animal models, but in humans its significance in eradicating malignant cells has been a controversial issue for many years. Animal studies by Eccles show an inverse correlation between immunogenicity and metastatic capacity (Eccles, 1982). The level of the immunogenic response also varies according to the type of carcinogen used. Chemically induced tumors seem to evoke stronger immunity than virally or spontaneously transformed tumors, as demonstrated by Kim *et al.* on rat mammary carcinomas (Kim, 1970; Kim *et al.*, 1975). The immune cell types thought to be involved in tumor cell destruction are T lymphocytes, natural killer (NK) cells, and macrophages. It is well established that T lymphocytes are required for generation of antitumor immunity (Plata, 1982; Yamauchi *et al.*, 1979). Noncytotoxic T cells can also participate in immunologic tumor rejection (Fernandez-Cruz *et al.*, 1982). NK cells, which are thought to be related to T lymphocytes (Grossman and Herberman, 1982), possibly play an important role in surveillance against circulating tumor cells. No studies to date have proven that NK cells can kill tumor cells outside of the circulation. The low incidence of metastasis in tumor-bearing nude mice that possess NK cells may suggest that these cells are important in preventing metastatic tumor spread (Hanna and Burton, 1981). The killing mechanism may be associated with the state of differentiation, and stimulation of differentiation makes the tumor cells less susceptible to lysis by NK cells (Gidlund *et al.*, 1981). Activated macrophages can destroy tumor cells *in vitro* and *in vivo* regardless of the method of activation (Hibbs, 1974; Liotta *et al.*, 1977a; Fidler and Raz, 1981). Data from diverse experimental systems indicate that macrophage-mediated cytolysis is independent of the metastatic potential, antigenicity, and drug sensitivity of the tumor cells (Fidler and Poste, 1982). The exact mechanism by which macrophages recognize and lyse tumor cells is still unknown, but it seems to be linked to the neoplastic phenotype, since nonneoplastic cells are less affected.

3. EXTRACELLULAR MATRIX

3.1. Structure and Function

Basement membranes are sheets of extracellular matrix found in every organ in which parenchymal cells interface with interstitial connective tissue (Vracko, 1974). Parenchymal cells include all types of epithelial cells, endothelial cells, mesothelial cells, endocrine cells, muscle fibers, adipocytes, and Schwann cells. BM may differ in structure and chemical composition depending on the tissue of origin (Madri *et al.*, 1983). Three layers of the BM have been identified by electron microscopy: lamina lucida (rara), which is an electrolucid zone directly below the cell membrane; lamina densa (basal lamina), which consists of a network of electrodense, randomly oriented fibrils; and finally the reticular layer, containing the anchoring fibrils, which blend into the collagen fibers of the underlying connective tissue (Kanwar and Farquhar, 1979). In most tissues, lamina lucida and lamina densa are of equal thickness (40–60 nm).

In adult tissues the main functions of the BM include serving as (1) tissue scaffolding, (2) a boundary between cell layers and underlying interstitial connective tissue, and (3) a filtration barrier to the passage of macromolecules. Traumatic disruption of the BM leads to scar formation and loss of normal architecture (Vracko, 1974). BM may play an important role in controlling cell proliferation, as is apparent when they become denuded of parenchymal cells and new ones continue to multiply until the cell-free gap is repopulated. It is possible that BM possess cell-specific markers that are recognized only by their tissue-specific epithelial cells.

Immunoelectronmicroscopic techniques, using antibodies against the major components of the BM, have been used to localize them within the BM. Some investigators have found that the BM components are zone-specific, while others have questioned this zone specificity. Three major BM components are type IV collagen, laminin, and proteoglycan. Type IV collagen has been visualized in the lamina densa (Laurie *et al.*, 1982), but laminin (Timpl et al., 1979) and heparan sulfate proteoglycan (Hassell et al., 1980) have both been seen in the lamina rara alone and throughout the BM. Fibronectin and type V collagen have also been found in the BM but are present as well in other tissues. Widespread changes occur in the distribution and amount of BM during the progression from benign to malignant tumors. The common human carcinomas all possess defective BM (Liotta et al., 1983; Barsky et al., 1983b). While benign neoplasms exhibit intact BM, the loss of BM by invading tumor cells may facilitate access of systemic antibodies to antigens on the tumor cell apical surface.

3.2. Basement Membrane Collagens

The major structural backbone of BM is type IV collagen, which is uniquely found in this matrix (Kefalides et al., 1979; Timpl et al., 1978, 1982a; Bornstein and Sage, 1980). Studies on isolation and characterization of the native type IV collagen have been hampered by its poor solubility owing to the presence of disulfide bonds. These difficulties were overcome by the discovery of the EHS tumor which contains large amounts of acid-soluble type IV collagen (Orkin et al., 1977; Kleinman et al., 1982). The PYS-2 endodermlike cell line has also been a good source for type IV procollagen (Lehman et al., 1974). Type IV procollagen, which is synthesized in organ cultures of EHS tumor and in PYS-2 cell cultures, is composed of two polypeptide chains with MW of about 170,000 and 185,000, designated as pro $\alpha1$(IV) and pro $\alpha2$(IV) (Tryggvason et al., 1980; Leivo et al., 1982; Garbisa et al., 1981). The conversion of type IV procollagen into the matrix form is not fully understood, but some data indicate that the procollagen is not substantially altered when deposited in the BM (Minor et al., 1976; Heathcote et al., 1980). Examination of type IV procollagen by rotary shadowing has revealed molecules consisting of 386-nm-long strands with globular end regions.

Type V collagen was first isolated in 1976 (Burgeson et al., 1976) and has been found in various tissues, including liver (Chung et al., 1976), synovial membrane (Brown et al., 1978), bone and placenta (Rhodes and Miller, 1978), embryonic tendons (Jimenez et al., 1978), lung (Madri and Furchtmayr, 1979), glomerular BM (Alexander et al., 1979), cornea (Welsh et al., 1980), aorta (Ooshima, 1981), and gingiva (Dabbous et al., 1981). Synthesis of this type of collagen in cultured cells has been demonstrated in fibroblasts, smooth muscle cells, and epithelial cells (Mayne et al., 1978; Stenn et al., 1979; Fessler et al., 1981). Type V collagen consists of three types of alpha chains—1(V), 2(V), and 3(V)—which have been separated by ion exchange chromatography (Burgeson et al., 1976; Chung et al., 1976; Rhodes and Miller, 1978). Type V collagen has been localized most consistently in pericellular spaces (Miller and Rhodes, 1982; Bailey et al., 1979; Sage et al., 1981). The structural and functional roles of type V collagen are still unclear and a unifying concept remains to be substantiated. It is resistant to the action of mammalian collagenase (Liotta et al., 1979; Welgus et al., 1981), but is degraded by thrombin (Sage et al., 1981) and type V collagenase.

3.3. Noncollagenous Components

Laminin is a main noncollagenous glycoprotein of BM produced by cells that normally produce a BM. It has been isolated and characterized from EHS tumor (Timpl et al., 1979, 1982b) and mouse endodermal cell cultures (Chung et al., 1979). Laminin is synthesized by a variety of normal epithelial, endothelial, and muscle cells in culture (Foidart et al., 1980), as well as by endodermal cells (Hogan, 1980; Sakashita and Ruoslahti, 1980; Howe and Solter, 1980) and tumor cells (Chung et al., 1979; Strickland et al., 1980; Leivo et al., 1982; Wewer et al., 1981; Martinez-Hernandez et al., 1982). It is a large protein with an MW of about 900,000 shown by ultracentrifugal analyses (Engel et al., 1981) and consists of at least two polypeptide chains with MW of 200,000 and 400,000. Rotary shadowing studies have demonstrated that laminin has a crosslike shape consisting of one long arm (75 mm) and three short arms (35 mm) with globular domains at the end of the arms. The intersection region of the short arms contains a disulfide-bonded protease-resistant domain (Liotta et al., 1981a,b; Engel et al., 1981; Rao et al., 1982a,b). The intersection region of the short arms may be derived from distinct chains that migrate in the 200,000-dalton range (Timpl et al., 1982a; Rao et al., 1982b).

A major biological function of laminin is to mediate attachment of epithelial and endothelial cells to the BM (Terranova et al., 1980; Hogan et al., 1980; Vlodavsky et al., 1980; Kleinman et al., 1981). It may also play an important role in embryogenesis, differentiation, and tissue remodeling (Howe and Solter, 1980; Strickland et al., 1980; Ekblom, 1981; Hogan, 1980; Leivo et al., 1980). Studies of the binding properties of different domains on the laminin molecule indicate that it binds to proteoglycan through the long arm, to the cell surface through the central cross portion, and to type IV collagen through the globular end regions, a process which requires an intact procollagen molecule (Rao et al., 1982a,b, 1983b). Laminin is used by highly metastatic tumor cells to attach to type IV collagen (Terranova et al., 1982). Tumor cells selected for their ability to use laminin for attachment produced more experimental metastases than the control tumor cells (Terranova et al., 1982). Furthermore, when laminin was preincubated with the tumor cells and then injected intravenously into mice, an increased number of metastases were observed (Barsky et al., 1984b). A study by Varani and co-workers using high- and low-metastatic tumor cells demonstrated that at least one line of high-metastatic cells expressed a lamininlike substance that facilitated adherence. A specific cell surface receptor for laminin was first identified on cultured MCF-7 human breast carcinoma cells (Terranova et al., 1983). The MW of the laminin receptor isolated either from MCF-7 cells or human breast carcinoma tissue is approximately 67,000 (Rao et al., 1983a). A fragment of laminin that contains the receptor binding domain blocks experimental metastases in a murine model (Barsky et al., 1984a,b). Monoclonal antibodies have been produced that recognize the binding domain for laminin on the human breast carcinoma laminin receptor (Liotta et al., 1985). Laminin receptor of the same MW has been isolated from metastatic murine B16 melanoma cells (Rao et al., 1983a) and murine fibrosarcoma cells (Malinoff and Wicha, 1983). The existence of laminin binding sites has also been reported on muscle cell membranes (Lesot et al., 1983) and mouse macrophages (Wicha and Huard, 1983). Blocking the laminin receptor may therefore be a feasible strategy to inhibit hematogenous metastases.

4. PROTEOLYTIC ENZYMES

Many investigators have suggested that proteolytic enzymes are a prerequisite for invasion (Liotta, 1985). Cellular proteases are a very diverse group of enzymes differing in specificity and conditions required for maximal activity. Proteases are classified as exopeptidases (peptidases) and endopeptidases (proteinases). Proteinases are grouped according to their catalytic sites, specific susceptibility to inhibitors, optimum pH, and cation requirements (Neurath and Walsh, 1976).

Other roles ascribed to proteinases in cancer include stimulation of cell division (Burger, 1970; Sefton and Rubin, 1970; Buchanan et al., 1976) and involvement in oncogenic transformation and tumorigenesis (Troll et al., 1970; Wigler and Weinstein, 1976; Kennedy and Little, 1978). The proteinases most commonly associated with malignant tumors and transformed cells are collagenases, plasminogen activators, and lysosomal proteinases (Sylven, 1974; Quigley, 1979b; Recklies et al., 1982).

4.1. Plasminogen Activators

Plasmin is a neutral proteinase capable of degrading many protein substrates such as fibrin and cell surface proteins (Astrup and Permin, 1947; Hynes, 1973; Blumberg and Robbins, 1975). Plasminogen is an inactive serum component that is catalytically converted to plasmin by plasminogen activator (PA). PA exists in multiple forms ranging in molecular mass from 28,000 to 165,000 daltons (Tucker et al., 1978; Naito et al., 1980; Markus et al., 1980). At least three groups of PA are known: urokinase, tissue PA, and circulating PA (Christman et al., 1977). PA may be important for a number of physiological processes since it is found in a variety of normal cells (E. Reich, 1978). Augmented PA activity has been observed in various biological processes associated with proteolysis and tissue breakdown, such as ovulation (Beers et al., 1975), trophoblast implantation (Strickland et al., 1976), inflammation (Unkeless et al., 1973), and mammary gland involution (Ossowski et al., 1979). Endothelial cells of different origin have also been shown to produce PA (Loskutoff and Edgington, 1977; Laug et al., 1980; Gross et al., 1980).

The association of enhanced fibrinolytic activity with malignant tumors was first made by Fischer in 1925 and has since been reported by many investigators (Tagnon *et al.*, 1952; Peterson, 1968; Peterson *et al.*, 1973; Wilson and Dowle, 1978; Tucker *et al.*, 1978; Webber *et al.*, 1981). Enhanced PA activity has been documented after neoplastic transformation with on-cogenic viruses, tumor promoters, and chemical carcinogens (Wigler and Weinstein, 1976; Wilson and Reich, 1978; Quigley, 1979a; Goldberg, 1974; Rifkin *et al.*, 1974; Christman *et al.*, 1977). However, other studies have failed to demonstrate a correlation between malignant transformation and elevated PA levels (Mott *et al.*, 1974; Wolf and Goldberg, 1976; Quigley, 1979b; Salo *et al.*, 1982).

4.2. Cysteine Proteinases

Lysosomal cysteine proteinases are ubiquitous in all mammalian tissues. Lysosomal enzymes together with a whole range of other proteinases have been implicated in the proteolytic activities that facilitate the multistep meta-static process, and increase in lysosomal enzymes has been detected in skin cancer and melanoma (Shamberger and Rudolph, 1967; Drewa *et al.*, 1978).

Cathepsin B is a cysteine proteinase that degrades pericellular proteins and thus facilitates cellular detachment. Cathepsin B also degrades proteo-glycan (Roughley and Barrett, 1977) and can convert procollagenase to its active form (Eeckhout and Vaes, 1977). High amounts of an enzyme similar to cathepsin B were demonstrated in human breast carcinoma in organ cul-ture compared to benign breast lesions (Poole *et al.*, 1978; Recklies *et al.*, 1980; Mort *et al.*, 1980). This enzyme, which is more stable at neutral pH and has a higher molecular weight than cathepsin B, is considered to be a precursor form of cathepsin B (Recklies and Poole, 1982).

Similarly, a precursor form of cathepsin B from ascites fluid from pa-tients with different types of neoplasms has been partially purified and characterized (Mort *et al.*, 1981, 1983). Some reports indicate that the highest levels of cathepsin B are found in the smallest and most rapidly growing tumors (Shamberger and Rudolph, 1967; Sloane *et al.*, 1981). An *in vivo* study using high and low metastatic variants of murine melanoma lines demonstrated a positive correlation of cathepsin B activity with metastatic potential but failed to detect any differences in the same cell lines cultured *in vitro* (Sloane *et al.*, 1982). A controversial point about lysosomal protein-ases such as cathepsin B has been the pH optimum of these enzymes, which is at acid pH. Many investigators doubt that these enzymes can function at the physiological pH of the extracellular spaces.

4.3. Metalloproteinases

4.3.1. Vertebrate (Mammalian) Collagenase

Since the discovery of the first vertebrate collagenase by Gross and Lapière (1962), it has been found to be produced by virtually all mesenchy-mal tissues, some epithelial cells, macrophages, and polymorphonuclear leukocytes (Gross, 1976; Perez-Tamayo, 1978; Woolley and Grafton, 1980).

Classic collagenase is a neutral metalloproteinase that requires Ca^{2+} or Zn^{2+} at physiological temperature for activity and is inhibited by chelating agents such as EDTA. Collagenase is the only proteolytic enzyme that cleaves the native triple helical portion of the collagen molecule, attacking approximately three quarters of the way from the C terminus of the alpha helix. Collagen types I, II, and III are all degraded in a similar manner by the vertebrate collagenase, although cleavage of type II collagen is much slower than that of the other two types (McCroskery et al., 1975; Woolley et al., 1978; T. Hayashi et al., 1980). Types IV and V collagen are not susceptible to the vertebrate collagenase (Liotta et al., 1979).

Disagreement exists among collagen researchers concerning whether the vertebrate collagenase is secreted in a latent or an active form. Some studies using tissue sections have only detected the active enzyme (Woolley et al., 1975), but other studies using tissue culture or direct tissue extractions have demonstrated the collagenase as a proenzyme (Stricklin et al., 1977). Latent collagenase can be activated with other proteinases such as plasmin or trypsin or organic mercurial compounds. The dilemma of whether or not activation involves removal of critical amino acid residues or inhibitor–enzyme complexes has not been resolved (Murphy and Sellers, 1980).

Augmented collagenase levels have been detected in organ cultures of tumor tissues (Dresden et al., 1972; Kuettner et al., 1977; Yamanishi et al., 1972; Biswas et al., 1978; Dabbous et al., 1977; Turpeenniemi-Hujanen et al., 1984). Tumor tissue collagenase can be derived from the host or the tumor cells. Immunofluorescent staining studies have shown in some tumor tissues that the collagenase is in the stromal cells and not in the tumor cells (Huang et al., 1976; Bauer et al., 1977). Other reports have suggested that tumor cells could stimulate fibroblasts to produce collagenase (Bauer et al., 1979; Matsumoto et al., 1979). Recent reports have demonstrated immunoreactive collagenase in the tumor cells themselves (Woolley and Grafton, 1980; Dabbous et al., 1983).

4.3.2. Basement Membrane (Type IV and V) Collagenases

BM collagen is specifically degraded by type IV collagenase, which is a neutral metalloproteinase inhibited by EDTA, α_2-macroglobulin, and cartilage inhibitors. It has been identified in polymorphonuclear leukocytes (Liotta et al., 1980; Mainardi et al., 1980a), fetal bovine endothelial cells (Kalebic et al., 1983), and cultured tumor cells (Liotta et al., 1977b, 1979, 1980; Thorgeirsson et al., 1982; Siegal et al., 1982). Type IV collagenase was first identified and purified from highly metastatic murine tumor cells (Liotta et al., 1981d; Salo et al., 1982). The purified enzyme appears as a doublet on polyacrylamide gel electrophoresis with molecular weights of about 68,000 and 62,000. The enzyme activity has a pH optimum of 7.6, requires trypsin for activation, and is reversibly inhibited by EDTA but not by N-ethylenemaleimide, phenylmethylsulfonyl fluoride, or Trasylol (Salo et al., 1983). Human type IV collagenase with comparable molecular weights has been purified from a fibrosarcoma cell line (HT-1080) and a metastatic melanoma line (A2058) (T. Turpeenniemi-Hujanen, unpublished results). Type IV collagenase produces specific cleavage fragments of type IV collagen at 25°C with a simple cleavage site forming fragments of a mass ratio 3:1. The cleavage site is at the NH_2 terminus of the collagen molecule, leaving the carboxy end regions intact (Fessler, 1984).

Type IV collagenase is secreted into the culture medium in a latent form (Liotta et al., 1979, 1980) that can be activated with trypsin or plasmin. Type IV collagenase immunoreactivity has been demonstrated in invasive breast carcinoma (Barsky et al., 1983a), and correlation has been shown between type IV collagenolytic activity and the metastatic potential of tumor cells (Liotta et al., 1980; Nakajima et al., 1984). A quantitative relationship has also been found between type IV collagenase activity and in vitro tumor cell invasion, using native BM of a human amnion as an invasion barrier (Thorgeirsson et al., 1982, 1984; Siegal et al., 1982). Further evidence for the significance of type IV collagenase in tumor cell invasion was found by using purified metalloprotease inhibitors, which greatly inhibited penetration of highly metastatic cells through a native BM of a human amnion in the invasion system (Thorgeirsson et al., 1982). Collagenase may be only one of many factors elevated in actively invading tumor cells. The metastatic process involves multiple cellular and host factors, and in some instances the host defenses, such as immune cell killing, can overcome the proteolytic activities of highly invasive tumor cells. Nevertheless, degradation of BM may be a critical step in the metastatic process.

4.4. Arrest of Metastases by Protease Inhibitors

The association of proteases with tumor invasion has led to the proposal that protease inhibitors could have therapeutic value. A significant study by Giraldi et al. (1984) has shown that a variety of certain protease inhibitors could significantly reduce tumor growth and metastases in an animal model system. This group injected (i.p.) protease inhibitors into mice bearing the transplantable Lewis lung carcinoma. An egg-white-derived inhibitor of cysteine proteinases (EWI) and phosphoramidon, a collagenase inhibitor, both significantly inhibited spontaneous metastases. The latter agent was more effective in these in vivo studies. Both inhibitors exhibited a dose-dependent effect. Phosphoramidon inhibited metastasis formation without depression of the primary tumor growth. Thus, this agent is not merely reducing the primary tumor mass, which could indirectly reduce metastases. These results support the concept that collagenase and cathepsin B may be involved in the metastatic process. They also provide incentive for further in vivo studies on the role of protease inhibitors as antimetastatic therapy. Antiinvasion factors with protease-inhibitory activity have been identified by Kuettner and Pauli (Kuettner et al., 1977; Pauli et al., 1981). The next phase of research for these factors may be in vivo testing.

Furthermore, in vitro tumor invasion studies using native human amnion BM have revealed that a purified metalloproteinase collagenase inhibitor inhibits tumor cell penetration of this barrier (Thorgeirsson et al., 1982). Extension of these encouraging results using protease inhibitors will undoubtedly be an important part of future work in the field of experimental cancer biology.

Type V collagenase has been identified in culture medium from various normal and malignant tumor cell types, such as pulmonary alveolar macrophages (Mainardi et al., 1980b), and from M5076 mouse reticulum sarcoma cells (Liotta et al., 1981c). This enzyme was partially purified from the M5076 cells by molecular sieve chromatography, was estimated to have a molecular weight of about 80,000 (Liotta et al., 1981c), and was found to degrade high-molecular-weight 1α and 2α cartilage collagens (Liotta et al., 1982).

5. CONCLUDING REMARKS

A number of biochemical factors—including cell surface antigens, proteolytic enzymes, and receptors—have now been discovered in association with metastatic tumor cells. Most investigators do not believe that these factors are tumor specific. They may be augmented only in the actively invading tumor cells. In benign or normal cells the genetic expression of the factors is reduced. This concept rests on the assumption that invasion and metastasis are active processes and a consequence of specific biochemical events. Attachment factors and cell surface receptors may play a role in the anchoring of tumor cells to the extracellular matrix. Local degradation of the matrix, including the BM, by tumor cells has been observed by many investigators. A cascade of enzymes undoubtedly facilitates this degradation. In vivo enzymes may be derived from both the tumor cells and the host. Among the most important proteases identified to date are collagenases, the plasminogen activators, the cathepsins, and the heparinases. In vivo studies using protease inhibitors provide the best evidence that these enzymes really play a role in the actual metastatic process.

REFERENCES

Abelev, G. I., 1974, α-Fetoprotein as a marker of embryo-specific differentiations in normal and tumor tissue, Transplant. Rev. 20:3–37.

Abelev, G. I., Perova, S. D., Khramkova, N. I., Postnikova, Z. A., and Irlin, I. S., 1963, Production of embryonal α-globulin by transplantable mouse hepatomas, Transplantation 1:174–186.

Alexander, W. F., Mills, B. K., and Lichtenstein, J. R., 1979, Isolation of collagen A and B chains from purified basement membranes, Fed. Proc. 38:1407.

Alpert, E., Coston, R. C., and Drysdale, J. W., 1973, Carcinofetal human isoferritins, Nature 242:194–196.

Anderson, L. C., Gahmberg, C. G., Nilsson, K., and Wigzell, H., 1977, Surface glycoprotein patterns of normal and malignant human lymphoid cells. I. T cells, T blasts and leukemic T cell lines, Int. J. Cancer 20:702–707.

Astrup, T., and Permin, P. M., 1947, Fibrinolysis in the animal organism, Nature 159:681–682.

Avis, P., Biol, M. I., and Lewis, M. G., 1973, Tumor associated fetal antigens in human tumors, J. Natl. Cancer Inst. 51:1063–1066.

Bailey, A. J., Shellswell, G. B., and Duance, V. C., 1979, Identification and change of collagen types in differentiating myoblasts and developing chick muscle, Nature 278:67–69.

Banwo, O., Versey, J., and Hobbs, J. R., 1974, New oncofetal antigen from human pancreas, Lancet 1:643–645.

Barsky, S. H., Togo, S., Garbisa, S., and Liotta, L. A., 1983a, Type IV collagenase immunoreactivity in invasive breast carcinoma, Lancet 1:296–297.

Barsky, S. H., Siegel, G. P., Jannotta, F., and Liotta, L. A., 1983b, Loss of basement membrane components by invasive tumors but not by their benign counterparts, Lab. Invest. 49:140–147.

Barsky, S. H., Rao, C. N., Hyams, D., and Liotta, L. A., 1984a, Characterization of a laminin receptor from human breast carcinoma tissue, Breast Cancer Res. Treat. 4:181–188.

Barsky, S. H., Rao, C. N., Williams, J. E., and Liotta, L. A., 1984b, Laminin molecular domains which alter metastasis in a murine model, J. Clin. Invest. 74:843–848.

Bauer, E. A., Gordon, J. M., Reddick, M. E., and Eisen, A. Z., 1977, Quantitation and immunocytochemical localization of human skin collagenase in basal cell carcinoma, J. Invest. Dermatol. 69:363–367.

Bauer, E. A., Uitto, J., Walders, R. C., and Eisen, A. Z., 1979, Enhanced collagenase production by fibroblasts derived from human basal cell carcinomas, Cancer Res. 39:4594–4599.

Baylin, S. B., 1982, Clonal selection and heterogeneity of human solid neoplasms, in: Design of Models for Testing Cancer Therapeutic Agents (I. J. Fidler and R. J. White, eds.), Van Nostrand, New York, pp. 50–64.

Beers, W. H., Strickland, S., and Reich, E., 1975, Ovarian plasminogen activator: Relationship to ovulation and hormonal regulation, Cell 6:387–394.

Bernstein, I. D., Tam, M. R., and Nowinski, R. C., 1980, Mouse leukemia: Therapy with monoclonal antibodies against a thymus differentiation antigen, Science 207:68–71.

Biswas, C., Moran, W. P., Bloch, K. J., and Gross, J., 1978, Collagenolytic activity of rabbit V2-carcinoma growing at multiple sites, Biochem. Biophys. Res. Commun. 80:33–38.

Björklund, B., 1976, Tissue polypeptide antigen (TPA) in cancer and other conditions, in: Oncodevelopmental Gene Expression (W. H. Fishman and S. Sell, eds.), Academic Press, New York, pp. 501–508.

Blumberg, P. M., and Robbins, P. W., 1975, Effect of proteases on activation of resting chick embryo fibroblasts and cell surface proteins, Cell 6:137–147.

Boon, T., and Kellerman, O., 1977, Rejection by syngeneic mice of cell variants obtained by mutagenesis of a malignant teratocarcinoma cell line, Proc. Natl. Acad. Sci. USA 74:272–275.

Bornstein, P., and Sage, H., 1980, Structurally distinct collagen types, Annu. Rev. Biochem. 49:957–1003.

Brown, R. A., Shuttleworth, C. A., and Weiss, J. B., 1978, Three new alpha-chains of collagen from a non-basement membrane source, Biochem. Biophys. Res. Commun. 80:866–872.

Buchanan, J. M., Bo Chen, L., and Zetter, B. R., 1976, Protease-related effects in normal and transformed cells, in: Cancer Enzymology (J. Schultz and F. Ahmad, eds.), Academic Press, New York, pp. 1–22.

Bumol, T. F., and Reisfeld, R. A., 1982, Unique glycoprotein–proteoglycan complex defined by monoclonal antibody on human melanoma cells, Proc. Natl. Acad. Sci. USA 79:1245–1249.

Bumol, T. F., Wang, Q. C., Reisfeld, R. A., and Kaplan, N. O., 1983, Monoclonal antibody and an antibody–toxin conjugate to a cell surface proteoglycan of melanoma cells suppress in vivo tumor growth, Proc. Natl. Acad. Sci. USA 80:529–533.

Burger, M. M., 1970, Proteolytic enzymes initiating cell division and escape from contact inhibition of growth, Nature 227:170–171.

Burgeson, R. E., El Adli, F. A., Kaitila, I. I., and Hollister, D. W., 1976, Fetal membrane collagens: Identification of two new collagen alpha chains, Proc. Natl. Acad. Sci. USA 73:2579–2583.

Butler, T. P., and Gullino, P. M., 1975, Quantitation of cell shedding into efferent blood of mammary adenocarcinoma, Cancer Res. 35:512–516.

Calabresi, P., Dexter, D. L., and Heppner, G. H., 1979, Clinical and pharmacological implications of cancer cell differentiation and heterogeneity, Biochem. Pharmacol. 28:1933–1941.

Ceriani, R. L., Thompson, K. E., Peterson, J. A., and Abraham, S., 1977, Surface differentiation antigens of human mammary epithelial cells carried on the human milk fat globule, Proc. Natl. Acad. Sci. USA 74:582–586.

Ceriani, R. L., Sasaki, M., Sussman, H., Wara, W. M., and Blank, E. W., 1982, Circulating human mammary epithelial antigens in breast cancer, Proc. Natl. Acad. Sci. USA 79:5420–5424.

Christman, J. K., Silverstein, S., and Acs, G., 1977, Plasminogen activation, in: Proteinases in Mammalian Cells and Tissues, Volume 2 (A. J. Barrett, ed.), Elsevier/North-Holland Biomedical Press, Amsterdam, pp. 91–149.

Chung, A. E., Rhodes, R. K., and Miller, E. J., 1976, Isolation of three collagenous components of probable basement membrane origin from several tissues, Biochem. Biophys. Res. Commun. 71:1167–1174.

Chung, A. E., Jaffe, R., Freeman, I. L., Vergnes, J. P., Braginski, J. E., and Carlin, B., 1979, Properties of a basement membrane-related glycoprotein synthesized in culture by a mouse embryonal carcinoma-derived cell line, Cell 16:277–287.

Dabbous, M. K., Roberts, A. N., and Brinkley, S. B., 1977, Collagenase and neutral protease activities in cultures of rabbit VX-2 carcinoma, Cancer Res. 37:3537–3544.

Dabbous, M. K., Hammouda, O., and Brinkley, S. B., 1981, Isolation and partial characterization of bovine gingival AB collagen, Mol. Cell. Biochem. 34:87–93.

Dabbous, M. K., El-Torky, M., Haney, L., Sobhy, N., and Brinkley, S. B., 1983, Separation of VX-2 rabbit carcinoma-derived cells capable of releasing collagenase, Exp. Mol. Pathol. 38:1–21.

Dresden, M. H., Heilman, S. A., and Schmidt, J. D., 1972, Collagenolytic enzymes in human neoplasms, Cancer Res. 32:993–996.

Drewa, G., Zbytniewski, Z., and Kanclerz, A., 1978, Activity of some lysosomal hydrolases in the homogenates of transplantable melanotic and amelanotic melanoma in golden hamster (Mesocricetus auratus, Waterhouse), Arch. Geschwulstforsch. 48:198–201.

Easty, G. C., and Easty, D. M., 1976, Mechanism of tumor invasion, in: Scientific Foundations of Oncology (T. Symington and R. L. Carter, eds.), Heinemann, London, pp. 167–172.

Eccles, S. A., 1982, Host immune mechanisms important in the control of tumor metastasis, in: Tumor Immunity in Prognosis: The Role of Mononuclear Cell Infiltration (J. S. Haskill, ed.), Marcel Dekker, New York, pp. 39–74.

Eeckhout, Y., and Vaes, G., 1977, Further studies on the activation of procollagenase, the latent precursor of bone collagenase: Effects of lysosomal cathepsin B, plasmin and kallikrein, and spontaneous activation, Biochem. J. 166:21–31.

Ekblom, P., 1981, Formation of basement membranes in the embryonic kidney: An immunohistological study, J. Cell Biol. 91:1–10.

Engel, J., Odermatt, E., Engel, A., Madri, J. A., Furthmayr, H., Rohde, H., and Timpl, R., 1981, Shapes, domain organizations and flexibility of laminin and fibronectin, two multifunctional proteins of the extracellular matrix, J. Mol. Biol. 150:97–120.

Fernandez-Cruz, E., Gilman, S. C., and Feldman, J. D., 1982, Immunotherapy of a chemically-induced sarcoma in rats: Characterization of the effector T cell subset and nature of suppression, J. Immunol. 128:1112–1117.

Fessler, L. I., Robinson, W. J., and Fessler, J. H., 1981, Biosynthesis of procollagen [(pro alpha 1 V) 2 (pro alpha 2 V)] by chick tendon fibroblasts and procollagen (pro alpha 1 V) 3 by hamster lung cell cultures, J. Biol. Chem. 256:9646–9651.

Fessler, L. I., Duncan, K. G., Fessler, J. H., Salo, T., and Tryggvason, K., 1974, Characterization of the procollagen IV cleavage products produced by a specific tumor collagenase, J. Biol. Chem. 259:9783–9789.

Fialkow, P. J., 1976, Clonal origin of human tumors, Biochim. Biophys. Acta. 458:283–321.

Fidler, I. J., 1970, Metastasis: Quantitative analysis of distribution and fate of tumor emboli labeled with ^{125}I-5 iodo-2'deoxyuridine, J. Natl. Cancer Inst. 45:733–782.

Fidler, I. J., and Kripke, M. J., 1977, Metastasis results from preexisting variant cells within a malignant tumor, Science 197:893–895.

Fidler, I. J., and Nicolson, G. L., 1981, Immunology of experimental metastatic melanoma, Cancer Biol. Rev. 2:171–234.

Fidler, I. J., and Poste, G., 1982, Macrophage mediated destruction of malignant tumor cells and new strategies for the therapy of metastatic disease, Immunopathology **5**:161–174.

Fidler, I. J., and Raz, A., 1981, The induction of tumoricidal rat macrophages by lymphokines, in: Lymphokines, Volume 3 (E. Pick, ed.), Academic Press, New York, pp. 345–363.

Fischer, A., 1925, Beitrag zur Biologie der Gewebszellen. Eine vergleichen-biologishe Gewebszellen in vitro, Arch. Entwicklungsmech. Org. **104**:210–261.

Fisher, M. S., and Cifone, M. A., 1981, Enhanced metastatic potential of murine fibrosarcomas treated in vitro with ultraviolet radiation, Cancer Res. **41**:3018–3023.

Foidart, J. M., Bere, E. W., Yaar, M., Rennard, S. I., Gullino, M., Martin, G. R., and Katz, S. I., 1980, Distribution and immunoelectron microscopic localization of laminin, a noncollagenous basement membrane glycoprotein, Lab. Invest. **42**:336–342.

Foulds, L., 1956, The histologic analysis of mammary tumors in mice. I. Scope of investigations and general principles of analysis, J. Natl. Cancer Inst. **17**:701–754.

Fritze, D., and Mach, J. P., 1975, Identification of new oncofoetal antigen associated with several types of human carcinomas, Nature **258**:734–737.

Gabbiani, G., 1979, The cytoskeleton in cancer cells in animals and humans, Meth. Achiev. Exp. Pathol. **9**:231–249.

Gahmberg, C. G., Jokinen, M., and Sandersson, L. C., 1979, Expression of the major red cell sialoglycoprotein, glycophorin A, in the human leukemic cell line K562, J. Biol. Chem. **254**:7442–7448.

Garbisa, S., Liotta, L. A., Tryggvason, K., and Siegel, G. P., 1981, Antibodies to collagenase resistant terminal regions of pro-type IV collagen recognize whole basement membrane and 7-S collagen, FEBS Lett. **127**:257–262.

Gershman, H., Katzin, W., and Cook, R. T., 1978, Motility of cells from solid tumors, Int. J. Cancer **21**:309–316.

Gidlund, M., Orn, A., Pattengale, P. K., Jansson, M., Wigzell, H., and Nilsson, K., 1981, Natural killer cells kill tumor cells at a given stage of differentiation, Nature **292**:848–850.

Giraldi, T., Sava, G., Perissin, L., and Zorzet, S., 1984, Primary tumor growth and formation of spontaneous lung metastases in mice bearing Lewis carcinoma treated with proteinase inhibitors, Anticancer Res. **4**:221–224.

Gold, P., and Freedman, S. O., 1965, Demonstration of tumor specific antigens in human colonic carcinomata by immunological tolerance and absorption techniques, J. Exp. Med. **121**:439–462.

Goldberg, A. R., 1974, Increased protease levels in transformed cells: A casein overlay assay for the detection of plasminogen activator production, Cell **2**:95–102.

Grimes, W. J., 1970, Sialic acid transferases and sialic acid levels in normal and transformed cells, Biochemistry **9**:5083–5092.

Gross, J., 1976, Aspects of animal collagenases, in: Biochemistry of Collagen (G. N. Ramachandran and A. H. Reddi, eds.), Plenum Press, New York, pp. 275–317.

Gross, J., and Lapière, C. M., 1962, Collagenolytic activity in amphibian tissues: A tissue culture assay, Proc. Natl. Acad. Sci. USA **48**:1014–1022.

Gross, J., Highberger, J. H., Johnsen-Wint, B., and Biswas, C., 1980, Role of action and regulation of tissue collagenases, in: Collagenase in Normal and Pathological Connective Tissues (D. E. Woolley and J. M. Evanson, eds.), John Wiley & Sons, New York, pp. 11–35.

Grossman, Z., and Herberman, R. B., 1982, Hypothesis on the development of natural killer cells and their relationship to T cells, in: NK Cells and Other Natural Effector Cells (R. B. Herberman, ed.), Academic Press, New York, pp. 229–238.

Häkkinen, I. P. T., 1974, FSA-foetal sulpho-glycoprotein antigen associated with gastric cancer, Transplant Rev. **20**:61–76.

Hakomori, S., and Kannagi, R., 1983, Glycosphingolipids as tumor-associated and differentiation markers, J. Natl. Cancer Inst. **71**:231–251.

Hanna, N., and Burton, R., 1981, Definitive evidence that natural killer (NK) cells inhibit experimental tumor metastasis in vivo, J. Immunol. **127**:1754–1758.

Hart, I. R., Talmadge, J. E., and Fidler, I. J., 1981, Metastatic behaviour of a murine reticulum cell sarcoma exhibiting organ specific growth, Cancer Res. **41**:1281–1287.

Hassell, J. R., Gehron-Robey, P., Barrach, H. J., Wilczek, J., Rennard, S. I., and Martin, G. R.,

1980, Isolation of a heparan sulfate-containing proteoglycan from basement membrane, *Proc. Natl. Acad. Sci. USA* **77**:4494–4498.

Hayashi, H., Yoshida, K., Ozaki, T., and Ushijima, K., 1970, Chemotactic factor associated with invasion of cancer cells, *Nature* **226**:174–175.

Hayashi, T., Nakamura, T., Hori, H., and Nagai, J., 1980, Degradation rates of type II and III collagens by tadpole collagenase are modulated by mutual presence, *J. Biochem. (Tokyo)* **87**:993–995.

Heathcote, J. G., Bailey, A. J., and Grant, M. E., 1980, Studies on the assembly of the rat lens capsule: Biosynthesis of a cross-linked collagenous component of high molecular weight, *Biochem. J.* **190**:229–237.

Hibbs, J. B., Jr., 1974, Discrimination between neoplastic and non-neoplastic cells *in vitro* by activated macrophages, *J. Natl. Cancer Inst.* **53**:1487–1492.

Hogan, B. L. M., 1980, High molecular weight extracellular proteins synthesized by endoderm cells derived from mouse teratocarcinoma cells and normal extraembryonic membranes, *Dev. Biol.* **76**:275–285.

Hogan, B. L. M., Cooper, A. R., and Kurkinen, M., 1980, Incorporation into Reichert's membrane of laminin-like extracellular proteins synthesized by parietal endoderm cells of the mouse embryo, *Dev. Biol.* **80**:289–300.

Howe, C. C., and Solter, D., 1980, Identification of noncollagenous basement membrane glycopolypeptides synthesized by mouse parietal endoderm and an entodermal cell line, *Dev. Biol.* **77**:480–487.

Huang, C. C., Abramson, M., Schilling, R. W., and Salorne, R. G., 1976, Collagenase activity in tumors of the head and neck, *Trans. Am. Acad. Ophthalmol. Otolaryngol.* **82**:138–141.

Hynes, R. O., 1973, Alteration of cell-surface proteins by viral transformation and by proteolysis, *Proc. Natl. Acad. Sci. USA* **70**:3170–3174.

Iannaccone, P. M., Gardner, R. L., and Harris, H., 1978, The cellular origin of chemically induced tumors, *J. Cell Sci.* **29**:249–269.

Jimenez, S. A., Yankowski, R., and Bashey, R. I., 1978, Identification of two new collagen alpha-chains in extracts of lathyritic chick embryo tendons, *Biochem. Biophys. Res. Commun.* **81**:1298–1306.

Kalebic, T., Garbisa, S., Glaser, B., and Liotta, L. A., 1983, Basement membrane collagen: Degradation by migrating endothelial cells, *Science* **221**:281–283.

Kanwar, Y. S., and Farquhar, M. G., 1979, Anionic sites in the glomerular basement membrane: *In vivo* and *in vitro* localization of the laminae rarae cationic probes, *J. Cell Biol.* **81**:137–153.

Kefalides, N. A., Alper, R., and Clark, C. C., 1979, Biochemistry and metabolism of basement membranes, *Int. Rev. Cytol.* **61**:167–228.

Kennedy, A. R., and Little, J. B., 1978, Protease inhibitors suppress radiation-induced malignant transformation *in vitro*, *Nature* **276**:825–826.

Kerbel, R. S., Dennis, J. W., Largarde, A. E., and Frost, P., 1982, Tumor progression in metastatis: An experimental approach using lectin resistant tumor variants, *Cancer Met. Rev.* **1**:99–140.

Kim, U., 1970, Metastasizing mammary carcinoma in rats: Induction and study of their immunogenicity, *Science* **67**:72–74.

Kim, U., Baumler, A., Carruthers, C., and Bielat, K., 1975, Immunological escape mechanism in spontaneously metastasizing mammary tumors, *Proc. Natl. Acad. Sci. USA* **72**:1012–1016.

Kleinman, H. K., Klebe, R. J., and Martin, G. R., 1981, Role of collagenous matrices in the adhesion and growth of cells, *J. Cell Biol.* **88**:473–485.

Kleinman, H. K., McGarvey, M. L., Liotta, L. A., Gehron-Robey, P., Tryggvason, K., and Martin, G. R., 1982, Isolation and characterization of type IV procollagen, laminin and heparan sulfate proteoglycan from the EHS sarcoma, *Biochemistry* **21**:6188–6193.

Koono, M., Ushijima, K., and Hayashi, H., 1974, Studies on the mechanisms of invasion in cancer. III. Purification of a neutral protease of rat ascites hepatoma cells associated with production of chemotactic factor for cancer cells, *Int. J. Cancer* **13**:105–115.

Koprowski, H., Steplewski, Z., Herlyn, D., and Herlyn, M., 1978, Study of antibodies against human melanoma produced by somatic cell hybrids, *Proc. Natl. Acad. Sci. USA* **75**:3405–3409.

Koprowski, H., Herlyn, M., and Steplewski, Z., 1981, Specific antigen in serum of patients with colon carcinoma, *Science* **212**:53–55.

Krueger, J. G., Garber, E. A., Goldberg, A. R., and Hanafusa, H., 1982, Changes in amino-terminal sequences of pp60^{src} lead to decreased membrane association and decreased *in vivo* tumorigenicity, *Cell* **28**:889–896.

Krupey, J., Gold, P., and Freedman, S. O., 1968, Physicochemical studies of the carcinoembryonic antigens of the human digestive system, *J. Exp. Med.* **128**:387–398.

Kuettner, K. E., Soble, L., Croxen, R. L., Marczynska, B., Hiti, J., and Harper, E., 1977, Tumor cell collagenase and its inhibition by a cartilage-derived protease inhibitor, *Science* **196**:653–654.

Laug, W. E., Tokes, Z. A., Benedict, W. F., and Sorgente, N., 1980, Anchorage independent growth and plasminogen activator production by bovine endothelial cells, *J. Cell Biol.* **84**:281–293.

Laurie, G. W., Leblond, C. P., and Martin, G. R., 1982, Localization of type IV collagen, laminin, heparan sulfate proteoglycan, and fibronectin to the basal lamina of basement membranes, *J. Cell Biol.* **95**:340–344.

Leavitt, J., Bushar, G., Kakunaga, T., Hamada, H., Hirakawa, T., Goldman, D., and Merril, C., 1982, Variations in expression of mutant beta actin accompanying incremental increases in human fibroblast tumorigenicity, *Cell* **28**:259–268.

Lehman, J. M., Speers, W. C., Swarzendruber, D. E., and Pierce, G. B., 1974, Neoplastic differentiation: Characteristics of cell lines derived from a murine teratocarcinoma, *J. Cell. Physiol.* **84**:13–27.

Leivo, I., Vaheri, A., Timpl, R., and Wartiovaara, J., 1980, Appearance and distribution of collagens and laminin in the early mouse embryo, *Dev. Biol.* **76**:100–114.

Leivo, I., Alitalo, K., Risteli, L., Vaheri, A., Timpl, R., and Wartiovaara, J., 1982, Basal lamina glycoproteins laminin and type IV collagen assembled into a fine-fibered matrix in cultures of a teratocarcinoma-derived endodermal cell line, *Exp. Cell Res.* **137**:15–23.

Lesot, H., Kuhl, U., and von der Mark, 1983, Isolation of a laminin-binding protein from muscle cell membranes, *EMBO J.* **2**:861–865.

Linzer, D. I., and Levine, A. J., 1979, Characterization of a 54K dalton cellular SV40 tumor antigen present in SV40-transformed cells and uninfected embryonal carcinoma cells, *Cell* **17**:43–52.

Liotta, L. A., 1985, Mechanisms of cancer invasion and metastasis, in: *Important Advances in Oncology* (V. T. DeVita, S. Hellman, and S. A. Rosenberg, eds.), Lippincott, Philadelphia, pp. 28–41.

Liotta, L. A., Kleinerman, J., and Saidel, G. M., 1974, Quantitative relationships of intravascular tumor cells, tumor vessels and pulmonary metastases following tumor implantation, *Cancer Res.* **34**:997–1004.

Liotta, L. A., Gattozzi, C., Kleinerman, J., and Saidel, G., 1977a, Reduction of tumor cell entry into vessels by BCG-activated macrophages, *Br. J. Cancer* **36**:639–641.

Liotta, L. A., Kleinerman, J., Catanzaro, P., and Rynbrandt, D., 1977b, Degradation of basement membrane by murine tumor cells, *J. Natl. Cancer Inst.* **58**:1427–1431.

Liotta, L. A., Abe, S., Gehron-Robey, P., and Martin, G. R., 1979, Preferential digestion of basement membrane collagen by an enzyme derived from a metastatic murine tumor, *Proc. Natl. Acad. Sci. USA* **76**:2268–2274.

Liotta, L. A., Tryggvason, K., Garbisa, S., Hart, I., Foltz, C. M., and Shafie, S., 1980, Metastatic potential correlates with enzymatic degradation of basement membrane collagen, *Nature* **284**:67–68.

Liotta, L. A., Goldfarb, R. H., Brundage, R., Siegal, G. P., Terranova, V., and Garbisa, S., 1981a, Effect of plasminogen activator (urokinase), plasmin, and thrombin on glycoprotein and collagenous components of basement membrane, *Cancer Res.* **41**:4629–4636.

Liotta, L. A., Goldfarb, R. H., and Terranova, V. P., 1981b, Cleavage of laminin by thrombin and plasmin: Alpha thrombin selectively cleaves the beta chain of laminin, *Thromb. Res.* **21**:663–673.

Liotta, L. A., Lanzer, W. L., and Garbisa, S., 1981c, Identification of a type V collagenolytic enzyme, Biochem. Biophys. Res. Commun. 98:184–190.

Liotta, L. A., Tryggvason, K., Garbisa, S., Gehron-Robey, P., and Abe, S., 1981d, Partial purification and characterization of a neutral protease which cleaves type IV collagen, Biochemistry 20:100–104.

Liotta, L. A., Kalebic, T., Reese, C. A., and Mayne, R., 1982, Protease susceptibilities of HMW 1α, 2α but not 3α cartilage collagens are similar to type V collagen, Biochem. Biophys. Res. Commun. 104:500–506.

Liotta, L. A., Rao, C. N., and Barsky, S. H., 1983, Tumor invasion and the extracellular matrix, Lab. Invest. 49:636–649.

Liotta, L. A., Horan-Hand, P., Rao, C. N., Bryant, G., Barsky, S. H., and Schlom, J., 1985, Monoclonal antibodies to the human laminin receptor recognize distinct structural domains, Exp. Cell Res. 156:117–126.

Loskutoff, D. J., and Edgington, T. E., 1977, Synthesis of a fibrinolytic activator and inhibitor by endothelial cells, Proc. Natl. Acad. Sci. USA 74:3903–3907.

McCroskery, P. A., Richards, J. F., and Harris, E. D., 1975, Purification and characterization of a collagenase extracted from rabbit tumor, Biochem. J. 152:131–142.

Madri, J. A., and Furchtmayr, H., 1979, Isolation and tissue localization of type AB2 collagen from normal lung parenchyma, Am. J. Pathol. 94:323–331.

Madri, J. A., Foellmer, H. G., and Furthmayr, H., 1983, Ultrastructural morphology and domain structure of a unique collagenous component of basement membranes, Biochemistry 22:2797–2804.

Mainardi, C. L., Dixit, S. N., and Kang, A. H., 1980a, Degradation of type IV (basement membrane) collagen by a proteinase isolated from human polymorphonuclear leukocyte granules, J. Biol. Chem. 255:5435–5441.

Mainardi, C. L., Seyer, J. M., and Kang, A. H., 1980b, Type specific collagenolysis: A type V collagen-degrading enzyme from macrophages, Biochem. Biophys. Res. Commun. 97:1108–1115.

Malinoff, H. L., and Wicha, M. S., 1983, Isolation of a cell surface receptor protein for laminin from murine fibrosarcoma cells, J. Cell Biol. 96:1475–1479.

Mareel, M., and de Brabander, M., 1978, Effect of microtubule inhibitors on malignant invasion in vitro, J. Natl. Cancer Inst. 61:787–792.

Mareel, M. M., Kint, J., and Meyvisch, C., 1979, Methods of study of the invasion of malignant C3H mouse fibroblasts into embryonic chick heart in vitro, Virchows Arch. Abt. B. Zellpathol. 30:95–111.

Markus, G., Takita, H., Camiolo, S. M., Corasanti, J. G., Evers, J. L., and Hobika, G., 1980, Content and characterization of plasminogen activators in human lung tumors and normal lung tissue, Cancer Res. 40:841–848.

Martinez-Hernandez, A., Miller, E. J., Damjanov, I., and Gay, S., 1982, Laminin-secreting yolk sac carcinoma of the rat: Biochemical and electron immunohistochemical studies, Lab. Invest. 47:247–257.

Matsumoto, A., Sakamoto, S., and Sakamoto, M., 1979, Stimulation of bone collagenase synthesis by mouse fibrosarcoma in resorbing bone in vitro culture, Arch. Oral Biol. 24:403–405.

Mayne, R., Vail, M. S., and Miller, E. J., 1978, Characterization of the collagen chains synthesized by cultured smooth muscle cells derived from rhesus monkey thoracic aorta, Biochemistry 17:446–452.

Miller, E. J., and Rhodes, R. K., 1982, Preparation and characterization of the different types of collagen, Meth. Enzymol. 82:33–64.

Minor, R. R., Clark, C. C., Strause, E. L., Koszalka, T. R., Brent, R. L., and Kefalides, N. A., 1976, Basement membrane procollagen is not converted to collagen in organ cultures of parietal yolk sac endoderm, J. Biol. Chem. 251:1789–1794.

Mort, J. S., Recklies, A. D., and Poole, A. R., 1980, Characterization of a thiol proteinase secreted by malignant human breast tumors, Biochim. Biophys. Acta 614:134–143.

Mort, J. S., Leduc, M. S., and Recklies, A. D., 1981, A latent thiol proteinase from ascites fluid of patients with neoplasia, Biochim. Biophys. Acta 662:173–180.

Mort, J. S., Leduc, M. S., and Recklies, A. D., 1983, Characterization of a latent cysteine proteinase from ascitic fluid as a high molecular weight form of cathepsin B, *Biochim. Biophys. Acta* **755**:369–375.

Mott, D. M., Fabisch, P. H., Sani, B. P., and Sorof, S., 1974, Lack of correlation between fibrinolysis and the transformed state of cultured mammalian cells, *Biochem. Biophys. Res. Commun.* **61**:621–627.

Murphy, G., and Sellers, A., 1980, The extracellular regulation of collagenase activity, in: *Collagenase in Normal and Pathological Connective Tissue* (D. E. Woolley and J. M. Evanson, eds.), John Wiley and Sons, New York, pp. 65–81.

Naito, S., Sueishi, K., Hattori, F., and Tanaka, K., 1980, Immunological analysis of plasminogen activators from cultured human cancer cells, *Virchows Arch. Abt. A. Pathol. Anat. Hist.* **387**:251–257.

Nakajima, M., Custead, S. E., Welch, D. R., and Nicolson, G. L., 1984, Type IV collagenolysis: Relation to metastatic properties of rat 13762 mammary adenocarcinoma metastatic cell clones, *Proceedings of the 75th Annual Meeting of the AACR*, Toronto, Canada, p. 62.

Neurath, H., and Walsh, K. A., 1976, Role of proteolytic enzymes in biological regulation, *Proc. Natl. Acad. Sci. USA* **73**:3825–3832.

Nicolson, G. L., and Poste, G., 1983, Tumor implantation and invasion of metastatic sites, *Int. Rev. Exp. Pathol.* **25**:77–181.

Nilsson, K., Andersson, L. C., Gahmberg, C. G., and Wigzell, H., 1977, Surface glycoprotein patterns of normal and malignant human lymphoid cells. II. B cells, B blasts, and Epstein–Barr virus (EBV)-positive and -negative B lymphoid cell lines, *Int. J. Cancer* **20**:708–716.

Nowell, P. C., 1976, The clonal evolution of tumor cell populations, *Science* **194**:23–28.

Ooshima, A., 1981, Collagen alpha B chain: Increased proportion in human atherosclerosis, *Science* **213**:666–668.

Orkin, E. R., Gehron-Robey, P., McGoodwin, E. B., Martin, G. R., Valentine, T., and Swarm, R. H., 1977, A murine tumor producing a matrix of basement membrane, *J. Exp. Med.* **145**:204–220.

Orr, F. W., Varani, J., Gondek, M. D., Ward, P. A., and Mundy, G. R., 1980, Partial characterization of a bone-derived chemotactic factor for tumor cells, *Am. J. Pathol.* **99**:43–52.

Ossowski, L., Biegel, D., and Reich, E., 1979, Mammary plasminogen activator: Correlation with involution, hormonal modulation and comparison between normal and neoplastic tissue, *Cell* **16**:929–940.

Pauli, B. U., Memoli, V. A., and Kuettner, K. E., 1981, Regulation of tumor invasion by cartilage-derived anti-invasion factor in vitro, *J. Natl. Cancer Inst.* **67**:65–73.

Perez-Tamayo, R., 1978, Pathology of collagen degradation: A review, *Am. J. Pathol.* **92**:508–566.

Peterson, H. L., 1968, Experimental studies on fibrinolysis in growth and spread of tumor, *Acta. Chir. Scand. Suppl.* **134**:394.

Peterson, H. L., Kjartansson, I., Korsan-Bengtsen, K., Rudenstam, C. M., and Zettergren, L., 1973, Fibrinolysis in human malignant tumors, *Acta. Chir. Scand.* **139**:219–223.

Plata, F., 1982, Specificity studies of cytolytic T lymphocytes against murine leukemia virus-induced tumors, *J. Exp. Med.* **155**:1050–1062.

Poole, A. R., Tiltman, K. J., Recklies, A. D., and Stoker, T. A. M., 1978, Differences in secretion of the proteinase cathepsin B at the edges of human breast carcinomas and fibroadenomas, *Nature* **273**:545–547.

Poste, G., Doll, J., and Fidler, I. J., 1981, Interactions among clonal subpopulations affect stability of the metastatic phenotype in polyclonal populations of B16 melanoma cells, *Proc. Natl. Acad. Sci. USA* **78**:6226–6230.

Poste, G., Greig, R., Tzong, J., Koestler, T., and Corwin, S., 1984, Interactions between tumor cell subpopulations in malignant tumors, in: *Cancer Invasion and Metastasis: Biologic and Therapeutic Aspects* (G. L. Nicolson and L. Milas, eds.), Raven Press, New York, pp. 223–243.

Quigley, J. P., 1979a, Phorbol ester-induced morphological changes in transformed chick fibroblasts: Evidence for direct catalytic involvement of plasminogen activator, *Cell* **17**:131–141.

Quigley, J. P., 1979b, Proteolytic enzymes of normal and malignant cells, in: *Surfaces of Normal and Malignant Cells* (R. O. Hynes, ed.), Wiley, New York, pp. 247–285.

Rao, C. N., Margulies, I. M., Goldfarb, R. H., Madri, J. A., Woodley, D. T., and Liotta, L. A.,

1982a, Differential proteolytic susceptibility of laminin alpha and beta subunits, *Arch. Biochem. Biophys.* **219**:65–70.

Rao, C. N., Margulies, I. M., Tralka, T. S., Terranova, V. P., Madri, J., and Liotta, L. A., 1982b, Isolation of a subunit of laminin and its role in molecular structure and tumor cell attachment, *J. Biol. Chem.* **257**:9740–9744.

Rao, C. N., Barsky, S. H., Terranova, V. P., and Liotta, L. A., 1983a, Isolation of a tumor cell laminin receptor, *Biochem. Biophys. Res. Commun.* **11**:804–808.

Rao, C. N., Goldstein, I. J., and Liotta, L. A., 1983b, Lectin-binding domains on laminin, *Arch. Biochem. Biophys.* **227**:118–124.

Raz, A., and Geiger, B., 1982, Altered organization of cell–substrate contacts and membrane-associated cytoskeleton in tumor cell variants exhibiting different metastatic capabilities, *Cancer Res.* **42**:5183–5190.

Recklies, A. D., and Poole, A. R., 1982, Proteolytic mechanisms of tissue destruction in tumor growth and metastasis, in: *Liver Metastasis* (L. Weiss and H. A. Gilbert, eds.), G. K. Hall, Boston, pp. 77–95.

Recklies, A. D., Tiltman, K. J., Stoker, A. M., and Poole, A. R., 1980, Secretion of proteinases from malignant and nonmalignant human breast tissue, *Cancer Res.* **40**:550–556.

Recklies, A. D., Poole, A. R., and Mort, J. S., 1982, A cysteine proteinase secreted from human breast tumours is immunologically related to cathepsin B, *Biochem. J.* **207**:633–636.

Reich, E., 1978, Activation of plasminogen: A widespread mechanismm for generating localized extracellular proteolysis, in: *Biological Markers for Neoplasia: Basic and Applied Aspects* (R. W. Ruddon, ed.), Elsevier, Amsterdam, pp. 491–500.

Reich, N., and Levine, A. J., 1982, Specific interaction of the SV40 T antigen–cellular p53 protein complex with SV40 DNA, *Virology* **117**:286–290.

Rhodes, R. K., and Miller, E. J., 1978, Physicochemical characterization and molecular organization of the collagen A and B chains, *Biochemistry* **17**:3442–3448.

Rifkin, D. B., Loeb, J. N., Moore, G., and Reich, E., 1974, Properties of plasminogen activators formed by neoplastic human cell cultures, *J. Exp. Med.* **139**:1317–1328.

Robertson, J. D., and Black, P. H., 1969, Changes in surface antigens of SV40 virus-transformed cells, *Proc. Soc. Exp. Biol. Med.* **130**:363–370.

Rohrschneider, L. R., 1980, Adhesion plaques of Rous sarcoma virus-transformed cells contain the src gene product, *Proc. Natl. Acad. Sci. USA* **77**:3514–3518.

Rohrschneider, L. R., Rosok, M., and Schriver, K., 1982, Mechanism of transformation by Rous sarcoma virus: Events within adhesion plaques, *Cold Spring Harbor Conf. Cell Prolif.* **46**:953–965.

Romualdez, A. G., and Ward, P. A., 1975, A unique complement derived chemotactic factor for tumor cells, *Proc. Natl. Acad. Sci. USA* **72**:4128–4132.

Roughley, P. J., and Barrett, A. J., 1977, The degradation of cartilage proteoglycans by tissue proteinases: Proteoglycan structure and its susceptibility to proteolysis, *Biochem. J.* **167**:629–637.

Sage, H., Pritzl, P., and Bornstein, P., 1981, Characterization of cell matrix associated collagens synthesized by aortic endothelial cells in culture, *Biochemistry* **20**:436–442.

Sakashita, S., and Ruoslahti, E., 1980, Basement membrane glycoprotein laminin binds to heparin or laminin-like glycoproteins in extracellular matrix of endodermal cells, *Arch. Biochem. Biophys.* **205**:283–290.

Salo, T., Liotta, L. A., Keski-Oja, J., Turpeenniemi-Hujanen, T., and Tryggvason, K., 1982, Secretion of basement membrane collagen degrading enzyme and plasminogen activator by transformed cells: Role in metastasis, *Int. J. Cancer* **30**:669–673.

Salo, T., Liotta, L. A., and Tryggvason, K., 1983, Purification and characterization of a murine basement membrane collagen degrading enzyme secreted by metastatic tumor cells, *J. Biol. Chem.* **258**:3058–3063.

Sasaki, M., Peterson, J. A., Wara, W. M., and Ceriani, R. L., 1981, Human mammary epithelial antigens (HME-Ags) in the circulation of nude mice implanted with a breast tumor and non-breast tumors, *Cancer* **48**:2204–2210.

Schirrmacher, V., 1980, Shifts in tumor cell phenotypes induced by signals from the microenvironment: Relevance for the immunobiology of cancer metastasis, *Immunobiology* **157**:89–98.

Schirrmacher, V., and Waller, C. A., 1982, Quantitative determination of disseminated tumor cells by ^{3}H thymidine incorporation *in vitro* by agar colony formation, *Cancer Res.* **42**:660–666.

Sears, H. F., Herlyn, M., Del Villano, B., Steplewski, Z., and Koprowski, H., 1982, Monoclonal antibody detection of a circulating tumor-associated antigen. II. A longitudinal evaluation of patients with colorectal cancer, *J. Clin. Immunol.* **2**:141–149.

Sefton, B. M., and Rubin, H., 1970, Release from density dependent growth inhibition by proteolytic enzymes, *Nature* **227**:843–845.

Shamberger, R. J., and Rudolph, G., 1967, Increase of lysosomal enzymes in skin cancers, *Nature* **213**:617–618.

Showell, H. J., Freer, R. J., Zigmond, S. H., Schiffmann, E., Aswanikumaar, S., Corcoran, B., and Becker, E. L., 1976, The structure activity relationship of synthetic peptides as chemotactic factors and inducers of lysosomal enzyme secretion for neutrophils, *J. Exp. Med.* **143**:1154–1169.

Siegal, G. P., Thorgeirsson, U. P., Russo, R. G., Wallace, D. M., Liotta, L. A., and Berger, S. L., 1982, Interferon enhancement of the invasive capacity of Ewing sarcoma cells *in vitro*, *Proc. Natl. Acad. Sci. USA* **79**:4064–4068.

Sloane, B. F., Dunn, J. R., and Honn, K. V., 1981, Lysosomal cathepsin B: Correlation with metastatic potential, *Science* **212**:1151–1153.

Sloane, B. F., Honn, K. V., Sadler, J. G., Turner, W. A., Kimpson, J. J., and Taylor, J. D., 1982, Cathepsin B activity in B16 melanoma cells: A possible marker for metastatic potential, *Cancer Res.* **42**:980–986.

Smith, J. B., and O'Neill, R. T., 1971, Fetal gut antigen: A substance in fetal gut and its relationship to gut carcinoma, *Commun. Chem. Pathol. Pharmacol.* **2**:1–15.

Steck, P. A., Luna, M. A., and Nicolson, G. L., 1984, Analysis of cell surface sialogalactoprotein isolated from lung metastases of rat 137562 NF and human mammary adenocarcinoma, *Proceedings of the 75th Annual Meeting of the AACR*, Toronto, Canada, p. 55.

Stenn, K. S., Madri, J. A., and Roll, F. J., 1979, Migrating epidermis produces AB$_2$ collagen and requires continual collagen synthesis for movement, *Nature* **277**:229–232.

Sträuli, P., 1980, A concept of tumor invasion, in: *Proteinases and Tumor Invasion* (P. Strauli, A. J. Barrett, and A. Baici, eds.), Raven Press, New York, pp. 1–15.

Strickland, S., Reich, E., and Sherman, E., 1976, Plasminogen activator in early embryogenesis: Enzyme production by trophoblast and parietal endoderm, *Cell* **9**:231–240.

Strickland, S., Smith, K. K., and Marotti, K. R., 1980, Hormonal induction of differentiation in teratocarcinoma stem cells: Generation of parietal endoderm by retinoic acid and dibutyryl cAMP, *Cell* **21**:347–355.

Stricklin, G. P., Bauer, E. A., Jeffrey, J. J., and Eisen, A. Z., 1977, Human skin collagenase: Isolation of precursor and active forms from both fibroblast and organ cultures, *Biochemistry* **16**:1607–1615.

Sylven, B., 1974, Biochemical factors involved in the cellular detachment from tumors, *Schweiz. Med. Wochenschr.* **104**:258–261.

Tagnon, H. J., Whitmore, W. F., and Shulman, N. R., 1952, Fibrinolysis in metastatic cancer of the prostate, *Cancer* **5**:9–12.

Tal, C., 1965, The nature of the cell membrane receptor for the agglutination factor present in the sera of tumor patients and pregnant women, *Proc. Natl. Acad. Sci. USA* **54**:1318–1321.

Talmadge, J. E., Starkey, J. R., Davis, W. C., and Cohen, A. L., 1979, Introduction of metastatic heterogeneity by short-term *in vivo* passage of a cloned transformed cell line, *J. Supramol. Struct.* **12**:227–243.

Talmadge, J. E., Kay, M. E., and Hart, I. R., 1981, Characterization of a murine ovarian reticulum cell sarcoma of histiocytic origin, *Cancer Res.* **41**:1271–1280.

Terranova, V. P., Rohrbach, D. H., and Martin, G. R., 1980, Role of laminin in the attachment of PAM 212 (epithelial) cells to basement membrane collagen, *Cell* **22**:719–726.

Terranova, V. P., Liotta, L. A., Russo, R. G., and Martin, G. R., 1982, Role of laminin in the attachment and metastasis of murine tumor cells, *Cancer Res.* **42**:2265–2269.

Terranova, V. P., Rao, C. N., Kalebic, T., Margulies, I. M., and Liotta, L. A., 1983, Laminin receptor on human breast carcinoma cells, Proc. Natl. Acad. Sci. USA **80**:444–448.

Thorgeirsson, U. P., Liotta, L. A., Kalebic, T., Margulies, I. M., Thomas, K., Rios-Candelore, M., and Russo, R. G., 1982, Effect of natural protease inhibitor and a chemoattractant on tumor cell invasion in vitro, J. Natl. Cancer Inst. **69**:1049–1054.

Thorgeirsson, U. P., Turpeenniemi-Hujanen, T., Neckers, L., Johnson, D. W., and Liotta, L. A., 1984, Protein synthesis but not DNA synthesis is required for tumor cell invasion in vitro, Invas. Met. **4**:73–83.

Timpl, R., Martin, G. R., Bruckner, P., Wick, G., and Widermann, H., 1978, Nature of the collagenous protein in a tumor basement membrane, Eur. J. Biochem. **84**:43–52.

Timpl, R., Rohde, H., Gehron-Robey, P., Rennard, S., Foidart, J. M., and Martin, G. R., 1979, Laminin—A glycoprotein from basement membranes, J. Biol. Chem. **254**:9933–9937.

Timpl, R., Oberbaumer, I., Furthmayr, H., and Kühn, K., 1982a, Macromolecular organization of type IV collagen, in: New Trends in Basement Membrane Research (K. Kühn, H. Schöne, and R. Timpl, eds.), Raven Press, New York, pp. 57–67.

Timpl, R., Rohde, H., Risteli, L., Ott, U., Gehron-Robey, P., and Martin, G. R., 1982b, Laminin, Meth. Enzymol. **82**:831–838.

Todaro, G. J., Green, H., and Goldberg, B. D., 1964, Transformation of properties of an established cell line by SV40 and polyoma virus, Proc. Natl. Acad. Sci. USA **51**:66–73.

Troll, W., Klassen, A., and Janoff, A., 1970, Tumorigenesis in mouse skin: Inhibition by synthetic inhibitors of proteases, Science **169**:1211–1213.

Tryggvason, K., Gehron-Robey, P., and Martin, G., 1980, Biosynthesis of type IV procollagens, Biochemistry **19**:1284–1289.

Tucker, W. S., Kirsch, W. M., Martinez-Hernandez, A., and Fink, L. M., 1978, In vitro plasminogen activator activity in human brain tumors, Cancer Res. **38**:297–302.

Turpeenniemi-Hujanen, T., Thorgeirsson, U. P., and Liotta, L. A., 1984, Collagenases in tumor cell extravasation, Annu. Rep. Med. Chem. **19**:231–239.

Unkeless, J. C., Tobia, A., Ossowski, L., Quigley, J. P., Rifkin, D. B., and Reich, E., 1973, An enzymatic function associated with transformation of fibroblasts by oncogenic viruses. I. Chick embryo fibroblast cultures transformed by avian RNA tumor viruses, J. Exp. Med. **137**:85–111.

Van Herendael, B. J., Oberti, C., Brosens, I., 1978, Microanatomy of the human amniotic membranes, Am. J. Obstet. Gynecol. **131**:872–880.

Varani, J., and Ward, P. A., 1982, Tumor cell chemotaxis, in: Tumor Invasion and Metastasis (L. A. Liotta and I. R. Hart, eds.), Martinus Nijhoff, The Hague, pp. 99–112.

Varani, J., Orr, W., and Ward, P. A., 1979, Cell-associated proteases affect tumor cell migration in vitro, Cancer Res. **39**:2376–2380.

Varani, J., Wass, J., Piontek, G., and Ward, P. A., 1981, Chemotactic factor-induced adherence of tumor cells, Cell. Biol. Int. Rep. **5**:525–530.

Vlodavsky, I., Lui, G. M., and Gospodarowicz, D., 1980, Morphological appearance, growth behavior and migratory activity of human tumor cells maintained on extracellular matrix versus plastic, Cell **19**:607–616.

Vracko, P., 1974, Basal lamina scaffold—Anatomy and significance for maintenance of orderly tissue structure, Am. J. Pathol. **77**:314–346.

Wang, E., and Goldberg, A. R., 1976, Changes in microfilament organization and surface topography upon transformation of chick embryo fibroblasts with Rous sarcoma virus, Proc. Natl. Acad. Sci. USA **457**:4065–4069.

Wass, J. A., Varani, J., and Ward, P. A., 1980, Size increase induced in Walker ascites cells by chemotactic factors, Cancer Lett. **9**:313–318.

Wass, J. A., Varandi, J., Pionter, G. E., Goff, D., and Ward, P. A., 1981, Characteristics of the chemotactic factor-mediated cell swelling response of tumor cells, J. Natl. Cancer Inst. **66**:927–933.

Watanabe, H., 1974, Purification and chemical characterization of α-fetoprotein from rat and mouse, Int. J. Cancer **13**:377–388.

Webber, M. M., James, G., Lucero, L., Van Buskirk, J. J., and Wettlaufer, J. M., 1981, Plasminogen activator: A marker for human prostatic epithelium and prostate cancer, In Vitro 17:249.

Weiss, L., 1980, Cancer cell traffic from the lungs to the liver: An example of metastatic inefficiency, Int. J. Cancer 25:385–392.

Weiss, L., Mayhew, E., Rapp, D. G., and Holmes, J., 1982, Metastatic inefficiency in mice bearing B16 melanomas, Br. J. Cancer 45:44–53.

Welgus, H. G., Jeffrey, J. J., and Eisen, A. Z., 1981, The collagen substrate specificity of human skin fibroblast collagenase, J. Biol. Chem. 256:9511–9515.

Welsh, C., Gay, S., Rhodes, R. K., Pfister, R., and Miller, E. J., 1980, Collagen heterogeneity in normal rabbit cornea. I. Isolation and biochemical characterization of the genetically-distinct collagens, Biochim. Biophys. Acta 625:78–88.

Wewer, U., Albrechtsen, R., and Ruoslahti, E., 1981, Laminin: A noncollagenous component of epithelial basement membranes synthesized by a rat yolk sac tumor, Cancer Res. 41:1518–1524.

Wicha, M. S., and Huard, T. K., 1983, Macrophages express cell surface laminin, Exp. Cell Res. 143:475–479.

Wigler, M., and Weinstein, I. B., 1976, Tumour promotor induces plasminogen activator, Nature 259:232–233.

Willingham, M. C., Jay, G., and Pastan, I., 1979, Localization of the ASV src gene product to the plasma membrane of transformed cells by electron microscopic immunocytochemistry, Cell 18:125–134.

Wilson, E. L., and Dowle, E., 1978, Secretion of plasminogen activator by normal, reactive and neoplastic human tissues cultured in vitro, Int. J. Cancer 22:390–399.

Wilson, E. L., and Reich, E., 1978, Plasminogen activator in chick fibroblasts: Induction of synthesis by retinoic acid; synergism with viral transformation and phorbol ester, Cell 15:385–392.

Wolf, B. A., and Goldberg, A. R., 1976, Rous-sarcoma-virus-transformed fibroblasts having low levels of plasminogen activator, Proc. Natl. Acad. Sci. USA 73:3613–3617.

Woolley, D. E., and Grafton, C. A., 1980, Collagenase immunolocalization studies of cutaneous secondary melanomas, Br. J. Cancer 42:260–265.

Woolley, D. E., Roberts, D. R., and Evanson, J. M., 1975, Inhibition of human collagenase activity by a small molecular weight serum protein, Biochem. Biophys. Res. Commun. 66:747–754.

Woolley, D. E., Glanville, R. W., Roberts, D. R., and Evanson, J. M., 1978, Purification, characterization and inhibition of human skin collagenase, Biochem. J. 169:265–276.

Yamanishi, Y., Dabbous, M. K., and Hashimoto, K., 1972, Effect of collagenolytic activity in basal cell epithelioma of the skin on reconstituted collagen and physical properties and kinetics of the crude enzyme, Cancer Res. 32:2551–2560.

Yamauchi, K., Fujimoto, S., and Tada, T., 1979, Differential activation of cytotoxic and suppressor T cells against syngeneic tumors in the mouse, J. Immunol. 123:1653–1658.

Yogeeswaran, G., and Salk, P. S., 1981, Metastatic potential is positively correlated with cell surface sialylation of cultured murine tumor cell lines, Science 212:1514–1516.

CHAPTER 3

MAMMARY TUMOR GROWTH ARREST BY COLLAGEN SYNTHESIS INHIBITORS

WILLIAM R. KIDWELL, MOZEENA BANO, and SUSAN J. TAYLOR

1. INTRODUCTION

The basal lamina is an extracellular matrix material that is deposited by mammary epithelium at the interface between the epithelium and surrounding stroma. It forms a limiting barrier and serves to maintain tissue organization. Recent experiments have indicated that production of the lamina is important for the growth and/or survival of the epithelium of the normal gland and for many well differentiated rate mammary tumors. Lamina deposition can be selectively blocked *in vivo* by proline analogues that are specific inhibitors of collagen production, with a consequent involution of the mammary epithelium and a regression of mammary tumors. Because of the importance of the lamina, the mechanisms and factors regulating its production have been sought. Current evidence indicates that endogenously produced growth factors regulate lamina production in an autocrine fashion. Very potent factors that differentially stimulate synthesis of the lamina proteins, type IV collagen and laminin, have been detected in rodent and human mammary tumors. Most interestingly, the responsiveness of mammary cells to these growth factors is potentiated when the mammary cells interact with stromal collagen. This seems to provide for the selective deposition of a lamina at the interface between the epithelium and stroma. The dependency of mammary tumors on lamina production can be lost by a process of se-

WILLIAM R. KIDWELL, MOZEENA BANO, and SUSAN J. TAYLOR • Laboratory of Pathophysiology, National Cancer Institute, National Institutes of Health, Bethesda, Maryland 20205.

lection or dedifferentiation. Some rat mammary tumors selected by serial transplantation no longer produce a lamina. Their growth *in vivo* becomes resistant to proline analogues and their production of the growth factor that enhances lamina protein production is lost. These tumors also do not contain myoepithelial cells, the cells believed to be responsible for most of the type IV collagen production by the normal epithelium and the epithelium of well differentiated mammary tumors.

2. STRUCTURE OF THE LAMINA

The three major constituents of the lamina have been purified to apparent homogeneity from a murine tumor that elaborates massive amounts of this substance (Timpl *et al.*, 1978, 1979; Hassell *et al.*, 1980). Type IV collagen is the major collagenous protein, with small amounts of type V collagen apparently present at the lamina–stromal interface (Martinez-Hernandez *et al.*, 1982). Type IV collagen is arranged in a chickenwire framework with overlapping tails that interact via disulfide bridges and a head-to-head interaction via an as yet incompletely understood mechanism (Furthmayr *et al.*, 1982). Type IV collagen is composed of two dissimilar peptide chains of molecular weight 185 and 170 kilodaltons. The two peptides apparently combine in a 2 : 1 ratio to form a triple helical structure that is the backbone of the lamina.

A second major component of the lamina is the glycoprotein laminin. Laminin is a protein containing two peptides of about 220,000 daltons and a third peptide about double this size. Rotary shadowing techniques show that laminin has a cross shape with globular ends (Rao *et al.*, 1982). Proteolytic cleavage has shown that there are cell binding sites at the intersection of the long and short arms, type IV collagen binding sites at the globular regions on the short arms of the cross, and a heparin sulfate proteoglycan binding site on the long arm of the cross. Laminin thus appears to be the glue that holds the lamina components together and also the attachment protein that anchors the epithelium to the basement membrane (Terranova *et al.*, 1982). Heparin sulfate proteoglycan, the third major component of the lamina, consists of a protein core with multiple heparin sulfate chains attached, giving a molecular weight approaching 10^6 daltons. The exact arrangement of the various components of the lamina and, indeed, whether there are other important components not yet identified, are areas of intense research and controversy (Leblond *et al.*, 1983). A more extensive presentation of lamina structure is given in Chapter 2 of this volume.

3. SYNTHESIS OF THE BASAL LAMINA BY THE MAMMARY EPITHELIUM

Although it has long been known that the mammary epithelium rests on a basal lamina, it was not until 1980 that it was shown that the lamina constituents are produced by the epithelium (Liotta et al., 1980). Utilizing a method developed by Janss et al. (1980) and modified by us, the isolation of pure mammary ducts and alveoli was achieved (Wicha et al., 1979a). These cells were cultured with a labeled amino acid and the constituent collagen purified and characterized. Type IV collagen was found to be the only collagenous protein made in detectable amounts. These studies were extended by analysis of well differentiated mammary tumor cells, which were shown to synthesize type IV collagen, and not any of the types of collagens (types I and III) that mammary stromal cells make (Liotta et al., 1980; Kidwell et al., 1980a; Lewko et al., 1981). Interestingly, poorly differentiated mammary tumors established by serial transplantation of adenocarcinomas did not make basement membrane collagen, but rather produced the collagenous types characteristic of the stromal cells (Lewko et al., 1981). This is shown in Figure 1. This switch in production of collagen types is very interesting and may prove to be a valuable marker of tumor progression if it is found to be a general characteristic of poorly differentiated tumors.

4. IDENTIFICATION OF THE MAMMARY CELL TYPES THAT PRODUCE TYPE IV COLLAGEN AND LAMININ

Indirect immunofluorescence studies of cultured epithelium and tissue slices suggested that most of the collagen IV was produced by a minority population of cells of the normal and neoplastic mammary epithelium. These cells appear to be the myoepithelial cells, which are present in both normal and adenocarcinoma tissues (Kidwell et al., 1980a,b; Strum et al., 1981). Recently, it has been possible to isolate and separately culture the epithelial and myoepithelial cell populations from 7,12-dimethylbenz(α)anthracene (DMBA)-induced rat mammary carcinoma (Figure 2). Radiolabeling exper-

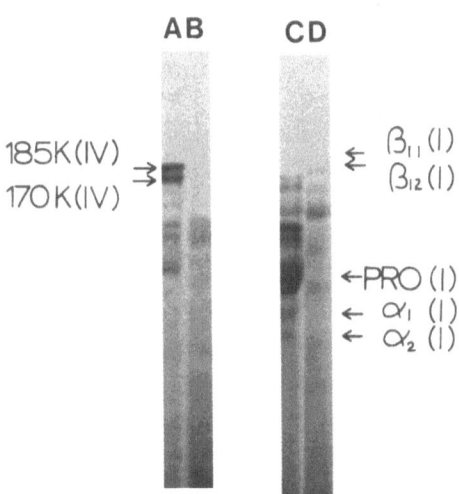

FIGURE 1. Types of collagens synthesized by rat mammary adenocarcinomas and carcinomas. Total collagen species were isolated after a brief culture in the presence of [^{14}C]proline. Proteins were electrophoresed on SDS gels and fluorographs developed. (A) Adenocarcinoma sample. (B) Same sample predigested with purified collagenase before electrophoresis. (C and D) Collagen samples from the carcinoma before and after collagenase digestion. The migration of collagen standards is depicted on the left (type IV collagen) and right (type I collagen) (from Lewko et al., 1981).

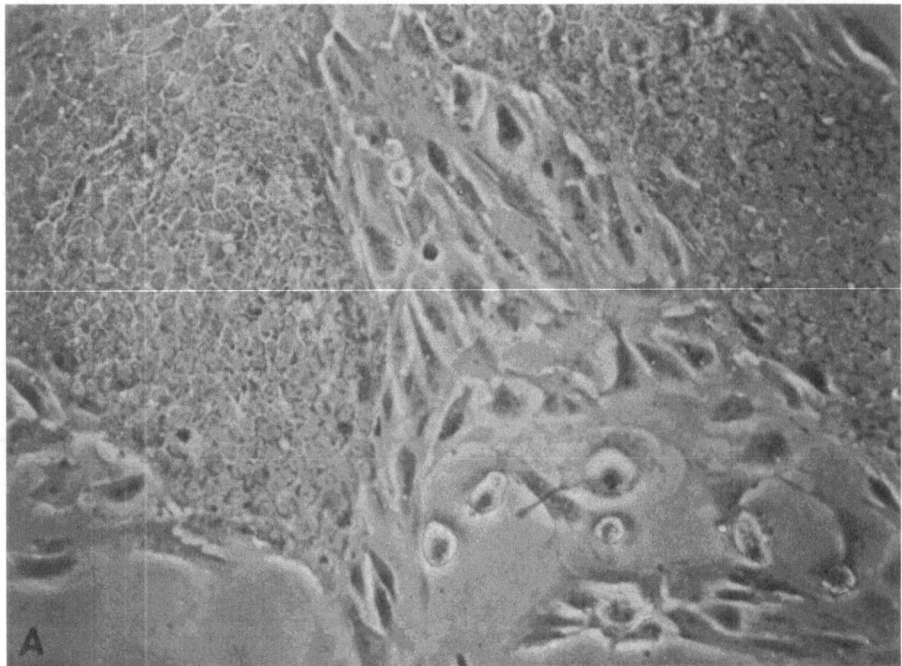

FIGURE 2. Separated cell types from the rat mammary adenocarcinoma. (A) Unseparated cell populations. Colonies of cuboidal epithelial cells are seen, surrounded by flattened, stellate basal cells. (B) Isolated basal cells. (C) Isolated epithelial cells. These separated cell populations were used for determining the collagen IV and laminin synthesis capabilities of the different cell types given in Table I (from Bano and Kidwell, 1984).

iments directly demonstrated that the isolated myoepithelial-like cell synthesized 50 times as much collagen as the epithelial cell population (Bano and Kidwell, 1984). Laminin production by the two cell populations in culture was also estimated. Using an enzyme-linked immunoassay technique, approximately equal amounts of laminin per cell were found in association with each cell type (Bano and Kidwell, 1984). These results are presented in Table I. They indicate that formation of the basal lamina by normal or neoplastic mammary epithelium requires the presence of the myoepithelial cells.

5. MECHANISMS FOR BLOCKING BASAL LAMINA FORMATION

Compositional analysis has indicated that about one quarter of the mass of the basement membrane is type IV collagen. This latter component is also the framework around which the lamina is assembled (see Section 2). In attempts to determine the consequences of blocking lamina formation on

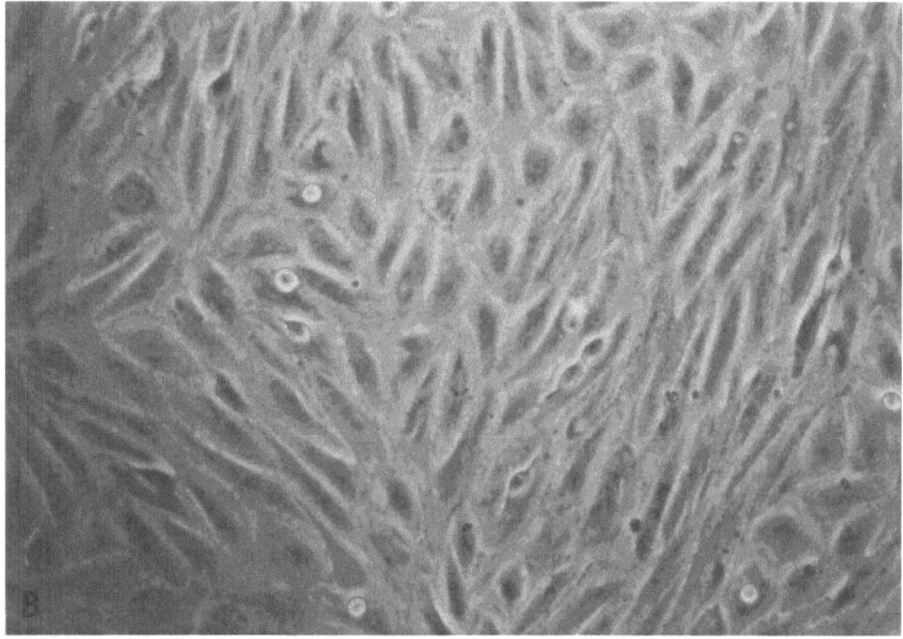

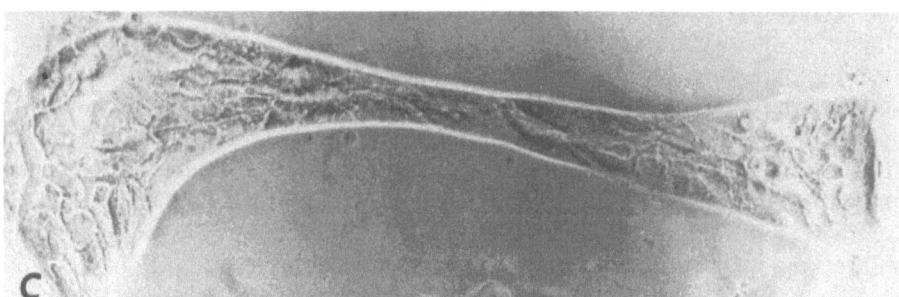

FIGURE 2. (continued)

mammary epithelium function, attention has focused on proline analogues such as cis-4-hydroxyproline, 4-thioproline, and azetidine carboxylate. These components (Figure 3) selectively block collagen production, as shown by several groups, but more extensively by Uitto and Prockop (1977). The proline analogues appear to affect collagen production selectively for two reasons. First, collagen is about eightfold richer in proline than the average cell protein (Peterkofsky and Diegelmann, 1971). Second, collagen is usually synthesized in much greater amounts than those in which it actually accumulates because of intracellular degradation (Bruckner et al., 1981; Bano et al., 1983a; and many others). Degradation of collagen inside the cell is, in part, regulated by the rate of assembly of the individual collagen peptide chains into a triple helical structure and apparently by the stability of the

TABLE I

Collagen IV and Laminin Production by Rat Mammary
Adenocarcinoma Cells

Cell type	Collagen IV[a]			Laminin[b] (ng/10^5 cells)
	cpm total protein	cpm collagen	Percent cpm in collagen	
Basal	1.4×10^5	3.9×10^4	27.9	13.7
Epithelial	1.2×10^6	4.2×10^3	0.4	16.3

[a]The amount of collagen IV produced was assessed by measuring amino acid incorporation into total protein and into collagen IV, which was purified by acid extraction
and gel electrophoresis (from Bano and Kidwell, 1984).
[b]Laminin was analyzed by enzyme-linked immunoassay by methods described by Liotta
et al. (1980).

triple helical structure after it forms (Bruckner *et al.*, 1981). *Cis*-hydroxy-
proline incorporation into collagen apparently reduces both the rate of formation as well as the stability of the collagen triple helix and therefore
facilitates the turnover of collagen intracellularly, at least in the fibroblast
cell types on which most such analyses have been made.

Whatever the mechanism, there is no doubt that the proline analogues
selectively block net collagen production in cultures of normal and neoplastic mammary epithelium. A comparison of the inhibitory effects of three
proline analogues on collagen synthesis by the epithelium in the DMBA-
induced mammary tumor is presented in Table II. Following 3 days in culture
in the presence of 25 μg/ml of the analogues there is a 27- to 7-fold differential
inhibition of collagen versus total cell protein synthesis. Therefore we tested
the ability of the analogues to block basement membrane deposition *in vivo*
by treating animals with various doses of the analogues followed by electron
microscopy of glandular tissue sections to visualize the integrity of the lamina. As seen in Figure 4, administration of *cis*-hydroxyproline for 3 days
was associated with a loss of basal lamina material and resulted in direct
contact of the mammary epithelium with the underlying stroma. The gaps
in the lamina were only seen if the glandular epithelium was proliferating

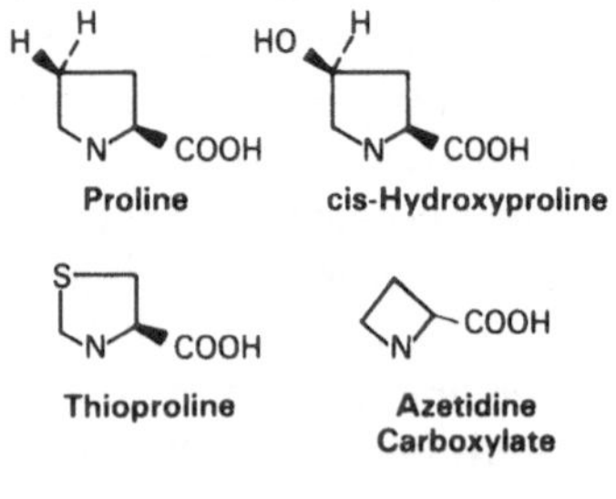

FIGURE 3. Structure of proline and proline analogues that selectively inhibit collagen production by mammary cells.

TABLE II

Selective Effects of Proline Analogues on the Biosynthesis of Collagen in Cultures of Rat Mammary Adenocarcinoma Cells

Analogue	Percent inhibition[a] of total protein	Percent inhibition[b] of collagen	Selective inhibition[c] of collagen
Azetidine carboxylate	3.3	89	27
Thioproline	3.2	71	14
cis-Hydroxyproline	9.9	69	7

[a]Expressed as the percent inhibition of [³H]lysine incorporation into total protein after 72 hr culture.
[b]The amount of collagen synthesized was estimated by digesting the total cell protein with purified, protease-free collagenase and determining the amount of radioactivity converted to an acid-soluble form.
[c]The ratio of inhibition of collagen labeling to total protein labeling (from Kidwell et al., 1984a).

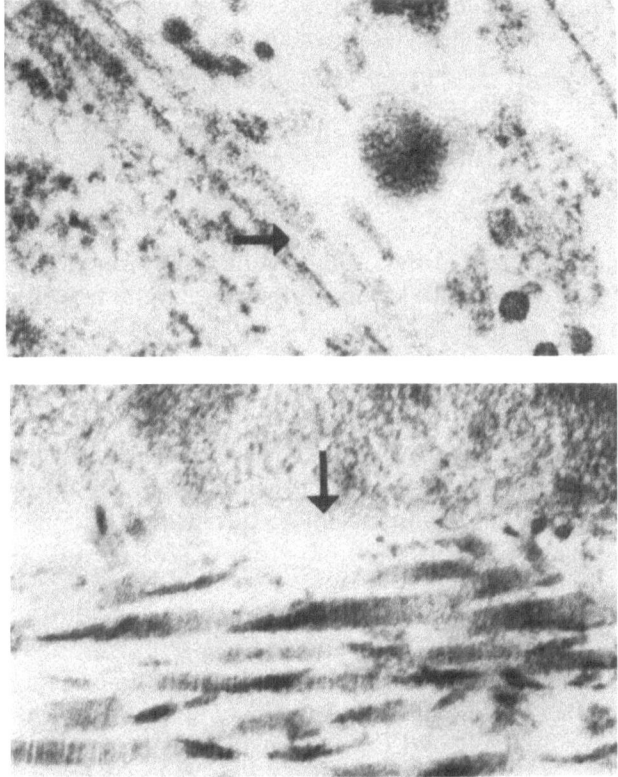

FIGURE 4. Effect of cis-hydroxyproline on the integrity of the basement membranes of the glandular epithelium of perphenazine-treated rats. (Top) Control animal glands. Note the basement membrane (arrow). (Bottom) Section of the gland on an animal receiving cis-hydroxyproline. Note the lack of a basement membrane and the juxtaposition of the stromal collagen fibers and the basal surface of an epithelial cell (from Wicha et al., 1980).

at the time of proline analogue administration, indicating that the gaps were produced at sites of new lamina synthesis (Wicha *et al.*, 1980).

6. EFFECTS OF PROLINE ANALOGUES ON MAMMARY TUMOR GROWTH

As shown in the previous section, proline analogues such as *cis*-hydroxyproline can block basal lamina formation *in vivo* in proliferating rat mammary epithelium. The direct or indirect consequences of this are an inhibition of the growth of mammary adenocarcinomas and an involutionlike process of the normal mammary epithelium (Wicha *et al.*, 1980; Lewko *et al.*, 1981). The effects on the normal proliferating gland are depicted in Figure 5. Animals were given perphenazine, which induces massive proliferation of the glands. Following 5–6 days with *cis*-hydroxyproline such animals develop a degenerated mammary epithelial cell population, a loss of most of the basal lamina except for segments of lamina that underlie the basal surface of the myoepithelial cells. When animals with nonproliferating glands are treated with *cis*-hydroxyproline there is no effect on the epithelium. This fact, plus the lack of general toxicity of *cis*-hydroxyproline and its highly specific effects on collagen production, strongly suggests that the proline analogue causes the proliferating epithelium to degenerate because it prevents the epithelium from producing a new lamina.

Since methylnitrosourea (NMU)-induced rat mammary adenocarcinomas are histologically well differentiated, with a continuous lamina encasing their epithelial structures, we surmised that these tumors would be affected by proline analogues, as is normal mammary epithelium. This is indeed the case. A summary of the effects of three proline analogues on adenocarcinoma growth *in vivo* is presented in Tables III–V. *Cis*-hydroxyproline treatment for 12 days reduced tumor growth by 95% ($p \leq 0.01$). Also shown in Table III is the lack of effect of this analogue on the growth of a transplantable, poorly differentiated NMU-induced rat mammary carcinoma. The latter tumor makes no basement membrane collagen (Lewko *et al.*, 1981). Its growth is completely unaffected by *cis*-hydroxyproline. These results are significant because they indicate that proline analogue sensitivity is not simply a consequence of the proliferation status of the tumor or whether the tumor synthesizes any types of collagen, but rather correlates with the degree of differentiation of the tumor and whether or not the tumor produces a basal lamina. A number of transplantable rat mammary tumors have also been tested for sensitivity to *cis*-hydroxyproline. The results found are consistent with the above conclusion (Kidwell *et al.*, 1984b), that is, sensitivity is roughly proportional to the amount of basal lamina produced by the tumors.

Thioproline and azetidine carboxylate are two other proline analogues that have a demonstrably selective effect on type IV collagen production by rat mammary adenocarcinoma cells, as previously shown in Table II. They

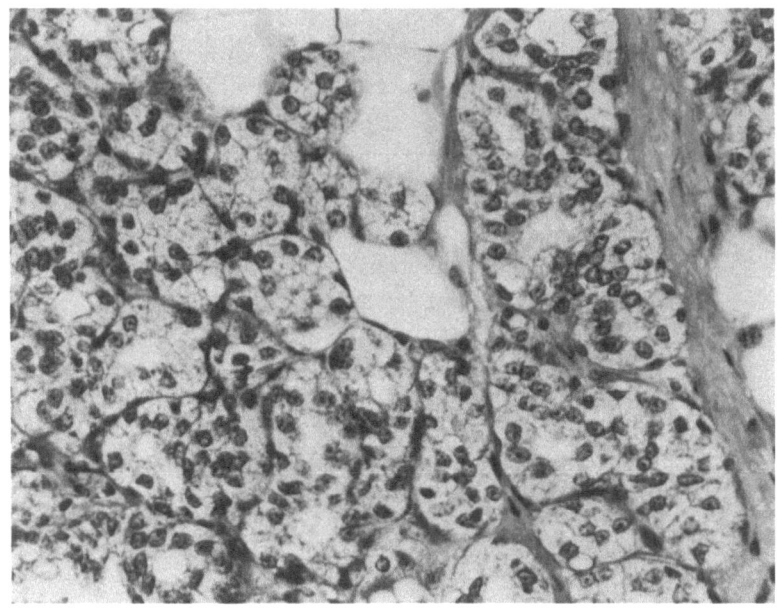

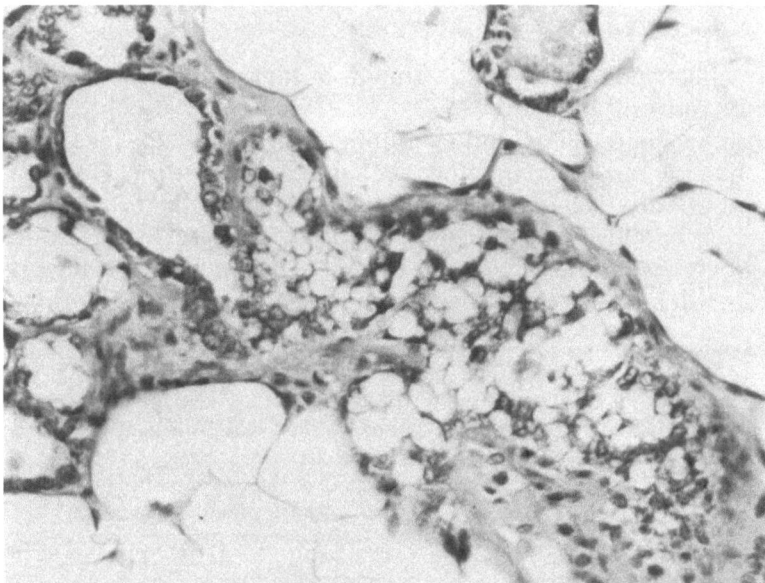

FIGURE 5. Effect of cis-hydroxyproline on the viability of the epithelium of normal mammary glands. The glandular epithelium was induced to proliferate by injecting the animals with perphenazine. Animals were then treated with or without cis-hydroxyproline for several days; the glands were then removed for histological examination. (Top) Gland of animal receiving perphenazine only. (Bottom) Gland of animal receiving both perphenazine and cis-hydroxyproline treatment (from Wicha et al., 1980).

TABLE III

Effect of cis-Hydroxyproline on the Growth of
NMU-Induced Mammary Tumors

Treatment	Tumor volume (cm³)	
Experiment 1: Primary tumors (adenocarcinomas)	Day 0[a]	Day 12[b]
Saline control (7)	3.1 ± 0.4	8.5 ± 2.0
cis-Hydroxyproline (9)[c]	2.7 ± 0.7	3.6 ± 0.8
Experiment 2: Transplantable NMU-induced tumors (carcinomas)	Day 0	Day 8
Saline control (8)	0.5 ± 0.1	10.5 ± 1.0
cis-Hydroxyproline (8)	0.4 ± 0.1	10.3 ± 0.9

[a]At day 0 there was no significant difference in the tumor volumes
of the tumors of the two groups in experiment 1 or between the two
groups in experiment 2.
[b]After 12 days of treatment the tumors in the saline control group
and in the cis-hydroxyproline treatment groups differed significantly
($p \leq 0.02$) but there were no significant differences between the two
groups in experiment 2.
[c]cis-Hydroxyproline was administered at 100 mg/kg, twice daily.

are also effective in blocking the growth of tumor cells in vivo, as seen in
Tables IV and V.

Treatment of the NMU-induced-tumor-bearing animals for 15 days with
thioproline (50 mg/kg) completely abolished tumor growth (Table V). This
treatment had no effect on total body weights, nor was there any abnormality
apparent on histological examination of bone, cartillage, gastrointestinal tract,
liver, or lung. Azetidine carboxylate treatment (50 mg/kg) for 21 days reduced
tumor growth by about one half; it was not as effective as cis-hydroxyproline

TABLE IV

Effects of Azetidine Carboxylate on NMU-Induced
Tumor Growth

Treatment	Tumor volume (cm³)	
	Day 0[a]	Day 21[b]
Saline control (10)[c]	4.3 ± 2.2	33.7 ± 15.6
Azetidine carboxylate (9)[d]	4.1 ± 3.2	19.6 ± 12.5

[a]The tumor volumes at day 0 were not different statistically ($p \leq 0.9$).
[b]The azetidine carboxylate treatment regimen reduced the growth
rate significantly ($p \leq 0.06$). In determining the significances between the groups all tumor values were considered so that $N \approx 60$.
[c]Numbers in parentheses indicate the number of animals per group.
There were about six tumors per animal.
[d]Azetidine carboxylate was administered s.c. at a dose of 50 mg/kg
twice daily for 21 days.

TABLE V
Effect of Thioproline on NMU-Induced
Tumor Growth

Treatment	Tumor volume (cm³)	
	Day 0[a]	Day 15[b]
Saline control (8)	3.0 ± 2.5	5.3 ± 3.2
Thioproline (10)[c]	3.2 ± 2.5	3.0 ± 1.8

[a]Starting tumor volumes were not significantly different.
[b]Thioproline totally arrested tumor growth. There were about six tumors per animal and all values were considered in the statistical analysis. The saline control tumor group approximately doubled over 15 days ($p \leq 0.05$), whereas the thioproline tumor group did not grow ($p \leq 0.9$).
[c]Thioproline was administered s.c. at a dose of 50 mg/kg twice daily for 15 days to animals bearing primary NMU-induced tumors.

at 100 mg/kg or as thioproline at 50 mg/kg (Table IV). These results may mean that there are differences in the clearance rates of the three proline analogues *in vivo*.

7. HOW THE PROLINE ANALOGUES PRODUCE THEIR EFFECTS

Previous studies suggested that normal mammary epithelium is dependent on contact with a basal lamina for growth and/or survival. Thus we showed that isolated mammary epithelium preferentially attaches to basement membrane collagen rather than stromal collagen (Wicha *et al.*, 1979b). On the latter substratum cells will not attach at all in the presence of *cis*-hydroxyproline. In fact, the cells are killed by *cis*-hydroxyproline on this substratum. However, the proline analogue does not affect attachment of normal mammary epithelium on basement-membrane-collagen-coated surfaces. Nor does the proline kill normal epithelium plated on the latter substratum. The conclusion reached is that interaction of the epithelium is needed for normal mammary cell survival (Wicha *et al.*, 1979b). This possibility cannot explain the growth-inhibitory effects of *cis*-hydroxyproline on mammary adenocarcinoma cells, however. These cells show no preferential attachment to basement membrane collagen relative to stromal collagen (Table VI). Also, the proline analogue sensitivity is the same on the two collagen types.

A recent observation of the proline dependency of both normal and tumor epithelium may explain their proline analogue sensitivities. A substantial growth stimulation of both normal and tumor epithelium is seen when proline at physiological concentrations is added to the culture medium

TABLE VI

Relative Attachment Efficiencies of Mammary Cells
from the Normal Gland and from Adenocarcinomas on
Type IV versus Type I Collagen Surfaces

Origin of epithelium	Percentage cells attached on IV[a] / Percentage cells attached on I
Normal gland	3.4
Adenocarcinoma	
NMU-induced	1.08
DMBA-induced	1.31

[a]Organoids were isolated from the normal and tumor tissues and the
percentage of cells attached after 15 hr in culture on dishes coated with
the two types of collagen was determined. Fibroblasts from the normal
mammary gland showed no preferential attachment on either substratum (adapted from Kidwell et al., 1980a).

and the cells are plated on a stromal collagen substratum. This is not the
case when the cells are cultured on a basement-membrane-collagen-coated
surface, as shown in Table VII.

A model that depicts our ideas of how this proline auxotrophy occurs
is presented in Figure 6. Proline is normally considered to be a nonessential
amino acid, one synthesized by almost all cells in sufficient quantities for
optimal growth. However, this is apparently not the case for the myoepithelial cells, which produce massive amounts of collagen IV. In our model,

TABLE VII

Proline Effects on Mammary Cell Growth
on Collagen Substrata

Source of epithelium	Growth stimulation[a]	
	Type I	Type IV
Normal mammary gland	+490%	−8%
Adenocarcinoma		
DMBA-induced	+180%	−10%
NMU-induced	+149%	−1%

[a]Proline was present at 0 or 50 μg/ml. Cell counts were
performed after 2 days in culture. The normal mammary
cell number increased approximately 10% on the type I
collagen substratum in the absence of proline supplementation and by 50% with proline added. On type IV
collagen substrata the cell number increased about 50%
with or without proline supplementation. Tumor cell
growth rates were higher than those for normal cells on
either substratum with or without proline present in the
culture medium. A significant increase in growth rate
($p \leq 0.05$) was seen in response to proline on the type
I collagen substratum, but no effect was produced by
proline on the type IV collagen substratum.

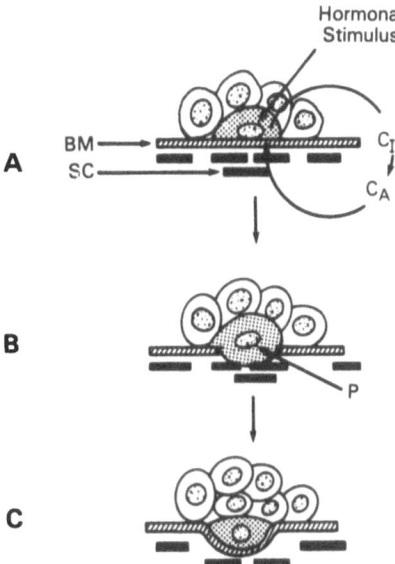

Hormonal
Stimulus

FIGURE 6. Model depicting the substratum effects
on proline requirements for cell growth. BM, basement membrane; C_A, type IV collagenase, active; C_I,
type IV collagenase, inactive; P, proline; SC, stromal
collagen.

the epithelium initially rests on a basement membrane substratum *in vivo*.
In this condition, the cells produce all the proline they require. Upon receiving a proliferation signal the cells penetrate through the basement membrane and come in contact with the underlying stromal collagen. Contact
with this surface triggers the cells, particularly the myoepithelial cells, to
begin to produce a new basement membrane containing the proline-rich
protein type IV collagen. This would increase the proline requirement beyond the cells' biosynthetic capacity, resulting in a proline auxotrophy.

There is some experimental evidence to support the model, other than
the fact that proline effects the proliferation rate of the epithelium. For
example, the addition of proline to the culture medium differentially amplifies collagen IV synthesis when the epithelium is plated on a stromal
collagen substratum but not when the cells are plated on type IV collagen
surfaces.

How would the latter observations explain the proline analogue effects
on mammary adenocarcinoma growth? We believe that in the adenocarcinomas the myoepithelial cell produces some factor that the epithelial cell
population requires for growth. Production of this factor is viewed as being
coupled to the production of collagen in the myoepithelial cells. Blocking
collagen production by proline analogues would thus block growth factor
production and result in the growth arrest of the tumor epithelial population.
Although they have not yet been characterized, candidates for such growth
factors have been detected (Bano and Kidwell, 1984). Epithelial and myoepithelial cells were isolated from the rat adenocarcinoma. A large stimulation of epithelial cell growth was seen when the two cell types were co-

cultured. Additionally, the medium from cultures of myoepithelial cells was strongly growth-promoting for the epithelial cells.

8. REGULATION OF COLLAGEN PRODUCTION BY MAMMARY TUMORS

8.1. Modulation of Collagenase Production by Steroids

Both anabolic and catabolic processes control basement membrane collagen production in cultures of normal mammary epithelium. Net production of collagen is dramatically enhanced by steroids such as hydrocortisone or dexamethasone. These hormones have been found to suppress the production of a collagenolytic activity by mammary cells and consequently the steroids modulate collagen production by blocking collagen turnover. A direct demonstration of this is presented in Figure 7. Mammary cell cultures were pulse-labeled with amino acids to measure newly synthesized collagen and the stability of the newly made collagen determined following a 24-hr chase period with labeled precursor removed from the culture medium. Very dramatic differences were seen when the chase was performed in the presence or absence of glucocorticoid hormones. When the hormone was present there was no collagen turnover. In the absence of the hormone, degradation was total (Liotta et al., 1980). The effect of the steroid was shown to be on extracellularly deposited collagen rather than on collagen inside the cell by demonstrating that hydrocortisone suppressed the ability of mammary cells to degrade a biosynthetically labeled collagen IV substratum on which the cells were plated (Salomon et al., 1981). These experiments demonstrate the importance of collagen turnover as a regulatory mechanism. Presumably this phenomenon applies to mammary tumor epithelium as well as to the normal epithelium, though this possibility has not been extensively assessed.

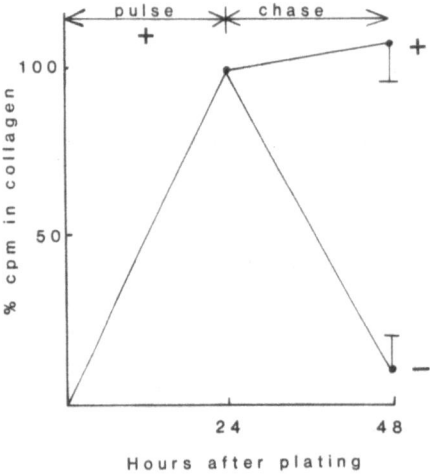

FIGURE 7. Modulation of basal lamina collagen turnover by hydrocortisone. Collagen was labeled in the presence of hydrocortisone then the precursor amino acid removed and the cultures of normal epithelium incubated for a further 24 hr with or without hydrocortisone. Note that the absence of the steroid during the chase period results in a near complete degradation of the newly synthesized collagen, whereas turnover is minimal if the steroid is present (from Liotta et al., 1980).

8.2. Amplification of Collagen Biosynthesis by Growth Factors

A large number of growth factors have been screened for their effects on collagen IV synthesis by mammary cells in culture. With corticosteroids present to block collagen degradation, a readily demonstrated effect of many growth factors on collagen biosynthetic rates has been shown (Kidwell *et al.*, 1984b). These are summarized in Table VIII, wherein effects on laminin are also presented. Of 16 factors tested, growth stimulation was produced by 12 in the mammary cell cultures. Of these 12, 11 also differentially amplified collagen IV production. The exception is insulin, which promotes mammary cell growth but does not differentially stimulate collagen synthesis. None of the growth factors tested that failed to stimulate cell growth had a stimulatory effect on collagen production. Among this latter category were estradiol-17β, progesterone, and prolactin. Although some cases were seen

TABLE VIII
Effects of Hormones and Growth Factors on Basal
Lamina Protein Synthesis

	Differential stimulation of production?	
	Collagen IV	Laminin
Growth-promoting factors[a]		
Insulin	No	Yes
Hydrocortisone	Yes	No
Epidermal growth factor	Yes	Yes
Multiplication growth factor	Yes	Yes
Transferrin	Yes	Yes
Prostaglandin E$_1$	Yes	Yes
Ascorbic acid	Yes	?[b]
Dibutyrl cAMP	Yes	Yes
Human-milk-derived growth factor	Yes	Yes
Human-mammary-tumor-derived growth factor	Yes	Yes
Rat-adenocarcinoma-derived growth factor	Yes	Yes
Mouse-adenocarcinoma-derived growth factor	Yes	?
Factors not stimulating mammary cell growth		
Estradiol-17β	No	No
Progesterone	No	No
Prolactin	No	No
Platelet-derived growth factor	No	No
Fibroblast growth factor	No	No
Prostaglandin E$_2$	No	?

[a]Determined on primary cultures of normal mouse mammary epithelium
(adapted from Kidwell *et al.*, 1984b).
[b]?, Assay not performed.

in which growth stimulation is produced in the absence of a differential amplification of laminin production, in general synthesis of this protein, like that of type IV collagen, is differentially stimulated by factors that promote mammary cell growth.

8.3. Tumor-Associated Growth Factors That Stimulate Collagen Synthesis

Included in Table VIII is a class of growth factors that we have discovered and purified from both human and rodent mammary tumors and from human milk. These growth factors are very potent in differentially stimulating collagen production by mammary epithelium, giving as much as a 10-fold amplification in amino acid incorporation into collagen IV compared to a 1.5- to 2-fold stimulation of total cell protein labeling (Kidwell *et al.*, 1982; Bano *et al.*, 1983a,b). These growth factors also differentially stimulate laminin production, though a more modest effect on synthesis of this protein is seen.

A summary of the properties of the growth factors and tissues where they have been detected is given in Table IX. A most interesting aspect of the tissues of origin of the growth factors is that they are present in differentiated tumors such as adenocarcinomas but low or absent in carcinomas. The two tumor types additionally differ from each other in that the former synthesizes a basal lamina and the latter does not (Lewko *et al.*, 1981; Kidwell *et al.*, 1984b). This suggests that the growth factor is an autocrine factor, made by tumors that produce a basal lamina. Definitive proof of this will require that we show that the mammary tumor factors are made by the tumor cells.

TABLE IX
Properties and Distribution of Mammary Tumor Factors

Tissue source	Abundance[a]	M.W. (daltons)	pI	Receptors
Human milk	High	62,000	4.8	$K_D = 5 \times 10^{-10}$
Human mammary adenocarcinoma	Moderate	62,000	4.8	N.D.[b]
Rat mammary adenocarcinoma	High	68,000	5.9	N.D.
Rat mammary carcinoma	Low to absent	—	—	—
Mouse mammary adenocarcinoma	Moderate to high	N.D.	N.D.	N.D.
Rat liver	Absent	—	—	—
Normal rat mammary gland	Very low	—	—	—

[a]Activity of factor assessed on basis of ability of crude extracts to stimulate collagen IV synthesis differentially in cultures of normal mammary epithelium.
[b]N.D., not done.

The fact that human milk contains a factor apparently identical to that in human mammary tumors (Table IX) suggests that basal lamina production by normal mammary epithelium might also be autocrinally regulated by factors synthesized by the normal epithelium. While this may be the case, current evidence suggests that adenocarcinomas produce much more growth factor than does the normal mammary gland (Bano et al., 1983a). In fact, the tumor factor isolated from the rat mammary adenocarcinoma does not stimulate collagen production in cultures of tumor epithelium while it is a very potent activator of collagen synthesis in cultures of normal epithelium (Kidwell et al., 1982). We presume that this means that the tumor cells in culture produce the growth factor optimally so that exogenously added factor gives no further stimulation, whereas the normal mammary epithelium produces the factor suboptimally and thus responds to exogenously added factor of the same type.

8.4. Substratum-Dependent Modulation of Growth Factor Responsiveness

As shown in Table IX, there is abundant growth factor present in milk. This factor is very potent in stimulating basal lamina protein production by cultures of normal mammary epithelium. However, the epithelium of the lactating mammary gland is quiescent insofar as proliferation and basal lamina production are concerned. From this fact it is clear that, while the presence of a specific growth factor such as the mammary tumor factor or mammary milk factor may be necessary for basal lamina production, it is not sufficient.

In attempts to understand this phenomenon we discovered that normal mammary epithelial cells differentially respond to growth factors depending on the type of substratum on which the cells are plated (Salomon et al., 1981). Specifically we found that the growth of the mammary epithelium is much more dramatically stimulated by epidermal growth factor (EGF) and hydrocortisone when the cells are plated on stromal-collagen-coated dishes than when they are plated on basement-membrane-collagen-coated dishes. This is not true for other growth factors such as insulin, however. When the rat mammary tumor factor and the human-milk-derived growth factor were tested, they were both found to be EGF- and hydrocortisonelike in regard to their substratum-potentiated action (Bano et al., 1985). For example, the growth factor from milk differentially stimulates collagen IV production fourfold in mammary cells plated on stromal-collagen-coated culture dishes but has little effect on synthesis of this protein when the cells are plated on basement-membrane-collagen-coated dishes.

The lack of response of the mammary epithelium to milk-derived growth factor, present in abundance and bathing the lactating gland epithelium, finds a ready explanation from the above observations. When the epithelium is in contact with the basement membrane on which it normally rests it is not responsive to such growth factors. When the epithelium comes in contact with the stroma it is sensitized to respond to the milk- or tumor-derived growth factors and to lay down a new basal lamina between itself and the stroma. This property of the epithelium provides a plausible mechanism by which the glandular epithelium might maintain itself as a continuum, separated from the stroma. Contact of the epithelium with the stroma presumably occurs as the epithelium invades the stromal compartment during proliferation, aided by the collagenolytic activity that the epithelium produces. Basal lamina production, then, is a process that is probably regulated by (1) autocrine growth factors, (2) the environment in which the normal and tumor epithelia finds themselves, and (3) the cell types present in the tissue, especially the basal or myoepithelial cell component. Mammary tumors may vary in one or more of these regulatory aspects. Carcinomas of the rat, for example, lack myoepithelial cells and contain no growth factors of the type detected in adenocarcinomas, and this tumor type thus far shows little sensitivity to proline analogues.

9. FEEDBACK INHIBITION OF BASAL LAMINA PRODUCTION

Although lamina production is differentially amplified in response to a large number of growth factors that promote mammary cell growth, it is possible to dissociate growth and lamina production. For example mammary cells cultured on stromal collagen substrata will grow rapidly as the same cells cultured on a basement membrane collagen substratum provided proline and mammary tumor factor are present in the culture medium. However, the amount of collagen IV produced is much greater on the former substratum than on the latter (Kidwell et al., 1982, 1984b). We have suggested that the difference in collagen IV production is in part due to a sensitization of mammary cells to the mammary tumor factor by contact with stromal elements such as stromal collagen (see Section 8.4).

There are probably two other controlling mechanisms and a stem cell effect. When the mammary epithelium is cultured on the two collagen substrata with proline present and without tumor factor, the cells still synthesize about two to three times as much collagen on the stromal as on the basement membrane collagen surfaces. The most likely explanation for this is that there is a negative feedback mechanism that regulates collagen production by the mammary cells. A suggestion of how this might work is provided by the observations of Werb's group, who have shown that when certain cells are plated on a sparsely charged polyhemin surface on which their flattening is minimized they greatly amplify their production of collagen (Werb et al., 1981). Mammary cells, which we showed attach and flatten more efficiently on a basement membrane collagen surface than on stromal collagen substrata (Wicha et al., 1979b; Kidwell et al., 1984b) would therefore be expected to synthesize less collagen on the basement membrane collagen substratum.

10. STEM CELLS AND THE PRODUCTION OF A
   BASAL LAMINA

Within the last few years a third controlling factor that may be involved in the production of a basal lamina has come to light from the studies of Rudland's and Daniel's groups. Both laboratories have presented evidence for a common precursor stem cell that can convert to either an epithelial or a myoepithelial cell (Warburton et al., 1981, 1982; Silberstein and Daniel, 1982; Williams and Daniel, 1983). These authors' results as well as those of Dulbecco et al. (1981) confirm our findings that the myoepithelial cell is the major mammary cell type responsible for the production of a basal lamina (Kidwell et al., 1982, 1984a). However, the existence of a stem cell precursor to the myoepithelial cell raises the possibility that a part of the control process for lamina production is in the rate of conversion of stem cells to myoepithelial cells. What, for example, would be the effect of the movement of such a stem cell from its resting position onto stromal collagen that lies underneath the lamina? Would it convert to a myoepithelial-like cell and then deposit a basal lamina? Are the mammary growth factors we have purified capable of facilitating such a conversion? Is it possible that the carcinoma is composed largely of stem cells that cannot convert to a myoepithelial cell type and therefore do not produce significant amounts of lamina, whereas the adenocarcinoma stem cell population efficiently undergoes this conversion?

At present we cannot isolate or absolutely identify a stem cell population in mammary tumors or the normal mammary gland, but the concept is nevertheless very realistic. How else can the heterogeneity of cell types within the gland be explained? What we do know with certainty is that the growth factors we have purified from the rodent and human mammary tumors and milk are capable of stimulating collagen synthesis and amplifying collagen mRNA production within 15 min of addition to cell cultures. So even if these factors can effect stem cell conversion to myoepithelial cells it is unlikely that they cannot also activate basal lamina synthesis in a preexisting myoepithelial cell population.

11. AMPLIFICATION OF COLLAGEN PRODUCTION AND
   PROLINE ANALOGUE SENSITIVITY

While these observations and proposals regarding the control of basal lamina may seem esoteric, in fact they may have a bearing on the relative sensitivity of mammary tumors to proline analogues. For example, the more activated the tumor cells are for producing a basal lamina, the more sensitive they may be to the proline analogues. This is not an unlikely proposition since we have found that several transplantable mammary tumors express different amounts of basal lamina production and that their sensitivity to *cis*-hydroxyproline is roughly proportional to their lamina content (Lewko *et al.*, 1981).

If the latter phenomena are causally related one would expect that hormonal, nutritional, or other factors that altered lamina deposition might also modify proline analogue sensitivity. This is an area of research that is currently being investigated. What, for example, would be the effect of ascorbate on proline analogue sensitivity of mammary tumor cells? This vitamin amplifies collagen production, apparently via enhancing proline hydroxylation posttranslationally in the collagen molecule. Increased hydroxylation facilitates triple helix formation and apparently facilitates processing and secretion of collagen via the Golgi. We would anticipate that a combined treatment of animals with ascorbate and *cis*-hydroxyproline would result in more faulty proline-analogue-containing collagen being formed, but that its accumulation inside the cell would be reduced and therefore that less cell kill would be obtained. Uitto *et al.* have suggested that it is the jamming up of the Golgi by *cis*-hydroxyproline-containing collagen that results in cell kill (Uitto *et al.*, 1977). Consequently the two effects of ascorbate might operate in different directions, one increasing proline analogue sensitivity and the other decreasing it. It has been proposed that ascorbate treatment alone might reduce tumor growth by facilitating tumor encapsulation (Cameron and Pauling, 1979) but the evidence for this is very controversial.

It is important to remember that proposals such as that of Uitto and Prockop (1977) on proline analogue killing have been formulated from studies on fibroblastic cells. It is not clear at present whether similar mechanisms apply to the mammary cells, which produce a completely different collagen type, because data regarding the processing of this collagen species (type IV collagen) intracellularly and extracellulary is fragmentary at present. For this reason we are most interested in elucidating various processes by which mammary cells elaborate basal lamina collagen.

12. SUMMARY

A model that summarizes our current concepts of the regulatory features of basal lamina production and plausibly explains the proline analogue sensitivity of lamina-producing mammary tumors is presented in Figure 8. The mammary epithelium rests on a basal lamina in a nonproliferating state and its production of lamina is turned off. Under the influence of a proliferative stimulus, the epithelium locally degrades the preformed lamina and migrates onto the underlying stroma. Contact with the stroma activates the cells (basal or myoepithelial) to synthesize new basal lamina containing the proline-rich protein type IV collagen. The increased collagen production requires more proline that the cells can synthesize or else there is an inhibition of *de novo* proline biosynthesis, which in effect produces a proline auxotrophy (and consequently an increased sensitivity to proline analogues). Providing exogenous proline supplies are adequate, the cells deposit a new lamina be-

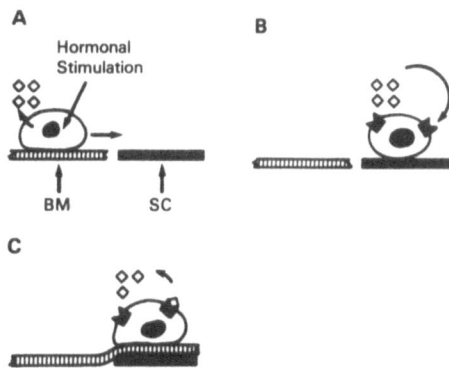

FIGURE 8. Model encompassing the regulatory features of basement membrane collagen production by normal epithelium and the epithelium of well differentiated mammary tumors. See text for explanation. BM, basement membrane; SC, stromal collagen; ◇, autocrine growth factor; ◖, receptor for autocrine growth factor.

tween themselves and the stroma in response to the growth factors made by the epithelium. The process repeats itself until proliferation is completed.

These characteristics are mostly retained by the rat mammary adenocarcinomas and consequently are likely to be the basis of their growth arrest by proline analogues. Carcinomas, on the other hand, have lost most of these properties, including their proline analogue sensitivity, by mechanisms that are not understood. Proline analogues may find a clinical application for the treatment of well differentiated mammary tumors, some of which are metastatic.

REFERENCES

Bano, M., and Kidwell, W. R., 1984, Characterization of subpopulations of rat mammary tumor cells, Cancer Res. **44**:3055–3062.

Bano, M., Zwiebel, J. A., Salomon, D. S., and Kidwell, W. R., 1983a, Detection and partial characterization of collagen synthesis stimulating activities in rat mammary adenocarcinomas, J. Biol. Chem. **258**:2729–2735.

Bano, M., Salomon, D. S., and Kidwell, W. R., 1983b, Control of basement membrane protein production by normal and neoplastic breast epithelium, J. Cell Biol. **97**:453a.

Bano, M., Salomon, D., and Kidwell, W. R., 1985. Isolation of a growth factor from human milk and human mammary tumors, J. Biol. Chem. **260**:5745–5750.

Bruckner, P., Eikenberry, E. F., and Procokop, D. J., 1981, Formation of triple helix of Type I procollagen in cells, Eur. J. Biochem. **118**:607–613.

Cameron, E., Pauling, L., and Leibovitz, B., 1979, Ascorbic acid and cancer: A review, Cancer Res. **39**:663–681.

Dulbecco, R., Henahan, M., Bowman, M., Okada, S., Battifora, H., and Unger, M., 1981, Generation of fibroblast-like cells from cloned epithelial mammary cells in vitro: A possible new cell type, Proc. Natl. Acad. Sci. USA **78**:2345–2349.

Furthmayr, H., Roll, F. J., Madri, J. A., and Foellmer, H. G., 1982, Composition of basement membranes as viewed with the electron microscope, in: New Trends in Basement Membrane Research (K. Kuhn, H. Schoene, and R. Timpl, eds.), Raven Press, New York, pp. 31–48.

Hassell, J. R., Robey, P. G., Barrach, H., Wilczek, J., Rennard, S. I., and Martin, G. R., 1980, Isolation of a heparin sulfate containing proteoglycan from basement membrane, Proc. Natl. Acad. Sci. USA **77**:4494–4498.

Janss, D. H., Hillman, E. A., Malan-Shibley, L. R., and Ben, T. L., 1980, Methods for the isolation and culture of normal human breast epithelial cells, Methods Cell Biol. **21**:108–135.

Kidwell, W. R., Wicha, M. S., Salomon, D. S., and Liotta, L. A., 1980a, Differential recognition of basement membrane collagen by normal and neoplastic breast epithelium, in: *Cell Biology of Breast Cancer* (M. Brennan, C. M. McGrath, and M. Rich, eds.), Academic Press, New York, pp. 17–32.

Kidwell, W. R., Wicha, M. S., Salomon, D. S., and Liotta, L. A., 1980b, Hormonal controls of collagen substratum formation by cultured mammary cells: Implications for growth and differentiation, in: *Control Mechanisms in Animal Cells* (L. Jiminez de Asua, R. Levi-Montakini, R. Shields, and S. Iacobelli, eds.), Raven Press, New York, pp. 333–340.

Kidwell, W. R., Salomon, D. S., Liotta, L. A., Zwiebel, J. A., and Bano, M., 1982, Effects of growth factors on mammary epithelial cell proliferation and basement membrane synthesis, in: *Growth of Cells in Hormonally Defined Media* (G. Sato, A. Pardee, and D. Sirbasku, eds.), Cold Spring Harbor Laboratory Press, Cold Spring Harbor, New York, pp. 807–818.

Kidwell, W. R., Taylor, S. J., and Bano, M., 1984a, Growth arrest of mammary tumors by proline analogs, in: *Progress in Cancer Research and Therapy*, Volume 31 (F. Bresciani, R. King, M. Lippman, M. Namer, and J.-P. Ragnaud, eds.), Raven Press, New York, pp. 129–136.

Kidwell, W. R., Bano, M., and Salomon, D. S., 1984b, Growth of normal mammary epithelium on collagen in serum-free medium, in: *Cell Culture Methods for Molecular and Cell Biology*, Volume 2 (D. Barnes, D. Sirbasku, and G. Sato eds.), Alan R. Liss, New York, pp. 105–125.

Leblond, C. P., Inoue, S., and Laurie, G. W., 1983, Ultrastructure of Reichert's membrane, a multilayered basement membrane in the parietal wall of the rat yolk sac, *J. Cell Biol.* **97**:1524–1532.

Lewko, W. M., Liotta, L. A., Wicha, M. S., Vonderhaar, B. K., and Kidwell, W. R., 1981, Sensitivity of N-nitrosomethylurea-induced rat mammary tumors to cis-hydroxyproline, an inhibitor of collagen production, *Cancer Res.* **41**:2855–2862.

Liotta, L. A., Wicha, M. S., Rennard, S. I., Foidart, J., Garbisa, S., and Kidwell, W. R., 1980, Hormonal requirements for basement membrane collagen deposition by cultured mammary epithelium, *Lab. Invest.* **41**:511–518.

Martinez-Hernandez, A., Gay, S., and Miller, E. J., 1982, Ultrastructural localization of type V collagen in the rat kidney, *J. Cell Biol.* **92**:343–349.

Peterkofsky, B., and Diegelmann, R., 1971, Use of a mixture of proteinase-free collagenase for the specific assay of radioactive collagen in the presence of other proteins, *Biochemistry* **10**:988–994.

Rao, C. N., Margules, I. M., Tralka, T. S., Terranova, V. P., Madri, J. A., and Liotta, L. A., 1982, Isolation of a subunit of laminin and its role in molecular structure and tumor cell attachment, *J. Biol. Chem.* **257**:9740–9744.

Salomon, D. S., Liotta, L. A., and Kidwell, W. R., 1981, Differential response to growth factors by rat mammary epithelium plated on different collagen substrata in serum free medium, *Proc. Natl. Acad. Sci. USA* **78**:382–386.

Silberstein, G. B., and Daniel, C. W., 1982, Glycosamino-glycans in the basal lamina and extracellular matrix of the developing mouse mammary duct, *Dev. Biol.* **90**:215–222.

Strum, J. M., Lewko, W. M., and Kidwell, W. R., 1981, Structural alterations within NMU-induced mammary tumors after *in vivo* treatment with cis-hydroxyproline, *Lab. Invest.* **45**:347–354.

Terranova, U. P., Liotta, L. A., Russo, R., and Martin, G. R., 1982, Laminin mediates the attachment of Pc epidermal cells to type IV collagen, *Cell* **22**:719–726.

Timpl, R., Martin, G. R., Bruckner, P., Wicha, G., Wideman, H., 1978, Nature of the collagenous protein in a tumor basement membrane, *Eur. J. Biol. Chem.* **84**:43–52.

Timpl, R., Rhode, H., Robey, P. G., Rennard, S. I., Foidart, J. M., and Martin, G. R., 1979, Laminin, a glycoprotein from basement membranes, *J. Biol. Chem.* **254**:9933–9937.

Uitto, J., and Prockop, D., 1977, Incorporation of proline analogs into procollagen, *Arch. Biochem. Biophys.* **181**:293–299.

Warburton, M. J., Ormerod, E. J., Monaghan, P., Ferns, S., and Rudland, P. S., 1981, Characterization of a myoepithelial cell line derived from a neonatal rat mammary gland, *J. Cell Biol.* **91**:827–836.

Warburton, M. J., Mitchell, D., Ormerod, E. J., and Rudland, P. S., 1982, Distribution of myoepithelial cells and basement membrane proteins in the resting, pregnant, lactating and involuting rat mammary gland, *J. Histochem. Cytochem.* **30**:667–676.

Werb, Z., Enders, G., and Friend, D. S., 1981, Differential effects of cell flattening on the synthesis of collagen and fibronectin in cultures of smooth muscle cells, *J. Cell Biol.* **91**:116a.

Wicha, M. S., Liotta, L. A., and Kidwell, W. R., 1979a, Effects of free fatty acids on the growth of normal and neoplastic mammary epithelial cells, *Cancer Res.* **39**:426–435.

Wicha, M. S., Liotta, L. A., Garbisa, S., and Kidwell, W. R., 1979b, Basement membrane collagen requirements for attachment and growth of mammary epithelium, *Exp. Cell Res.* **124**:181–190.

Wicha, M. S., Liotta, L. A., Vonderhaar, B. K., and Kidwell, W. R., 1980, Effects of inhibition of basement membrane collagen deposition on rat mammary gland development, *Dev. Biol.* **80**:253–266.

Williams, J. M., and Daniel, C. W., 1983, Mammary ductal elongation: Differentiation of myo-epithelium and basal lamina during branching morphogenesis, *Dev. Biol.* **97**:274–290.

CHAPTER 4

THE EVOLUTION OF PHENOTYPIC DIVERSITY IN METASTATIC TUMOR CELLS

GARTH L. NICOLSON

1. INTRODUCTION

It has been approximately one hundred years since Paget (1889) proposed the "seed and soil" hypothesis of tumor spread. This hypothesis was developed to explain the nonrandom occurrence of metastases in particular organs. Paget proposed that the microenvironment in unique organs or tissues ("soil") influenced the extravasation, survival, and growth of particular tumor cells ("seeds"). This hypothesis has remained one of the most important concepts of tumor metastasis. We now know that malignant neoplasms are composed of diverse cell "seeds" that are heterogeneous for a multitude of cellular properties, including cellular morphology, surface antigens, glycolipids, glycoproteins, recognition and adhesion components, and degradative and biosynthetic enzymes. They are also quite variable in their abilities to communicate with other cells, invasiveness, and metastatic properties, and, as expected, heterogeneity also exists in their sensitivities to various therapeutic agents (such as drugs, radiation, and hyperthermia), as well as host–response mechanisms (reviewed in Hart and Fidler, 1981; Fidler and Hart, 1982; Nicolson, 1982, 1984a; Nicolson and Poste, 1982, 1983a,b). Heterogeneity in cellular properties is also present in normal cells and tissues, but the range of diversity may not be as extensive as in malignant neoplasms (Peterson *et al.*, 1981, 1983).

The presence of unique organ environments and microenvironments also lends support to Paget's proposal. Differences in vascular endothelium,

GARTH L. NICOLSON • Department of Tumor Biology, The University of Texas–M. D. Anderson Hospital and Tumor Institute, Houston, Texas 77030.

parenchymal cells, innervation, and endocrine status may differentially affect tumor "seeds" or cell subpopulations and allow selective implantation, invasion, survival, and growth at particular sites (Nicolson, 1984b,c).

In this brief review I will consider the evolution of tumor heterogeneity and the possible effect that unique "soils" may have on the diversity of neoplastic cell "seeds."

2. ORIGINS OF NEOPLASTIC CELL HETEROGENEITY

Fialkow (1979) has reviewed the data on the origin of spontaneous and induced neoplasms and has concluded that they develop overwhelmingly from single cells. Even late in the pathogenesis of tumors, when diversification to heterogeneous cellular phenotypes has already occurred, evidence of such clonal origin exists (Nowell, 1976, 1983).

To explain the evolution of tumor cells from a single phenotype to diverse phenotypes, several processes have been invoked. The most important of these is that, as tumors progress in their host, they undergo cellular phenotypic diversification, and this occurs concomitant with host selection, resulting in neoplastic cells with heterogeneous characteristics and behaviors (Foulds, 1975; Nowell, 1976, 1983; Nicolson, 1984b,c). Essentially any property of tumor cells can evolve through phenotypic change and host selection to eventually yield highly malignant cells with enhanced autonomy, survival, growth, and metastatic behaviors.

Another important factor determining the diversity of cells within a neoplasm is the unique microenvironment of each tumor cell. To survive and grow as part of a heterogeneous cell population under limiting nutrient, hormonal, or other conditions, tumor cells must have selective growth and survival properties over the remaining cells in the tumor. Under such conditions some tumor cell subpopulations may cease to proliferate and become dormant, if they are inhibited by host mechanisms or are unresponsive to microenvironmental signals provided by hormones, growth factors, extracellular matrix, and other factors. Thus certain tumor cell subpopulations may eventually become dominant, and the resulting tumor can then evolve with variant phenotypic characteristics. Such a neoplasm can be considered a "dynamic ecosystem" (Heppner, 1984) in which alterations in the compositions of tumor cell subpopulations and their properties can vary with time (Heppner et al., 1984).

Tumor cell phenotypic diversification probably occurs at variable rates. In the simplistic scheme shown in Figure 1, a benign tumor would show minimal phenotypic diversity with time compared to a malignant neoplasm (Figure 1, A), while malignant neoplasms may diversify phenotypically at various times after transformation and at various rates (Figure 1, B–E). Some neoplasma may diversify slowly, beginning early after transformation (Figure 1, C), while others may diversify late in the natural history of the tumor (Figure 1, B). Malignant neoplasms may also change in their apparent rates

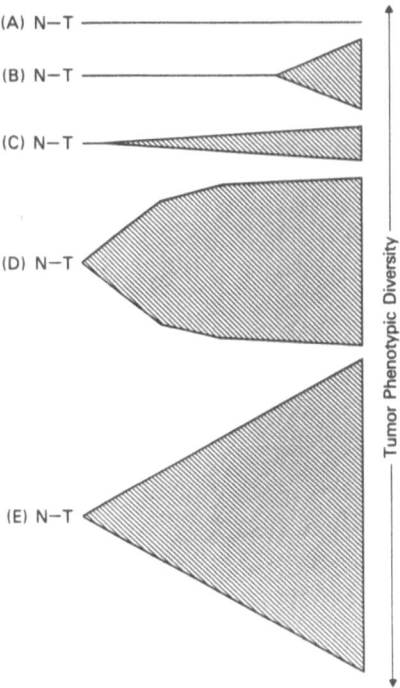

FIGURE 1. Evolution of tumor phenotypic diversification. (A) Transformation (N-T) does not result in detectable tumor phenotypic diversity (for example, a low-grade benign lesion); (B) transformation does not initially result in tumor phenotypic diversification; however, late in the natural history of the neoplasm, diversification occurs; (C) transformation results in a slow rate of progression and a gradual increase in the number of more diversified phenotypes; (D) phenotypic diversification occurs at a rapid rate until "interactions" between tumor cell subpopulations limit the rate at which new metastatic variants are generated; (E) tumor phenotypic diversification occurs at a rapid rate that is not limited by "interactions" between tumor cell subpopulations (from Nicolson, 1984c).

of phenotypic diversification in response to microenvironmental changes or subpopulation interactions (Figure 1, D) (Poste, 1982; F. A. Miller, 1983; Nicolson and Poste, 1983b; Nicolson, 1984c).

Not all tumor cell properties may diversify with time in malignant neoplasms. In particular, characteristics that are unrelated to cell response, survival, growth, and malignancy may actually be lost at certain stages of tumor evolution. In some cases this has been interpreted as "loss of differentiation," but it should be noted that the relationships between differentiation, tumor progression, and malignancy are unclear (Nicolson, 1984a–c).

3. INSTABILITY OF MALIGNANT NEOPLASMS

As tumor cells progress, they are thought to be subject to increasing genetic alterations that are generated by random, somatic mutational events (Nowell, 1976). This process allows the eventual dominance of emerging tumor cell subpopulations that show alterations in malignant and other phenotypic properties (Figure 2) (Nowell, 1976; Nicolson, 1984b,c). Tumor cell subpopulations that have the property of rapid diversification should display enhanced genetic instability, and in addition those properties that are the most favorable for cell survival, growth, and malignancy.

Cytogenetic and genetic data support the hypothesis that malignant neoplasms that grow progressively, invade, and metastasize possess enhanced

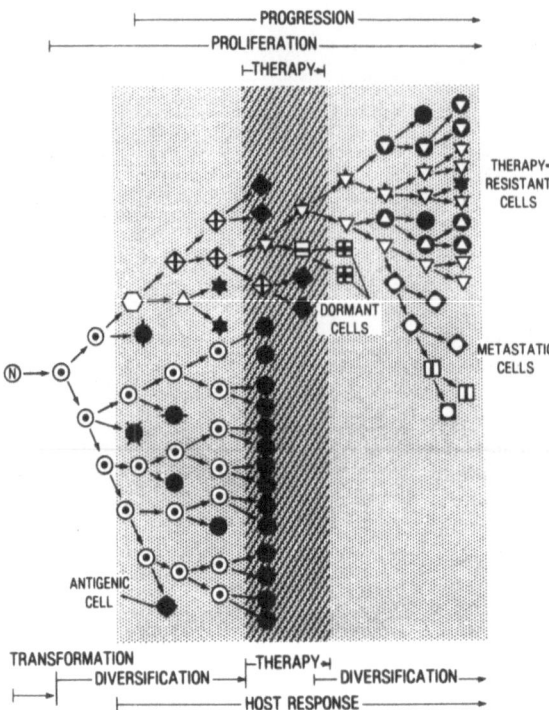

FIGURE 2. Tumor phenotypic diversification and progression and the effect of antitumor therapy. Transformation of a normal cell (N) into a tumor cell can lead to cellular diversification in malignant neoplasms. Some of these variant tumor cells die (solid symbols) owing to lethal mutations or host responses, or they fail to grow and become dormant, while other tumor cells become more competitive and malignant as they undergo phenotypic diversification. Cytotoxic therapy results in the death of most tumor cells (solid symbols) and restriction of phenotypic diversity. However, some malignant cells escape randomly or as a result of therapeutic resistance and continue to diversify phenotypically. Eventually a malignant subpopulation arises that possesses the correct phenotypic properties for metastasis (from Nicolson, 1984b).

genetic instability. This has been shown in studies in which gross chromosomal alterations, mitotic errors, and rates of spontaneous mutation have been compared between highly malignant cells and normal or less malignant counterparts. The data indicate that the former are genetically less stable (Nowell, 1983; Wolman, 1983). During the evolution of malignant neoplasms, chromosomal abnormalities and alterations in their morphologies or banding patterns may progressively increase, although this is not always seen (Wolman, 1983). For example, in chronic granulocytic leukemia (CGL) chromosomal analysis and banding reveal that most patients have a minute chromosome, the Ph[1] chromosome, in addition to trisomy in chromosome 8 and a translocation of a portion of chromosome 22 to chromosome 9 (reviewed in Nowell, 1983). In approximately two-thirds of leukemia patients with CGL who do not have progressive disease and in whom years pass before the terminal phase of accelerated CGL growth, the above changes are additionally associated with other chromosome alterations (Nowell, 1983).

During the progression of malignant animal tumors, gross chromosome changes have also been seen. For example, in Rous-sarcoma-virus-transformed fibroblasts, consistent chromosome changes are associated with neoplastic progression. One of the first changes noted is the appearance of an extra chromosome 7, followed by the acquisition of an additional chromosome 13, and finally an extra chromosome 12 (Mitelman, 1974). In rat mammary adenocarcinomas Pearce et al. (1984) have identified a number of chromosome markers that correlate with the primary or secondary origin of the tumor cells. In this system the most metastatic cell clones obtained from secondary sites possessed a particular set of Giemsa-stained chromosome markers at high frequency.

A more precise way to determine the instability of malignant neoplasms is to determine their spontaneous rates of gene mutation. Cifone and Fidler (1981) have examined the rates of spontaneous mutation to drug resistance in animal tumor cells of differing metastatic potentials. Using cell lines and clones of murine melanomas and fibrosarcomas, they measured the rates of spontaneous mutation to drug resistance and found that the more metastatic cells possessed six to seven times higher rates of spontaneous mutation than cells of low metastatic potential.

Nowell (1983) has proposed a number of different possible mechanisms for generating increased genotypic instability, including inherited defects in DNA repair or maintenance genes; acquired defects in specialized genes, such as "mutator" genes or genes involved in synthesizing DNA; chromosomal alterations, such as aneuploidy, transpositions, and abnormal sister chromatid exchanges; chromosome amplification regions, such as homogeneously staining regions and double minute chromosomes; integrated virus sequences, oncogenes, or protooncogenes; mutagenic agents, such as radiation or chemotherapeutic drugs; and microenvironmental alterations, such as nutritional differences. These mechanisms are not mutually exclusive and may produce differing end results in particular neoplasms residing in certain "soils."

One mechanism that may alter genomic stability is the incorporation of viral regulatory genes (oncogenes) or their cellular prototypes (protooncogenes) into cellular DNA (Cooper, 1982). However, we appear to know more about the role of oncogenes in the induction or maintenance of neoplastic transformation (Blair et al., 1981; DeFeo et al., 1981; Cooper, 1982) than in malignancy. In certain studies ligation of cellular oncogenes to transcriptional promoter sequences of viral origin has induced neoplastic transformation. The actual mechanism of cellular gene activation by oncogenes in such studies has been determined by inserting a viral long-terminal repeat sequence containing a viral promoter upstream in the cellular DNA, resulting in activation of a cellular oncogene and expression of the transformed phenotype (Hayward et al., 1981). This may not be the only mechanism for cellular oncogene amplification or activation, resulting in induction of transformation. In other studies, gross chromosomal changes have been linked to genetic alterations induced by oncogene insertion or activation. Schwab et al. (1983) found that the homogeneously staining regions and double minutes of a murine adrenocortical tumor and a human neuroblastoma contained amplified copies of particular cellular oncogenes.

The relationship of oncogene insertion into host genomes and neoplastic transformation is clearer than the possible relationship of such alterations to tumor phenotypic diversification or tumor progression (Nicolson, 1984b,c).

In one study low- and high-metastatic-potential sublines of a murine large cell lymphoma induced by Abelson leukemia virus were examined for expression of the *abl* oncogene by examining *abl*-encoded mRNA and cytoplasmic protein p160 (Rotter *et al.*, 1985). However, in this case differences in the expression of *abl* oncogene products could not be detected in large cell lymphoma sublines of various metastatic potentials. Therefore, the highly malignant phenotype need not be associated with increased expression of a transforming oncogene. It seems more likely that the insertion of oncogenes in proper genomic location(s) could activate previously cryptic genes and initiate the process of neoplastic diversification and progression (Nicolson, 1984b,c).

4. MODULATION OF NEOPLASTIC PHENOTYPIC INSTABILITY

Phenotypic instability and host selection fail to explain the high rates of tumor diversification and progression in many tumor systems. The highest known rates of spontaneous gene mutation in metastatic cells (i.e., $5–7 \times 10^{-5}$ mutations/cell per generation; Cifone and Fidler, 1981) are orders of magnitude less than rates of phenotypic variation observed in malignant neoplasms. A possible explanation is that gene mutation occurs at regulatory genome sites that are capable of generating rapid heterogeneity in cellular phenotypes. Modifications in regulatory genes of malignant cells could explain the fact that most changes in gene products associated with the malignant phenotype are quantitative rather than qualitative in their nature (Nicolson, 1982, 1984a).

In the instances in which phenotypic changes in tumor markers have been determined, malignant neoplasms show much higher rates of diversification than normal or benign cells. For example, the rate of appearance of quantitative variants in the expression of a surface glycoprotein on breast cancer cells was significantly higher in malignant than in normal epithelial cells (Peterson *et al.*, 1983). In this example, quantitative variants appeared in the breast tumor cell population at a mean rate of approximately 2.2×10^{-2} variants/cell per generation compared to a rate of approximately 0.36×10^{-2} variants/cell per generation in normal cells. Rapid rates of phenotypic diversification have been seen in a variety of tumor systems (Talmadge *et al.*, 1979; Chow and Greenberg, 1980; Neri and Nicolson, 1981; Nicolson *et al.*, 1982; Stackpole, 1983). In the ESb/Eb lymphoma system Bosslet and Schirrmacher (1982) noted a high frequency of generation of new immunoresistant tumor variants in the more metastatic ESb subline *in vivo*. They calculated that T-cell-resistant ESb lymphoma cells arose at a frequency of 10^{-3} variants/cell per generation, a rate that was too high to be explainable by sequential selection mechanisms. A somewhat slower rate of variant appearance ($\sim 10^{-5}$ variants/cell per generation) was found by Harris *et al.* (1982) using the metastatic KHT sarcoma system. These authors found that many of the KHT sarcoma cell clones were unstable and rapidly diversified in their lung colonization potentials. When these same cell clones were analyzed for their rates of spontaneous mutation to ouabain resistance, a much lower mutation rate ($\sim 3 \times 10^{-8}$ mutants/cell per generation) was found (Harris et al., 1982).

The generation of phenotypic diversity in tumor cell populations should result in the generation of tumor cells that have increased, as well as decreased, malignant properties, a result that has been confirmed in a number of tumor systems (Fidler and Nicolson, 1981; Neri and Nicolson, 1981; Poste et al., 1981; Miner et al., 1982; Nicolson et al., 1982). When malignant cells change to more benign phenotypes in vivo, they should be more susceptible to host controlling mechanisms, resulting in their dimunition with time and the appearance of more dominant phenotypes in the tumor (Nicolson, 1984b,c). In one study using a lectin-resistant variant of the MDAY tumor, Dennis et al. (1981) selected a wheat-germ-agglutinin-resistant subline that was much less metastatic than the original parental tumor. The wheat-germ-agglutinin-resistant subline still formed a few rare metastases, and when they formed tumor cells were recovered and their lectin sensitivities examined in vitro. After recovery, the metastatic cells were found to be lectin sensitive, suggesting that the highly malignant phenotype was rapidly generated in vivo, and that these highly malignant cells were the ones that metastasized in their host. Dennis et al. could calculate that the rate of spontaneous reversion to the more metastatic phenotype was $\sim 2 \times 10^{-5}$ variants/cell per generation.

A useful system to examine the phenotypic instability of a variety of cellular phenotypes is a series of rat mammary adenocarcinoma cell clones obtained from the 13762NF tumor and its spontaneous lung metastases (Neri and Nicolson, 1981; Neri et al., 1982). These 13762NF clones were found to vary reproducibly in their metastatic properties during in vitro growth (Neri et al., 1982; Welch et al., 1983b). Interestingly, changes in the metastatic properties of these clones were accompanied by changes in a number of phenotypic characteristics, such as cell and tissue morphologies (Neri and Nicolson, 1981; Neri et al., 1982), chromosome markers (Pearce et al., 1984), and cell surface glycoproteins (Neri and Nicolson, 1981; Steck and Nicolson, 1983), and they were also paralleled by shifts in cellular sensitivities to hyperthermia (Tomasovic et al., 1982), gamma radiation (Welch et al., 1983a), and chemotherapeutic drugs (Welch and Nicolson, 1983). These changes occurred at predictable tissue culture passage numbers in vitro, if the change occurred. In this system phenotypic change occurred for some, but not all, cellular properties, suggesting that phenotypic variation can be nonrandom and reproducible and can occur at unique rates. More recently this phenomenon has been seen in subclones generated from these same clonal 13762NF cell populations. When a panel of such subclones was examined at specific tissue culture passage numbers, the rates of change in sensitivities to hyperthermia, gamma radiation, and chemotherapeutic drugs were different (Welch et al., 1984).

Another technique for examining rates of clonal phenotypic diversification is the clonogenic assay, in which single cells are grown in semisolid medium (Hamburger and Salmon, 1977). When Raz (1982) examined the emergence of metastatic variants in B16 melanoma cell clones during growth in semisolid agarose, he found that each subclone had different metastatic properties. In a similar experiment performed with cell clones of the 13762NF system (Nicolson et al., 1983), it was found that a series of subclones diversified in their spontaneous metastatic properties, cell surface properties, and sensitivities to chemotherapeutic drugs. These results indicate that rapid phenotypic changes can occur during cellular growth in the semisolid medium of the clonogenic assay.

The high rates of phenotypic change seen in malignant tumor cells are not always maintained during clonal expansion. For example, Poste et al. (1981) found that although B16 melanoma cell clones grown in vitro diversified at a rapid rate, mixing several different cell clones in vitro stabilized the resulting polyclonal population and reduced their normally rapid rates of phenotypic change. It was previously noted that polyclonal lines of B16 melanoma were quite stable during prolonged in vitro growth, while clonal populations rapidly generated cell subpopulations with differing metastatic properties (Fidler and Nicolson, 1981). Stabilization of phenotypic properties has also been seen in cell clones of brain-colonizing subline B16-B14b (Miner et al., 1982). Although cell clones of B16-B14b were relatively unstable during in vitro growth, co-culturing three unstable clones resulted in phenotypic stabilization and maintenance of metastatic properties, compared to mixing the same three separately grown clones just prior to tumor cell inoculation (Figure 3). Also, the expression of a fetal-like cell surface glycoprotein (gp90) correlated with these phenotypic changes. Cell surface gp90 was expressed in higher amounts on brain-colonizing clones of high brain colonization potential, but when these brain-colonizing clones lost their potential to implant and grow in the brain meninges during in vitro growth, the amounts of gp90 decreased concomitantly with the decrease in brain colonization behavior (Miner et al., 1982).

The stabilization and subsequent destabilization of tumor cell phenotypes by polyclonal interactions has been documented in vitro by depleting the polyclonal cell populations of specific clones by drug treatment (Poste et al., 1982). In this experiment, mixing several B16 clones with unstable metastatic phenotypes but stable drug-resistant markers in vitro resulted in stabilization of the clones and their phenotypes (Poste et al., 1982). However, when all but a few of these clonal subpopulations were killed by drug treatment, the surviving cell subpopulations rapidly diversified (Figure 4). This diversification occurred until polyclonal interactions again stabilized the population as a whole and apparently reduced the rate of phenotypic diversification. If this new "equilibrium" was disturbed by exposure to another drug, which killed most of the cells in the new heterogeneous population, again restricting subpopulation diversity, then a new round of phenotypic diversification occurred (Figure 4).

Phenotypic stability may also be modulated by fusion of normal with neoplastic cells (Goldenberg et al., 1974). The ability of tumor cells to undergo

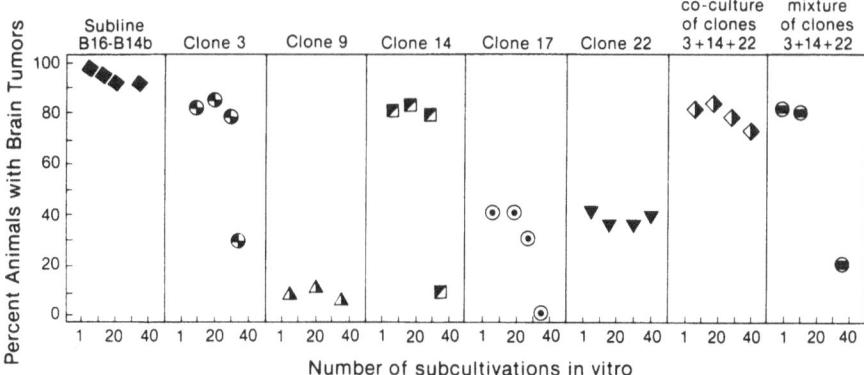

FIGURE 3. The instability of individual brain-colonizing B16 melanoma cell clones and their polyclonal stabilization. Cell clones were derived from the murine B16-B14b melanoma subline and cultured for various intervals *in vitro*, after which they were assayed for their metastatic properties according to Miner *et al.* (1982). Some cultures were established with equal numbers of cells from three different clones (co-culture of clones), and these were subcultured for various intervals and tested for their biologic properties. As a control for this type of experiment, equal numbers of cells from the three clones grown separately were combined (mixture of clones) immediately before the *in vivo* assays. Experimental metastatic brain colonization was assessed by intravenous injection of 2×10^4 singly suspended melanoma cells and determination of brain colonization 5–8 weeks later (data are from Miner *et al.*, 1982; figure from Nicolson and Poste, 1983b).

fusion *in vivo* with normal host cells to form hybrids could result in modulation of phenotypic properties, such as tumor progression, and the emergence of more malignant phenotypes. Indeed, DeBaetselier *et al.* (1981) used hybridization of nonmetastatic plasmacytoma cells with normal B cells to generate hybrids that were metastatic. Increases in cell ploidy occur often during tumor progression, and this could be the result of normal cell fusion with neoplastic cells *in vivo*. Lagarde *et al.* (1983) have proposed that the emergence of highly metastatic cells from a low metastatic tumor line during growth *in vivo* is at least consistent with cell fusion of tumor cells with some unknown normal host cells, resulting in the generation of cell hybrids with altered phenotypes. These authors found that cells obtained from metastases were hyperdiploid, and thus they may have been generated by hybridization followed by extensive chromosome segregation. Cell fusion with normal host cells could be an important mechanism for causing increased ploidy and phenotypic instability.

5. THE PHENOTYPIC DIVERSIFICATION OF MALIGNANT NEOPLASMS

The most important implication of tumor phenotypic diversification is that as malignant tumors diversify, the chance that any antitumor therapy

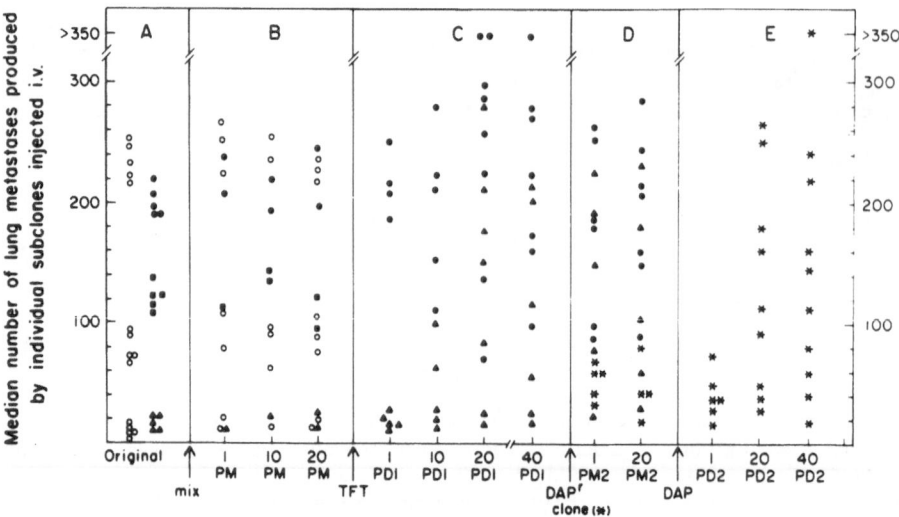

Number of subcultivations in vitro after mixing (PM) of clones and after first (PDI) and second (PD2) drug treatments

FIGURE 4. The influence of clonal diversity on the stability of the metastatic phenotype in B16-F10 melanoma clones. Three wild-type clones (O) and clones resistant to trifluorothymidine (TFT) (▲), ouabain (■), or trifluorothymidine and ouabain (●) with defined metastatic abilities were mixed and co-cultivated *in vitro* (panel A). Subclones were isolated after a further 10 or 20 subcultivations (panel B) and assayed for their metastatic properties and drug sensitivities. After 20 subcultivations the cultures were treated with TFT. The surviving cells were then passaged (panel C), and subclones were isolated and tested for metastatic properties and for resistance to TFT (▲) or TFT and ouabain (●). After 40 subcultivations a new clone of dia-minopurine-resistant (DAP^r) cells (*) was added. Subclones were isolated from this mixed cell population after 20 subcultivations (panel D) and their metastatic properties and susceptibility to TFT, ouabain, and DAP evaluated. The surviving cells were passaged (panel E), and subclones were isolated at the indicated intervals and tested for their metastatic properties and their ability to grow [DAP^r variants (*) grow; TFT^r variants fail to grow] in HAT medium (from Poste, 1982).

will succeed is diminished accordingly. This is because antitumor therapies must eliminate the highly metastatic cell subpopulations in a tumor or its metastatic lesions. Thus, the ability of malignant cells to undergo rapid phenotypic changes could account for the large number of therapeutic fail-ures in highly malignant diseases (Nicolson and Poste, 1982; Poste, 1982; Nicolson, 1984c). In addition, malignant tumors are known to possess het-erogeneous sensitivities to antitumor therapies, and this could result in the emergence of resistant subpopulations after treatment (Goldin and Johnson, 1977). Similarly, heterogeneous sensitivities to cytolysis or cytostasis by natural killer cells (Gorelik *et al.*, 1979, 1982; Hanna and Fidler, 1981), T cells (Gorelik *et al.*, 1979; F. R. Miller and Heppner, 1979; Schirrmacher and Bosslet, 1982), or macrophages (Miner *et al.*, 1983; Miner and Nicolson, 1983) may also result in the evolution of tumor cells that are more refractory to host responses.

As described in Section 4, tumor cell subpopulation interactions may modulate phenotypic diversification and the emergence of variant cells (Poste, 1982; Poste et al., 1982; Miner et al., 1982). In addition to modulating metastatic phenotypic diversification, certain mammary tumor cell subpopulations can modulate cell growth interactions, as well as drug sensitivities (B. E. Miller et al., 1981; F. R. Miller, 1983), suggesting that after antitumor treatment surviving cell subpopulations may display different types of cellular interactions, resulting in phenotypic stabilization or diversification during the regrowth of the surviving tumor cells. In addition to eliminating the rare, highly metastatic cells in a tumor, the success of antitumor therapy could also depend upon the ability of such therapy to control the highly unstable cell subpopulations that have the potential to diversify phenotypically to eventually yield some highly metastatic cells (Nicolson and Poste, 1982, 1983a,b; Poste, 1982).

The rapid rates of phenotypic diversification seen in malignant tumors cannot be explained solely by genetic mutation and host selection. Additional proposals include modifications in regulatory genes, alterations in tumor chromosomal arrangements (recombination), or integration of oncogenes or protooncogenes, among others (Nicolson, 1984b,c). Individually or collectively these changes could modulate phenotypic stability.

Epigenetic mechanisms resulting in nonmutational DNA modifications can alter gene expression, and these modifications can persist for a few generations before reversion back to the unmodified phenotype (Frost and Kerbel, 1983). Alterations in DNA methylation, such as hypomethylation, can result in epigenetic modulation of phenotypic diversity (Frost and Kerbel, 1983). For example, Kerbel et al. (1984) found that the nucleotide analogue 5-aza-cytidine (5-aza-C) could produce relatively stable, short-term modifications in mammalian cells. In these studies 5-aza-C modulated the tumorigenicity and metastatic properties of several murine tumor cell lines. In every case the modified cells reverted back to their original phenotypes a few generations after removal of 5-aza-C, concomitant with a return to the normal levels of DNA methylation. A variety of other mechanisms may also be involved in regulating gene expression and gene product activities that do not lead to permanent DNA modification (Nicolson, 1984b,c); however, the role of these epigenetic processes in modulating phenotypic diversification is not known.

The microenvironment of a tumor can have a profound influence on phenotypic stability and the resulting cellular diversity (Heppner et al., 1984). Since individual cells within a tumor are exposed to variable concentrations of nutrients, oxygen, enzymes, growth factors, ions, inducers, and other regulatory molecules, phenotypic diversification may be determined, in part, by microenvironmental heterogeneity (Figure 5). Once extracellular signals are transferred into cells, they may modify genetic programs or cause epigenetic modifications. Microenvironmental signals could cause differential activation of specific genes, as is apparent when cells interact with stromal components (Bissell et al., 1983). Stromal components, such as extracellular matrix, include basal lamina or basement membranes,

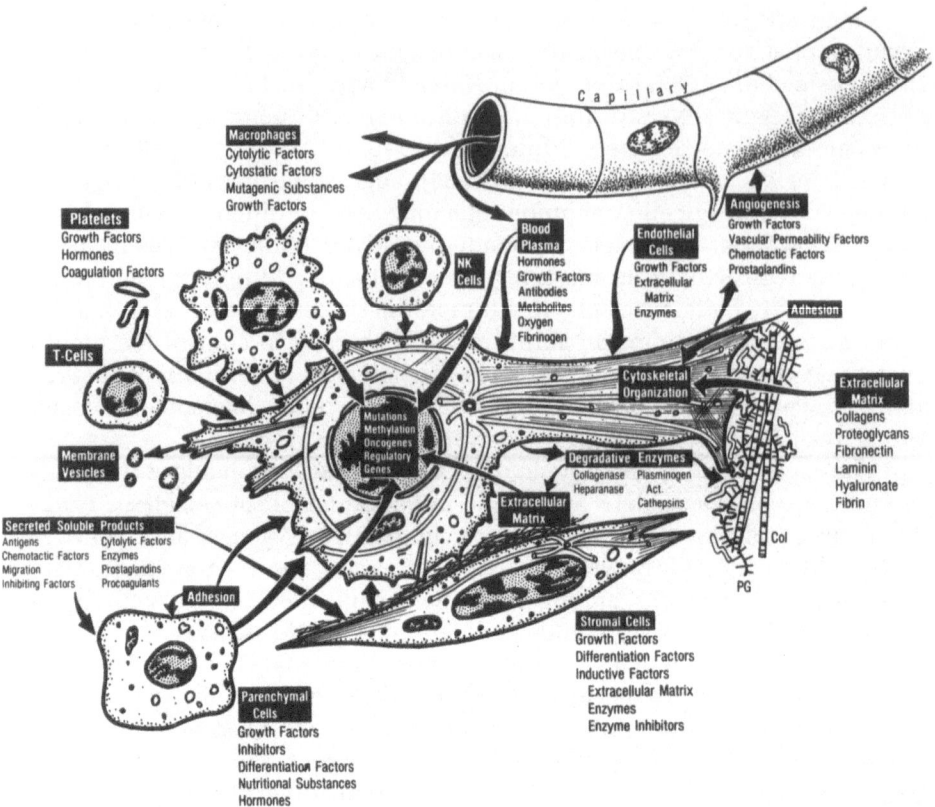

FIGURE 5. Microenvironmental influences on malignant tumor cells. Soluble components, cells, extracellular matrix, and other factors affect individual tumor cells differentially (from Nicolson, 1984b).

tissue matrix and stroma synthesized by fibroblasts, mesothelial cells, and other cells capable of nonimmune "host reactions" against tumors. Cell–extracellular matrix interactions are known to be important in maintaining states of gene activation and differentiation of normal cells and tissues (Bissell et al., 1983). Although tumor cells are not normal, they may be capable of responding to their stromal microenvironments to various degrees, and their responses may mimic certain events that occur during differentiation or development.

Cellular differentiation is controlled, in part, by microenvironmental signals that act differentially in tissues. Under certain conditions the malignant phenotype could be modulated by such signals, resulting in reversion or partial reversion of the malignant phenotype to a more "normal" or more "benign" cellular phenotype (Sachs, 1980). For example, certain myeloid leukemia cells can be modulated to more "normal" phenotypes using macrophage/granulocyte inducer or colony-stimulating factors (Metcalf, 1969;

Landau and Sachs, 1971). In an extreme case of such modulation by microenvironment, certain malignant teratocarcinoma cells can be inserted into normal blastocysts, which, after implantation, will develop into phenotypically normal progeny (Pierce et al., 1979; Mintz and Illmensee, 1975). The normal blastocyst microenvironment is thought to modulate the malignant teratocarcinoma cells, and the result is a normal developing embryo. However, not all malignant teratocarcinomas develop normally when implanted into normal blastocysts (Pierce et al., 1979). Thus, microenvironment can modulate tumor cell phenotype, but there is tremendous heterogeneity in the ability of malignant cells to revert to a normal phenotype through microenvironmental signaling.

Extensive infiltration of tumors by normal host cells, such as lymphocytes, granulocytes, and macrophages, can be seen in some neoplasms in vivo. Presumably this occurs when chemotactic factors are released by tumor cells that can stimulate normal cell infiltration. When such normal cells infiltrate into tumors, they can have profound effects on tumor growth and other properties (Heppner et al., 1984). Factors can be released by infiltrating cells that cause tumor cell cytolysis or cytostasis, and some host cells, such as macrophages, can release mutagenic substances that could change DNA programs by spontaneous mutation events (Heppner et al., 1984). However, not all phenotypic changes occurring at tumor primary or secondary sites are necessarily related to tumor progression.

Recently a model was proposed to explain the diversification of malignant neoplasms (Nicolson, 1984b,c). The basic rationale utilized in the model is that the phenotypic diversification of a malignant neoplasm shows a striking similarity to the somatic generation of antibody diversity in normal lymphocytes. In the somatic diversification of lymphocyte stem cells, plasma cells are generated until that process produces 10^7–10^8 different cells, each synthesizing unique immunoglobulin molecules (Hood et al., 1977a,b).

Plasma-cell-secreted immunoglobulin molecules are composed of two identical light and two identical heavy polypeptide chains with variable (V) regions of extensive amino acid sequence diversity and constant (C) regions of limited sequence diversity. Immunoglobulin V and C regions can be further divided into homology units based on similarities in sequence. For example, heavy chains can be divided into four homology units (V_H, C_H1, C_H2, and C_H3), and light chains can be divided into two such units (V_L and C_L). The actual domains of globular units in immunoglobulin molecules arise from pairs of homology units, such as V_H-V_L, C_H1-C_L, and others, that fold into the correct globular units of the immunoglobulin molecule (Hood et al., 1977a).

Another important consideration in the synthesis of immunoglobulins is that these molecules are encoded by multigene families. V and C immunoglobulin regions are encoded by separate germlike genes that are present in multiple gene segments scattered along a specific chromosome (Tonegawa et al., 1977). These gene families are separated and must undergo rearrangement to form a single, continuous V-C gene before translation. In the mature plasma cell there is a DNA-joining mechanism that results in recombination of the V and C gene families and the synthesis of a complete gene segment (Tonegawa, 1983).

Molecular diversification of immunoglobulin molecules occurs at different levels. At the genetic level there are specific V-gene regions that have very high mutation rates and yield diversification via DNA sequence. At another level the V and C genes can be joined in various combinations to produce the immunoglobulin homology units. For example, each gene may be joined with the same C gene or with different C genes, allowing genetic diversification to be amplified through combinational diversification. The amalgamation of these two diversification mechanisms can allow for the rapid generation of immunoglobulin molecular diversity (Tonegawa, 1983).

Experimental work on the diversification mechanisms for immunoglobulin molecules has resulted in hypotheses on the generation of diversity (GoD) of other recognition and signaling molecules important in differentiation, development, and other cellular interactions. Such recognition and signaling molecules have been called "area code" molecules by Hood et al. (1977a), and they have speculated that the GoD of structure, function, and regulation of cell surface developmental and recognition units is controlled by area code molecules. Area code molecules are probably also important in determining many of the properties of malignant cells (Nicolson, 1982, 1984a; Nicolson and Poste, 1982, 1983a,b). Thus, the diversification of tumor cell neoplasms could be mediated by GoD mechanisms similar to those that control the GoD of immunoglobulin and other area code molecules.

The generation of diversified sets of complete genes from a limited number of inherited gene segments through the use of developmentally regulated gene rearrangements is an attractive model to explain the GoD of tumor phenotype diversification and modifications in area code molecules. During plasma cell diversification the activation of specific V-gene segments occurs when they are rearranged near a transcriptional enhancer element that is located upstream from the C-region gene segments. The V-gene segments are inserted between the joining segments in the switch region in the immunoglobulin gene family (Tonegawa, 1983; Gillies et al., 1983). Therefore, immunoglobulin gene rearrangements may be linked to enhancer elements in phenotypic diversification.

The relationship of enhancer elements to neoplastic transformation has been confirmed in avian-leukosis-virus-transformed cell lines. In these cells the integration of a transcriptional promoter or enhancer element adjacent to the cellular oncogene is thought to be involved in maintenance of the transformed phenotype (Hayward et al., 1981). The importance of cellular oncogenes in the induction and/or maintenance of the transformed phenotype has been confirmed in a number of neoplastic systems (Nicolson, 1984c), and the activation of cellular oncogenes or their viral analogues may occur when these genes are translocated into a locus of area code genes. For example, characteristic translocations exist in human non-Hodgkin's lymphomas, where the c-myc gene has been recombined into the immunoglobulin gene locus (Adams *et al.*, 1983). This can result in activation of the cellular or viral oncogenes. In other neoplastic systems, "silent" cellular oncogenes can be translocated next to enhancer elements, resulting in their activation. Alternatively, activation of cellular oncogenes could occur by accumulation of mutations in regulatory regions not associated with immunoglobulin genes (Pincus *et al.*, 1983), and, finally, cellular oncogenes may regulate their own transcription after translocation by escaping gene repression mechanisms (Nishikura *et al.*, 1983).

The activation of cellular oncogenes within other multigene families could possibly occur with or without diversification mechanisms, in contrast to the immunoglobulin gene family. The misuse of developmentally regulated enhancer elements resulting in the activation of cellular oncogenes is an intriguing mechanism for maintenance of neoplastic transformation, but this alone probably does not explain the GoD seen in malignant neoplasms. The use of normal hypermutable genes and gene combinational GoD systems could, however, initiate the sequence of events resulting in quantitative and qualitative alterations in gene expression through either regulatory genes or their promoters/enhancers. The insertion of cellular oncogenes or protooncogenes at specific sites in such regions of the host DNA could turn on GoD mechanisms that ultimately result in phenotypic heterogeneity (Nicolson, 1984b,c).

One might expect that increases in cellular oncogene transcription and in their gene products might correlate with phenotypic diversification and ultimately tumor progression. Although this could be important in certain tumors, it is certainly not universal. Recent evidence indicates that metastatic lymphoma variants transformed by Abelson murine leukemia virus possess the *abl* oncogene and express this gene and its gene products similarly in cells of low or high metastatic potential (Rotter *et al.*, 1985). Although the expression of oncogenes at higher levels may not be essential in determining degrees of malignancy or metastatic potential, they may be critical in initiating and maintaining states of neoplastic transformation (Nicolson, 1984b,c). Other possibilities include the insertion or activation of promoters at certain sites of the genome near regulatory genes that could initiate GoD through processes of hypermutation and recombination. Once this mechanism has been initiated after transformation, additional changes in the genome might be unnecessary to generate phenotypic variants within the cell population. Of course, the differential control of multigene families in individual cells may be modulated by microenvironmental signals. Since each cell within a tumor is in a slightly different microenvironment and receives a unique array of extracellular signals, this could result in differential expression of certain genes and diversification of others. As cells divide, grow, and invade, they would be exposed to new microenvironments, and they would also be continually exposed to host selection pressures, resulting in the evolution of phenotypic variants in the tumor cell population. Eventually some of these variants would be expected to possess the characteristics essential to complete the metastatic process.

The striking similarity of phenotypic diversification of tumor cells and normal differentiation and development has been demonstrated in certain neoplasms, such as teratocarcinomas. It is probably not an accident that the genes that program a variety of normal cell processes could be activated, amplified, or modified, resulting in the properties necessary for malignant cell behavior. Since many, if not all, of the malignancy-associated properties are probably also important during certain stages of normal development, virtually all of the molecules produced after neoplastic transformation may be normal, albeit inappropriately expressed, gene products.

ACKNOWLEDGMENTS. I thank A. Brodginski and E. Felonia for assistance in preparing this manuscript. The author's studies are supported by USPHS grants RO1 CA28844, CA28867, and CA29571 from the U.S. National Cancer Institute.

REFERENCES

Adams, J. M., Gerondakis, S., Webb, D., Corcoran, L. M., and Corry, S., 1983, Cellular myc oncogene is altered by chromosome translocation to an immunoglobulin in locus in murine plasmacytomas and is rearranged similarly in human Burkitt lymphomas, Proc. Natl. Acad. Sci. USA 80:1982–1986.

Bissell, M. J., Hall, H. G., and Parry, G., 1983, How does the extracellular matrix direct gene expression, J. Theor. Biol. 99:31–68.

Blair, D. G., Oskarsson, M., Wood, T. G., McClements, W. L., Fischinger, P. J., and van De Woude, G., 1981, Activation of the transforming potential of a normal cell sequence: A molecular model for oncogenesis, Science 212:941–943.

Bosslet, K., and Schirrmacher, V., 1982, High-frequency generation of new immunoresistant tumor variants during metastasis of a clone murine tumor line (ESb), Int. J. Cancer 29:195–202.

Chow, D. A., and Greenberg, A. H., 1980, The generation of tumor heterogeneity in vivo, Int. J. Cancer 25:261–265.

Cifone, M. A., and Fidler, I. J., 1981, Increasing metastatic potential is associated with increasing genetic instability of clones isolated from murine neoplasms, Proc. Natl. Acad. Sci. USA 78:6949–6952.

Cooper, G. M., 1982, Cellular transforming genes, Science 218:801–806.

DeBaetselier, P., Gorelik, E., Eshhar, Z., Ron, Y., Katzav, S., Feldman, M., and Segal, S., 1981, Metastatic properties conferred on nonmetastatic tumors by hybridization of spleen β-lymphocytes with plasmacytoma cells, J. Natl. Cancer Inst. 67:1079–1087.

DeFeo, D., Gonda, M. A., Young, H. A., Chang, E. H., Lowy, D. R., Scolnick, E., and Ellis, R. W., 1981, Analysis of divergent rat genomic clones homologous to the transforming gene of Harvey murine sarcoma virus, Proc. Natl. Acad. Sci. USA 78:3328–3332.

Dennis, J., Donaghue, T., Florian, M., and Kerbel, R. S., 1981, Apparent reversion of stable in vitro genetic markers detected in tumour cells from spontaneous metastases, Nature 292:242–245.

Fialkow, P. J., 1979, Clonal origin of human tumors, Annu. Rev. Med. 30:135–176.

Fidler, I. J., and Hart, I. R., 1982, Biological diversity in metastatic neoplasms: Origins and implications, Science 217:998–1003.

Fidler, I. J., and Nicolson, G. L., 1981, Immunobiology of experimental metastatic melanoma, Cancer Biol. Rev. 2:171–234.

Foulds, L. (ed.), 1975, Neoplastic Development, Academic Press, New York.

Frost, P., and Kerbel, R. S., 1983, On the possible epigenetic mechanism(s) of tumor cell heterogeneity, Cancer Metastasis Rev. 2:375–378.

Gillies, S. D., Morrison, S. L., Oi, V. T., and Tonegawa, S., 1983, A tissue-specific transcription enhancer element is located in the major intron of a rearranged immunoglobulin heavy chain gene, Cell 33:717–728.

Goldenberg, D. M., Pavia, R. A., and Tsao, M. C., 1974, In vivo hybridization of human tumor and normal hamster cells, Nature 250:649–651.

Goldin, A., and Johnson, R. K., 1977, Resistance to antitumor agents, in: Recent Advances in Cancer Treatment (H. J. Tagnon and M. J. Staquet, eds.), Raven Press, New York, pp. 155–169.

Gorelik, E., Fogel, M., Feldman, M., and Segal, S., 1979, Differences in resistance of metastatic tumor cells and cells from local tumor growth to cytotoxicity of natural killer cells, J. Natl. Cancer Inst. 63:1397–1404.

Gorelik, E., Feldman, M., and Segal, S., 1982, Selection of a 3LL tumor subline resistant to natural effector cells concomitantly selected for increased metastatic potency, Cancer Immunol. Immunother. 12:105–109.

Hamburger, A. W., and Salmon, S. E., 1977, Primary bioassay of human tumor stem cells, Science 197:461–463.

Hanna, N., and Fidler, I. J., 1981, Relationship between metastatic potential and resistance to natural killer cell-mediated cytotoxicity in three murine tumor systems, J. Natl. Cancer Inst. 66:1183–1190.

Harris, J. F., Chamber, A. F., Hill, R. P., and Ling, V., 1982, Metastatic variants are generated spontaneously at a high rate in mouse KHT tumor, Proc. Natl. Acad. Sci. USA 79:5547–5551.

Hart, I. R., and Fidler, I. J., 1981, The implications of tumor heterogeneity for studies on the biology and therapy of cancer metastasis, Biochim. Biophys. Acta 651:37–50.

Hayward, W. S., Neel, B. G., and Astrin, S. M., 1981, Activation of a cellular onc gene by promoter insertion in ALV-induced lymphoid leukosis, Nature 290:475–480.

Heppner, G. H., 1984, Tumor heterogeneity, Cancer Res. 44:2259–2265.

Heppner, G. H., Loveless, S. E., Miller, M. F. R., Mahoney, K. H., and Fulton, A. M., 1984, Mammary tumor heterogeneity, in: Cancer Invasion and Metastasis: Biologic and Therapeutic Aspects (G. L. Nicolson and L. Milas, eds.), Raven Press, New York, pp. 209–221.

Hood, L., Loh, E., Hubert, J., Barstad, P., Eaton, B., Early, P., Fuhrman, J., Johnson, N., Kronenberg, M., and Schilling, J., 1977a, The structure and genetics of mouse immunoglobulins: An analysis of NZB myeloma proteins and sets of BALB/c myeloma proteins binding particular haptens, Cold Spring Harbor Symp. Quant. Biol. 41:817–836.

Hood, L., Huang, H. V., Dreyer, W. J., 1977b, The area-code hypothesis: The immune system provides clues to understanding the genetic and molecular basis of cell recognition during development, J. Supramol. Struct. 7:531–559.

Kerbel, R. S., Frost, P., Liteplo, R., Carlow, D., and Elliott, B. E., 1984, Possible epigenetic mechanisms of tumor progression: Induction of high frequency heritable but phenotypically unstable changes in the tumorigenic and metastatic properties of tumor cell populations by 5-azacytidine treatment, J. Cell. Physiol. Suppl. 3:87–97.

Lagarde, A. E., Donaghue, T. P., Dennis, J. W., and Kerbel, R. S., 1983, Genotypic and phenotypic evolution of a murine tumor during its progression in vivo toward metastasis, J. Natl. Cancer Inst. 71:183–191.

Landau, T., and Sachs, L., 1971, Characterization of the inducer required for the development of macrophage and granulocyte colonies, Proc. Natl. Acad. Sci. USA 68:2540–2544.

Metcalf, D., 1969, Studies on colony formation in vitro by mouse bone marrow cells. I. Continuous cluster formation and relation of clusters to colonies, J. Cell. Physiol. 74:323–332.

Miller, B. E., Miller, F. R., and Heppner, G. H., 1981, Interactions between tumor subpopulations affecting their sensitivity of the antineoplastic agents cyclophosphamide and methotrexate, Cancer Res. 41:4378–4381.

Miller, F. R., 1983, Tumor subpopulation interactions in metastasis, Invasion Metastasis 3:234–242.

Miller, F. R., and Heppner, G. H., 1979, Immunologic heterogeneity of tumor cell subpopulations from a single mouse mammary tumor, J. Natl. Cancer Inst. 63:1457–1463.

Miner, K. M., and Nicolson, G. L., 1983, Differences in the sensitivities of murine metastatic lymphoma/lymphosarcoma cells to macrophage-mediated cytolysis and/or cytostasis, *Cancer Res.* **43**:2063–2071.

Miner, K. M., Kawaguchi, T., Uba, G. W., and Nicolson, G. L., 1982, Clonal drift of cell surface, melanogenic and experimental metastatic properties of *in vivo*-selected, brain meninges-colonizing murine B16 melanoma, *Cancer Res.* **42**:4631–4638.

Miner, K. M., Klostergaard, J., Granger, G. A., and Nicolson, G. L., 1983, Differences in the cytotoxic effects of activated peritoneal macrophages and J774 monocytic cells on metastatic variants of B16 melanoma, *J. Natl. Cancer Inst.* **70**:717–724.

Mintz, B., and Illmensee, K., 1975, Normal genetically mosaic mice produced from malignant teratocarcinoma cells, *Proc. Natl. Acad. Sci. USA* **72**:3585–3589.

Mitelman, F., 1974, The Rouse sarcoma virus story: Cytogenetics of tumor induced by RSV, in: *Chromosomes and Cancer* (J. German, ed.), Wiley, New York, pp. 675–693.

Neri, A., and Nicolson, G. L., 1981, Phenotypic drift of metastatic and cell surface properties of mammary adenocarcinoma cell clones during growth *in vitro*, *Int. J. Cancer* **28**:731–738.

Neri, A., Welch, D., Kawaguchi, T., and Nicolson, G. L., 1982, The development and biologic properties of malignant cell sublines and clones of a spontaneously metastasizing rat mammary adenocarcinoma, *J. Natl. Cancer Inst.* **68**:507–517.

Nicolson, G. L., 1982, Cancer metastasis: Organ colonization and the cell surface properties of malignant cells, *Biochim. Biophys. Acta* **695**:113–176.

Nicolson, G. L., 1984a, Cell surface molecules and tumor metastasis: Regulation of metastatic diversity, *Exp. Cell Res.* **150**:3–22.

Nicolson, G. L., 1984b, Generation of phenotypic diversity and progression in metastatic tumors, *Cancer Metastasis Rev.* **3**:25–42.

Nicolson, G. L., 1984c, Tumor progress, oncogenes and the evolution of metastatic phenotypic diversity, *Clin. Exp. Metastasis* **2**:85–106.

Nicolson, G. L., and Poste, G., 1982, Tumor cell diversity and host responses in cancer metastasis. I. Properties of metastatic cells, *Curr. Probl. Cancer* **7**(6):1–83.

Nicolson, G. L., and Poste, G., 1983a, Tumor cell diversity and host responses in cancer metastasis. II. Host immune responses and therapy of metastases, *Curr. Probl. Cancer* **7**(7):1–43.

Nicolson, G. L., and Poste, G., 1983b, Tumor implantation and invasion at metastatic sites, *Int. Rev. Exp. Pathol.* **25**:77–181.

Nicolson, G. L., Mascali, J. J., and McGuire, E. J., 1982, Metastatic RAW117 lymphosarcoma as a model for malignant–normal cell interactions: Possible roles for cell surface antigens in determining the quantity and location of secondary tumors, *Oncodev. Biol. Med.* **4**:149–159.

Nicolson, G. L., Steck, P. A., Welch, D. R., and Lembo, T., 1983, Heterogeneity and instability of phenotypic and metastatic properties of local tumor- and metastasis-derived clones of a mammary adenocarcinoma, in: *Understanding Breast Cancer: Clinical and Laboratory Concepts* (M. Rich, J. Hager, and P. Furmanski, eds.), Marcel Dekker, New York, pp. 145–166.

Nishikura, K., Ar-Rushdi, A., Erikson, J., Watt, R., Rovera, G., and Croce, C. M., 1983, Differential expression of the normal and of the translocated human *c-myc* oncogenes in B-cells, *Proc. Natl. Acad. Sci. USA* **80**:4822–4826.

Nowell, P. C., 1976, The clonal evolution of tumor cell populations, *Science* **194**:23–28.

Nowell, P. C., 1983, Tumor progression and clonal evolution: The role of genetic instability, in: *Chromosome Mutation and Neoplasia* (J. German, ed.), Alan R. Liss, New York, pp. 413–432.

Paget, S., 1889, The distribution of secondary growth in cancer of the breast, *Lancet* **1**:571–573.

Pearce, V., Pathak, S., Mellard, D., Welch, D. R., and Nicolson, G. L., 1984, Chromosome and DNA analysis of rat 13762NF mammary adenocarcinoma cell lines and clones of different metatatic potentials, *Clin. Exp. Metastasis* **2**:271–286.

Peterson, J. A., Bartholomew, J. C., Stamper, M., and Ceriani, R. L., 1981, Analysis of expression of human mammary epithelial antigens in normal and malignant breast cells at the single level by flow cytofluorimetry, *Exp. Cell Biol.* **49**:1–14.

Peterson, J. A., Ceriani, R. L., Blank, E. W., and Osvaldo, L., 1983, Comparison of rates of phenotypic variability in surface antigen expression in normal and cancerous breast epithelial cells, *Cancer Res.* **43**:4291–4296.

Pierce, G. B., Lewis, S. H., Miller, G. J., Motitz, E., and Miller, P., 1979, Tumorigenicity of embryonal carcinoma as an assay to study control of malignancy blastocyst, *Proc. Natl. Acad. Sci. USA* **76**:6649–6655.

Pincus, M. R., van Renswoude, J., Harford, J. B., Chang, E. H., Carty, R. P., and Klausner, R. D., 1983, Prediction of the three-dimensional structure of the transforming region of the EJ/T24 human bladder oncogene product and its normal cellular homologue, *Proc. Natl. Acad. Sci. USA* **80**:5253–5257.

Poste, G., 1982, Experimental systems for analysis of the malignant phenotype, *Cancer Metastasis Rev.* **1**:141–199.

Poste, G., Doll, J., and Fidler, I. J., 1981, Interactions among clonal subpopulations affect stability of the metastatic phenotype in polyclonal populations of B16 melanoma cells, *Proc. Natl. Acad. Sci. USA* **78**:6226–6230.

Poste, G., Bucana, C., Raz, A., Bugelski, P., Kirsh, R., and Fidler, I. J., 1982, Analysis of the fate of systemically administered liposomes and implications for their use in drug delivery, *Cancer Res.* **42**:1412–1422.

Raz, A., 1982, Clonal emergence of metastatic heterogeneity in a growing tumor, *Cancer Lett.* **17**:153–160.

Rotter, V., Wolf, D., Blick, M., and Nicolson, G. L., 1985, Expression of the *abl* and other oncogenes is independent of metastatic potential in malignant murine lymphoma cells, *Clin. Exp. Metastasis* (in press).

Sachs, L., 1980, Constitutive uncoupling of pathways of gene expression that control growth and differentiation in myeloid: A model for the origin and progression of malignancy, *Proc. Natl. Acad. Sci. USA* **77**:6152–6156.

Schirrmacher, V., and Bosslet, K., 1982, Clonal analysis of expression of tumor associated transplantation antigens and of metastatic capacity, *Cancer Immunol. Immunother.* **13**:62–68.

Schwab, M., Alitalo, K., Klempnauer, K. H., Varmus, H. E., Bishop, J. M., Gilber, F., Brodeur, G., Goldstein, M., and Trent, J., 1983, Amplified DNA with limited homology to *myc* cellular oncogene is shared by human neuroblastoma cell lines, and a neuroblastoma tumour, *Nature* **305**:245–248.

Stackpole, C. W., 1983, Generation of phenotypic diversity in the B16 mouse melanoma relative to spontaneous metastasis, *Cancer Res.* **43**:3057–3065.

Steck, P. A., and Nicolson, G. L., 1983, Cell surface glycoproteins of 13762NF mammary adenocarcinoma clones of differing metastatic potentials, *Exp. Cell Res.* **147**:255–267.

Talmadge, J. E., Starkey, J. R., Davis, W. C., and Cohen, A. L., 1979, Introduction of metastatic heterogeneity by short-term *in vivo* passage of a cloned transformed cell line, *J. Supramol. Struct.* **12**:227–243.

Tomasovic, S. P., Thames, H. D., Jr., and Nicolson, G. L., 1982, Heterogeneity in hyperthermic sensitivities of rat 13762NF mammary adenocarcinoma cell clones of differing metastatic potentials, *Radiat. Res.* **91**:555–563.

Tonegawa, S., 1983, Somatic generation of antibody diversity, *Nature* **302**:575–581.

Tonegawa, S., Hozumi, N., Matthyssens, G., Schuller, R., 1977, Somatic changes in the content and context of immunoglobulin genes, *Cold Spring Harbor Symp. Quant. Biol.* **41**:877–889.

Welch, D. R., and Nicolson, G. L., 1983, Phenotypic drift and heterogeneity in response of metastatic mammary adenocarcinoma cell clones to adriamycin, 5-fluoro-2'-deoxyuridine and methotrexate treatment *in vitro*, *Clin. Exp. Metastasis* **1**:317–325.

Welch, D. R., Milas, L., Tomasovic, S. P., and Nicolson, G. L., 1983a, Heterogeneous response and clonal drift of sensitivities of metastatic 13762NF mammary adenocarcinoma clones to gamma radiation *in vitro*, *Cancer Res.* **43**:6–10.

Welch, D. R., Neri, A., and Nicolson, G. L., 1983b, Comparison of "spontaneous" and "experimental" metastasis using rat 13762 mammary adenocarcinoma metastatic cell clones, *Invasion Metastasis* **3**:65–80.

Welch, D. R., Evans, D. P., Tomasovic, S. P., Milas, L., and Nicolson, G. L., 1984, Multiple phenotypic divergence of mammary adenocarcinoma cell clones. II. Sensitivity to radiation, hyperthermia and FUdR, *Clin. Exp. Metastasis* **2**:357–371.

Wolman, S. R., 1983, Karyotypic progression in human tumors, *Cancer Metastasis Rev.* **2**:257–293.

CHAPTER 5

FACTORS INFLUENCING THE GENERATION OF PHENOTYPIC HETEROGENEITY IN MAMMARY TUMORS

UNTAE KIM

1. INTRODUCTION

The concept of tumor heterogeneity (tumors composed of genetically poly-morphic subpopulations) has been well recognized by cancer researchers for many years (see Furth, 1959; Kim and Depowski, 1975), and by physicians whose patients have experienced a recurrence of cancers that had initially responded to certain anticancer drugs. Indeed, the recognition of phenotypic heterogeneity of tumors is the rational basis for the development of modern multiple-drug modalities in the treatment of advanced cancer patients (see Skipper, 1983). Lately, interest on this topic seems to have been rekindled by the demonstration of various phenotypic traits in clones of cells isolated *in vivo* or *in vitro* from tumors of diverse origin (Heppner, 1984). In addition to the difference in drug sensitivity, tumor heterogeneity includes variations in cellular structure and functional differentiation, growth pattern, hormone dependence, antigenic expression, metastatic potential, and stem cell kar-yotype. With the availability of more sensitive markers, coupled with the refinement of detection techniques, an even greater genetic diversity of tumor cells is likely to be discovered in the future. However, knowledge as to the mechanism by which neoplastic cells acquire such heritable characteristics during the oncogenic process, as well as to the evolution of each trait in the course of tumor progression, it still quite limited. A critical review of the

UNTAE KIM ● Department of Pathology, Roswell Park Memorial Institute, Buffalo, New York 14263.

natural history of various experimental mammary tumors developed in our laboratory, including a systematic tracing of their acquisition of new characteristics, may shed some light on the subject.

2. PATHOGENESIS OF MAMMARY TUMORS

Of all research on malignant human diseases, that on breast cancer could be considered the most advanced. Our ignorance on its etiology notwithstanding, experimental mammary tumors can be readily induced in laboratory animals with viruses, chemicals, ionizing radiation, or hormones. Nearly 90 years ago, Beatson (1896) was the first to link mammary cancer in women with the ovary and in the decades that followed, virtually all studies on this disease revolved around the ovary and its hormones. The discovery of a mouse mammary tumor virus (MMTV) by Bittner (1940) ushered in the second epoch. Along with his colleagues at the Jackson Laboratories, he recognized the triad of factors essential for the development of mammary tumors in mice: genetics, hormones, and a virus (Bittner, 1942), laying down the foundation for the molecular biology of tumors. Subsequently, all three factors have been demonstrated to hold for most mammals. In man the existence of tumor viruses still rests on indirect evidence, despite the recent findings of protooncogenes or cellular oncogenes in various human tumors (Weinberg, 1981; Cooper, 1982). Huggins et al. (1959, 1961) popularized a method for the rapid induction of mammary carcinomas in rats with polycyclic aromatic hydrocarbons. Radiation mammary tumorigenesis was first discovered by Furth and Furth (1936) in mice, followed by Cronkite et al. (1957) in rats. However, there is no solid evidence as yet that chemicals or radiation play a causal role in human breast cancer. These factors vary greatly in the development of mammary tumors not only among species, but also among their respective strains. It is believed that carcinogenic agents alter the genetic code, while hormones are homeostatic regulators of the target cell, and that a complex interaction of these factors produces tumors with individual mosaics of secondary characteristics.

The factors responsible for or contributing to the development of secondary heritable characteristics that render tumors heterogeneous are now reviewed.

2.1. Oncogenic Agents

There are four agents known to cause mammary carcinomas in laboratory animals: MMTV; polycyclic aromatic hydrocarbons, the most commonly used being 3-methylcholanthrene (MCA), 7,12-dimethylbenz(a)anthracene (DMBA), and N-methylnitrosourea (NMU); total-body X-irradiation; and estrogens.

2.1.1. MMTV

MMTV is the B-type retrovirus that causes mammary adenocarcinomas in certain inbred strains of mice. It is usually transmitted to the newborn through the mother's milk during suckling, with the tumors appearing in most mice at 8–10 months of age. Although it has a unique tropism for the alveolar cells of the mammary gland, it neither contains a viral oncogene equivalent nor transforms the target cell *in vitro*. The development of tumors is a rare event considering the number of putatively infected cells in the host animal. The tumor is probably composed of clonal outgrowths derived from single phenotypically transformed cells that generally contain one or more integrated provirus elements (Cohen *et al.*, 1979; Cardiff and Young, 1980; Nusse and Varmus, 1982; Peters *et al.*, 1983). MMTV-induced mammary tumors are not usually hormone responsive, nor do they require hormonal stimulation for their growth (Bern and Nandi, 1961). Even those induced by a combination of the virus and sustained mammotropic hormonal stimulation are found to be mostly autonomous (Yokoro and Furth, 1962). Whether the insertion of a viral genome into the endocrinologically primitive, rudimentary mammary cells of newborn mice is the reason for their hormone indifference is not known. The strain of mice from which the MMTV is obtained seems to be relevant, for there are significant qualitative as well as quantitative differences in the incidence, latency, and even morphology of tumors in BALB/cf mice infected with MMTV from C3H versus RIII mice (Squartini and Bostocchi, 1977; Bostocchi *et al.*, 1977; Pingitore and Squartini, 1982). As to their metastatic potential, those tumors with extraordinarily long latency periods (496–517 days, as compared to the usual 242–327 days) tend to metastasize to the lung via embolization (Severi *et al.*, 1958; Squartini and Bostocchi, 1977; Bostocchi *et al.*, 1977).

2.1.2. Chemical Carcinogens

Polycyclic aromatic hydrocarbons, e.g., MCA, DMBA (Huggins *et al.*, 1959, 1961), or NMU (Gullino *et al.*, 1975), readily produce mammary adenocarcinomas in young-adult female rats, whether fed or injected i.v. Although the molecular mechanism of chemical carcinogenesis is not fully understood, it is commonly believed that the covalent binding of the initiating carcinogen or its metabolites to target cell DNA causes a simple random point mutation due to errors in DNA replication at the site of carcinogenic damage, followed by a series of selection processes that eventually lead to clonal outgrowth of malignant tumors. However, considering the high efficiency of carcinogen-induced target cell transformation, the lengthy latency period required for the expression of neoplastic state, and the multistage nature of chemical carcinogenesis, the mutation-selection hypothesis would seem too simplistic. An alternative mechanism was proposed by Weinstein (1981; Weinstein *et al.*, 1984) suggesting that the carcinogen-induced DNA

damage may bring about complex genomic changes, such as gene rearrangement or amplification during the normal embryological development of the
target organ in which new stem cell populations emerge and develop into
specialized cells and tissues, and that such a multistep carcinogenesis scheme
may involve qualitatively different events that are enhanced or inhibited by
various environmental and host factors. Indeed, such events may lead to the
generation of tumor cells with diverse phenotypic characteristics. In contrast
to oncogenic viruses, chemical carcinogens and ionizing radiation are thought
to be incapable of introducing new genetic information into target cells and,
therefore, they must call on genes already present in the cell to bring about
and maintain the neoplastic state during the transformation process. The
chemical carcinogens and MMTV have been found to act synergistically by
enhancing mammary tumorigenesis *in vivo* (Faulkin, 1966) as well as *in
vitro* (Howard *et al.*, 1983). It is interesting to note, however, that most
mammary carcinomas induced in rats by chemical carcinogens are hormone
dependent (Kim and Furth, 1960a,b; Gullino *et al.*, 1975; Arafah *et al.*, 1982),
whereas the MMTV-induced mammary adenocarcinomas in mice are hormone independent, despite the fact that both species require at least a physiological hormonal milieu during the carcinogenic period. The mechanism
of such contrasting hormonal characteristics is completely unknown, but
the genetic background of the species may contribute to the phenomenon.
With respect to the carcinogenic hydrocarbons, they have built-in estrogenic
and progestinlike properties (Jull, 1958) by virtue of the similarity in their
molecular configuration with gonadal steroid hormones (Yang *et al.*, 1961).

2.1.3. Ionizing Radiation

Total-body ionizing radiation is also a potent mammary oncogen (Shellabarger *et al.*, 1960; Yokoro *et al.*, 1961). The incidence of mammary tumors
in young-adult female rats induced by a single dose of 400 rads is more than
30% within 3 months, which can be increased to 100% by mammary gland
stimulation with either prolactin or estrogen (Yokoro *et al.*, 1961). However,
unlike chemically induced rat mammary tumors, the radition-induced ones
are autonomous, even when induced in combination with sustained mammotropic stimulation. They are also unresponsive to hormonal treatment
upon transplantation into syngeneic rats.

2.1.4. Estrogen

The basic physiological role of hormones in the mammary gland is to
regulate growth and function. However, estrogen is a unique hormone that
can be carcinogenic in various organs of seemingly "virus-free" rodents
without the aid of any established carcinogen, for it produces tumors in the
anterior pituitary, mammary gland, uterus, cervix, vagina, adrenal, kidney,
and hematopoietic tissue (Burrows and Horning, 1952; Gardner, 1957). The
growth of these tumors in laboratory animals is usually dependent upon a

continuous supply of estrogen (conditioned neoplasms) (Noble and Collip, 1941), at least in the original hosts and during the first few transplantation generations, after which they become independent or autonomous. Cutts and Noble (1964) and Cutts (1969) reported that some of the mammary tumors induced by chronic administration of estrogen were stimulated by androgen and that a few even metastasized. The mechanism of such conversion to metastatic phenotype is not known. On the other hand, excessive and prolonged exposure to estrogen, whether of endogenous or exogenous origin, tends to cause more endometrial than breast cancer in women (Ross et al., 1980; Cowan et al., 1981) and, when taken during pregnancy, a synthetic estrogen (diethylstilbestrol) often causes vaginal cancer in daughters (Bibbo et al., 1978).

Estrogen Receptor. Our current understanding on the mode of action of steroid hormones on target cells is that when they bind to their specific cytosol receptor, the complex is translocated to the nucleus, attaches itself to chromatin, and initiates a series of molecular events leading to the production of mammary-associated proteins (Gorski et al., 1968; Jensen et al., 1968). This receptor appears to be a biological requirement for the initiation of hormonal perturbations in the target cell. Normal human and animal mammary cells contain receptor-specific proteins for estrogen, progesterone, glucocorticoids, and androgens in varying quantities, depending on the stage of mammary gland differentiation, and their levels are used for assessing the hormone sensitivity of tumors (Jensen et al., 1971; Wittliff, 1979). The concentration of estrogen receptors (ER) in human breast cancer differs greatly, ranging from 0 to 6000 fmoles/mg cytosol protein (Wittliff, 1984) with no histological feature found so far to explain such variation, although the endocrine status of the host has been inferred (Kiang and Kennedy, 1977; Bland et al., 1981). About 55% of mostly postmenopausal women with either primary or metastatic ER-positive breast tumors respond to endocrine therapy, with the hormone-insensitivity of the rest probably due to a defect in the intracellular cascade of events that normally control biological responsiveness to a hormonal stimulus. Of the patients with ER-negative tumors, only 3% respond to the therapy. One of the approaches for evaluating the intactness of the estrogen-response mechanism in mammary cancer is the determination of progesterone receptors (PR) (Horwitz and McGuire, 1975). The assumption is that PR formation in mammary tumor cells is regulated by ER, in a manner similar to that in rodent uterine tissue as first described by Rao and Meyer (1977). By simultaneously determining ER and PR, a more accurate selection of hormone-responsive tumors can be made. Indeed, 78% of the patients with tumors containing both receptors have objective response to hormonal treatment. However, the fact that more than 20% of the remaining tumors do not respond indicates that the interrelationship between hormone receptors and hormone sensitivity is extremely complex.

In reviewing the autopsy findings of 25 breast cancer patients, De la Monte et al. (1984) postulated that ER-positive tumors metastasize more frequently to the thyroid and/or parathyroid glands, ER-negative ones to the leptomeninges, and PR-positive ones to the myocardium, suggesting a possible relationship between the steroid receptors and the tumor cells in their affinity for a given tissue or organ. After long-term follow-up of 233 breast cancer patients, Aamdal et al. (1984) concluded that an ER-positive status does influence the disease in those patients with metastases in the auxillary lymph node (Stage II), i.e., postmenopausal women have a longer disease-free and survival rate than ER-negative ones, although only during the first few years. In premenopausal women with Stage II disease, the ER status has no influence on the short-term prognosis and, unexpectedly, seems to affect adversely the long-term prognosis. It appears that the percentage of patients having occult metastases at the time of primary surgery is independent of the ER status, and thus the receptor level is not helpful in long-term prognostication. It has not been determined whether the level of ER is a reflection of a heterogeneous cell population in which the tumor cells exhibit different estrogen sensitivity, or that of a more homogeneous one in which individual cells contain a variable number of ER molecules (Wittliff, 1984).

2.2. Genetic Susceptibility

Recognition of a possible interrelationship between mammary tumor incidence in certain close-bred laboratory animals and their genetic susceptibility to the disease led to the development of a number of genetically homogeneous strains of mice through successive sister–brother matings at the Jackson Laboratories, from which resulted the discovery of the Bittner milk agent or MMTV (Bittner, 1940). Among inbred mice, the strain with the greatest hereditary susceptibility to the development of spontaneous mammary tumors is the C3H of Bittner. Comparative analyses of inbred and hybridized mice indicated that tumor susceptibility and MMTV are interrelated (Bittner, 1962). It seems doubtful, however, that any strain of mice is completely free of the virus, even those that do not develop tumors.

In recent years, molecular biologists have learned that normal cells in inbred strains of mice harbor several MMTV proviruses (Varmus et al., 1972), perhaps representing "endogenous viral genes" transmitted through the germ line as part of the normal gene complement. The expression of these endogenous proviruses is believed to be tightly regulated, since viral RNA production varies widely depending on the tissue, the mouse strain, and the hormonal status of the animal (Bentvelzen and Hilgers, 1980). For example, in some strains the tumor incidence is high in both virgin and breeding females, while in others only in the breeders, requiring hormonal promotion (Medina et al., 1970). The highest MMTV production usually occurs in the lactating mammary gland in which, together with milk protein, MMTV RNA induction is regulated by glucocorticoid hormones (Ringold et al., 1983). This is probably the reason why many investigators had attributed the difference in MMTV susceptibility among strains of inbred mice to the hormonal sensitivity of their mammary gland, e.g., estrogen, progesterone, cortisone, growth hormone (Nandi and Bern, 1960; Rivera, 1966; Medina et al., 1970; Singh et al., 1970), and prolactin (Yanai and Nagasawa, 1970; Sinha et al., 1974). Irrespective of heritable or nonheritable host factors, viruses with low infectivity has also been isolated (Bern and Nandi, 1961). As discussed previously, despite the critical role of hormones in the initiating period of viral mammary tumorigenesis in mice, the tumors lose their hormone responsiveness after they have become established. A similar strain difference in susceptibility to chemical carcinogenesis has been observed in the random-bred Sprague–Dawley and the inbred Wistar/Furth and Fischer rats. The first two strains are highly susceptible, whereas the third is resistant (Huggins et al., 1959; Kim and Furth, 1960a; Gullino et al., 1975).

Epidemiological studies on breast cancer incidence among different races or ethnic groups, although often obscured by demographic factors, also suggest the existence of genetic susceptibility (MacMahon et al., 1973; Henderson et al., 1974; Thomas, 1980). In India, endogamous Parsee women, who are known to have an extremely high incidence of the disease, show elevated levels of the reverse transcriptase and other biochemical markers considered to indicate the presence of retroviruses homologous to MMTV (Spiegelman, 1974; Spiegelman et al., 1980). In Israeli women, in which breast cancer is also the most common neoplasm (Katz et al., 1981), an antigen related to the envelope protein (gp52) of MMTV was detected in 60–78% of the cases tested (Keydar et al., 1982), suggesting a possible viral etiology, hence an unfavorable prognosis. Abnormal patterns of estrogen and androgen metabolism have been reported as "risk factors" in individuals (Bulbrook et al., 1971; Fishman et al., 1979), and elevated serum prolactin levels as "breast cancer prone" in families (Anderson, 1973; Kwa et al., 1974; Henderson et al., 1975). More recently, Lynch et al. (1984) identified a mutant breast cancer-prone genotype in patients with or at risk for hereditary breast cancer, manifested in skin fibroblasts in vitro as hyperdiploidy. Incidence of such cellular abnormality, when observed in consecutive generations, is presumably due to an in vitro expression of germinal mutations, indicating a vertical transmission similar to that of MMTV in mice. Thus, there seems to be a distinct hereditary susceptibility for breast cancer in both laboratory animals and women associated with the quality and quantity of oncogens and the hormonal milieu of the host in rendering the target cells more receptive to oncogenic agents.

2.3. Age

The highest susceptibility of mice to MMTV is at birth (see Bittner, 1947) and during the nursing period (Moore et al., 1970), whereas the mammary tumor incidence in newborn (3 days of age) female rats receiving 400 rads of total-body irradiation is 18%, decreasing slightly at 21 days, and increasing to a peak of 30% at 52 days of age (late puberty) (Huggins and Fukunishi,

1963). MCA fed to 23- and up to 50-day-old rats rapidly produces tumors in all rats (Huggins et al., 1961). In all cases the susceptibility or incidence decreases with age.

The elevated lactogenic hormone levels in newborn rats and mice may be the reason for their high susceptibility to radiation and to MMTV infection, respectively. The serum prolactin levels of human newborns are reported to be nearly 17-fold those of normal adults, or as high as the maternal levels at term (Hwang et al., 1971), but there is no evidence linking breast cancer to such levels. In young-adult female rats (40–65 days old), the peak susceptibility to carcinogenesis by either chemicals or ionizing radiation coincides with the eruptive proliferation and maturation of the rudimentary mammary gland, which contains many mitotic figures (Furth, 1973) and corresponds to the period of biochemical maturation of the human breast (Smithline et al., 1975). The rapid decline in mammary tumor incidence from chemical carcinogens in virgin rats older than 70 days of age is puzzling. These age variations could not be correlated with plasma estrogen or prolactin levels.

In women, a higher incidence of breast cancer exists among those who experienced menarche at a yonger age, gave birth to a first child at an older age, or had delayed menopause (MacMahon et al., 1973; Henderson et al., 1974). Pregnancy (Dao et al., 1960; Shellabarger et al., 1960), graft of a functional pituitary mammotropic tumor (Kim and Furth, 1976), or the combined administration of progesterone and estradiol-17β (Huggins et al., 1962), which brings about the full growth, differentiation, and function of the mammary gland prior to carcinogenic exposure, are known to suppress mammary tumor development. These facts suggest that cells are susceptible to carcinogens only during their growth, becoming resistant when fully mature and functional.

2.4. Nutrition

The role of nutrition and diet in the causation and prevention of human cancer is a subject of great public interest. Among many dietary ingredients that have been found to influence mammary tumor development in man and laboratory animals (Carroll, 1973; Gridley et al., 1983; Cancer Research Supplement, 1983), the following four are evaluated as to their influence in the generation of tumor heterogeneity.

2.4.1. Dietary Fat

Epidemiological surveys on breast cancer patients (Drasar and Irving, 1975; Armstrong and Doll, 1975; Hirayama, 1978; Gray et al., 1979) and mammary tumor induction experiments in rats and mice (Silverstone and Tannenbaum, 1950; Carroll and Khor, 1970; Ip and Sinha, 1981; Gridley et al., 1982) have established a positive correlation between high dietary fat intake and incidence of mammary cancer, independent of genetic factors, obesity, possible chemical contaminants in the diet, or other environmental factors. The promoting effect of this diet, however, may be hormone mediated, since steroid hormones and prostaglandins are derived from essential dietary fatty acid. Indeed, elevated serum prolactin levels (Chan et al., 1975; Ip et al., 1980) and increased prostaglandin synthesis (Kollmorgen et al., 1979; Erickson et al., 1980; Wagner et al., 1982) have been found in mammary tumor-bearing rats. The indirect hormonal influence notwithstanding, tumors are not necessarily more responsive to hormones, for their ER and PR levels are equivalent to those of control tumors in rats fed a conventional diet (Ip and Ip, 1981). Furthermore, the diet has no effect on either the growth or the ER levels of the established, transplantable rat mammary carcinoma MT-W9B (Ip et al., 1978, 1979, 1980; Ip and Ip, 1981).

As to the influence of a prostaglandin-mediated high-fat diet on the cells, Rao and Abraham (1975) showed that the growth rate of transplanted mammary tumors in C3H mice fed a polyunsaturated fat diet was directly correlated with the arachidonic acid level in tumor cells. It is possible, therefore, that a large amount of diet-induced arachidonate made availaable for membrane phospholipid biosynthesis in an appropriate hormonal environment would enhance tumor growth directly, or through interaction with the host immune system indirectly. In addition, Guffy et al. (1982) altered the membrane fatty acid composition of L1210 mouse leukemia cells in vitro by the addition of docosahexaenoic and oleic acid to the medium, rendering the cells more sensitive to heat, as well as to the anticancer drug adriamycin (Guffy et al., 1984). Thus, although a dietary supplement of fat may not modify the hormone sensitivity of the mammary tumor cells, it could make them more vulnerable to heat and drugs.

2.4.2. Vitamin A

A principal function of vitamin A, both in natural and synthetic forms collectively called retinoids, is to regulate the differentiation and maintain the stuctural integrity of several epithelial tissues. The pioneering work of Mori (1922) and Wolbach and Howe (1925) independently demonstrated that a vitamin A-deficient diet causes hyperkeratinization, squamous metaplasia, and even the development of tumors in various organs of laboratory animals. These observations were confirmed by a number of investigators who demonstrated an increased incidence of chemically induced tumors in these animals (Rogers et al., 1973; Cohen et al., 1976). A dietary supplement of retinoids in large doses, on the other hand, prevents or reduces the tumor incidence, or prolongs its latency period in various organs, including the mammary gland in rats and mice, be it during chemical or viral tumorigenesis (Bollag, 1972; Rogers et al., 1973; Cohen et al., 1976; Moon et al., 1976, 1977; Sporn et al., 1977; Thompson et al., 1979; Maiorana and Gullino, 1980), indicating that (1) some animals are more sensitive to the retinoid treatment than others; (2) after the tumor develops, the vitamin has no further effect on its growth; and (3) in order to achieve an antitumor effect, the vitamin supplement has to be continued during the carcinogenic period, for its premature discontinuation will result in the prompt appearance of tumors.

Retrospective analyses of the dietary habits of various cancer patients and those of matching noncancerous individuals have repeatedly established a negative correlation between vitamin A intake and cancer incidence of the skin, larynx, lung, colon, urinary bladder, and breast (Bjelke, 1975; Mettlin et al., 1981).

The mechanism by which retinoids inhibit carcinogenesis is not clear. Nevertheless, Moon et al. (1983) have provided valuable insights into the subject, particularly on their mechanism of action on the mammary gland and mammary tumors. The vitamin exerts an antiproliferative effect by inhibiting ductal branching and end-bud growth via inhibition of DNA synthesis in the cells. It also reduces the number of MMTV-induced hyperplastic alveolar nodules in the mammary gland of C3H mice by as much as 50% Such inhibitory action does not seem to be mediated by either pituitary or ovarian function (Moon et al., 1976; Welsch et al., 1980). However, hormones may regulate the level of cytosolic retinoic acid-binding protein (CRABP) in the mammary gland at various stages of differentiation (Moon and Mehta, 1982). One of the most interesting findings is that the levels of CRABP in mammary tumors and their hormone dependence may be correlated, for the hormone-independent tumors seem to be more sensitive to retinoid inhibition in vivo than the hormone-dependent ones (Mehta et al., 1982). If that were the case, the few slow-growing tumors that survive through the hostile, vitamin A-rich environment would be highly selected clones of well-differentiated adenocarcinoma cells with marked hormone responsiveness. Experimental verification of this supposition is needed.

2.4.3. Selenium

This trace element is essential in all mammalian species. It catalyzes glutathione peroxidase to detoxify lipid and organic peroxidases in the cell, thereby preventing damage to cellular macromolecules (Ganther et al., 1976). At high doses it becomes toxic in animals and suppresses their growth, causes DNA fragmentation, and may increase mitosis (Lo et al., 1978), while at subcellular levels it has been reported to inhibit various enzyme systems, such as mitochondrial succinate dehydrogenase and cytochrome c oxidase activities, as well as protein and DNA synthesis (Klug et al., 1953). At low concentrations, on the other hand, it stimulates protein synthesis and cell growth (McKeehan et al., 1976; Lewko and McConnell, 1982). A dietary supplement of selenium inhibits chemical and viral mammary tumorigenesis in rats and mice (Thompson and Becci, 1980; Medina and Shepherd, 1980, 1981; Ip and Sinha, 1981), as well as chemical carcinogenesis in other organs, including the skin, liver, and colon (Harr et al., 1973; Shamberger et al., 1978; M. M. Jacobs, 1980). Ip and Sinha (1981) reported that during the induction of tumors with DMBA, the incidence was much greater in rats fed a high polyunsaturated fat diet lacking selenium and that the mammary gland of the hosts showed increased lipid peroxidation, which is believed to facilitate the initiation phase of chemical carcinogenesis, and hence the mammary tumor-promoting effect of selenium deficiency (Ip, 1981). This mechanism is not yet well understood, for there is no information on the biological or biochemical characteristics of mammary tumor cells arising in animals whose diets have been deprived of or supplemented with selenium.

2.4.4. Iodine

It has been reported that thyroid hormones are capable of influencing the development of the mammary gland by altering the metabolism of prolactin and growth hormone (Moon, 1962), and that there is a possible relationship between thyroid dysfunction and the development of mammary tumors (Gruenstein et al., 1968; Kellen, 1972; Itoh and Maruchi, 1975; Kapdi and Wolf, 1976; Mittra and Haywood, 1977), with some skepticism (Cave et al., 1979). The discovery of a higher incidence of breast cancer in those regions of endemic goiter (Eskin, 1970) seems to support such a notion. Iodine deficiency, by virtue of a negative homeostatic feedback mechanism, most probably stimulates the hypothalamus to produce increased amounts of thyrotropin-releasing hormone (TRH), which in turn elevates the pituitary thyroid-stimulating hormone (TSH) and raises the level of serum triiodothyronine (Chopra et al., 1976), although such increase is not always detectable in goitrous patients (Vagenakis et al., 1973). Since the brilliant work of Guillemin et al. (1963) and Schally and Bowers (1963), which led to the identification, synthesis, and clinical use of TRH, this hormone has been found to release not only TSH but prolactin as well (Bowers et al., 1971; Tashjian et al., 1971). Therefore, the sequence of chronic iodine deficiency, sustained mammary gland stimulation, and development of breast cancer in women of endemically goitrous areas seems a distinct possibility. Theoretically, a similar reasoning could be applied to the low breast cancer rate in Japan where the dietary intake of iodine is known to be high, although this low incidence is commonly attributed to the low consumption of animal fat (Wynder et al., 1960; Nagataki et al., 1967). Perhaps iodine deficiency and a high dietary fat intake combine to become the critical factors in "endemic" breast cancer.

2.5. Hormonal Factors

There is a great deal of information on the experimental hormonal requirement for the growth and differentiation of the mammary gland in vivo (Lyons et al., 1958; Nandi, 1958; Talwalker and Meites, 1961) and in vitro (Ichinose and Nandi, 1966; Wood et al., 1975; Rudland et al., 1979; Tonelli and Sorof, 1980, 1981), e.g., prolactin, growth hormone, insulin, epidermal growth factor (EGF), estrogen, progesterone, and glucocorticoids. For mammary tumor induction in laboratory animals with carcinogens, the minimum requirement is a functional ovary or pituitary. With the exception of estrogen, hormones always play the role of promoter and carcinogens that of initiator, with the balance between the two determining the secondary characteristics of the transformed cells, e.g., the greater the promoting influence, the stronger their reliance on hormonal stimulation for their growth, and vice versa.

2.5.1. Prolactin

There are a number of procedures to raise the serum prolactin levels (hyperprolactinemia) that may lead to the development of mammary tumors in rats and mice (Welsch and Nagasawa, 1977): (1) repeated injections of homologous or even heterologous prolactin preparations (Boot et al., 1962; Brock and Sutcliffe, 1972; Lorber et al., 1973); (2) ectopic or extra-cellular pituitary grafts (Loeb and Kirtz, 1939; Mühlbock and Boot, 1959; Bruni and Montemurro, 1971); (3) syngeneic mammotropic tumor (MtT) grafts (Kim and Furth, 1961; Yokoro and Furth, 1962); (4) induction of specific hypothalamic lesions (Welsch et al., 1970); and (5) administration of dopamine antagonists, such as reserpine or bromocryptine (Lacassagne and Duplan, 1959; Welsch and Meites, 1969; Armstrong et al., 1974). Prolactin at high doses can overcome a subthreshold dose of chemical carcinogen, radiation, or MMTV by effectively inducing mammary tumors in rats and mice (Kim and Furth, 1960a; Yokoro et al., 1961; Yokoro and Furth, 1962), and even resuscitating dormant ones that have seemingly regressed completely following hypophysectomy or precancerous lesions (Kim and Furth, 1960a). These tumors are prolactin and/or estrogen dependent (Kim and Furth, 1961; Kim et al., 1963; Kim and Depowski, 1975), and in many aspects resemble the pregnancy-dependent mouse mammary tumors of Foulds (1949). With respect to the prolactin receptor, it is generated by the hormone itself, but interferred with by estrogen (Costlow et al., 1975).

2.5.2. Insulin

The role of insulin in the differentiation and function of mammary cells in vivo as well as in vitro seems to be well established (Ichinose and Nandi, 1966; Topper and Oka, 1974). Heuson and colleagues (1970, 1972) demonstrated, and Hilf et al. (1978) confirmed, that alloxan-induced diabetes or insulin deficiency is as effective in inhibiting the growth of hormone-dependent, DMBA-induced mammary tumors as oophorectomy, with the difference that the tumors in diabetic rats contain abundant insulin-binding protein but low ER, while in those from ovariectomized hosts the insulin receptor is decreased. Insulin treatment of diabetic rats usually reactivates the hormone-dependent tumor growth, accompanied by the restoration of ER to its original levels. Hormone-independent tumors, on the other hand, have insulin-binding capacity. Rhomberg (1975) reported an analogous situation in diabetic, advanced breast cancer patients who responded better than nondiabetic ones to endocrine therapy. It seems, therefore, that a hypoglycemic environment promotes the selection of hormone-dependent mammary tumor cell clones.

2.6. Immunological Factors

All carcinogens have an immunosuppressive effect on laboratory animals (Haughton and Whitmore, 1976). Further immunological intervention, such as neonatal thymectomy, enhances tumorigenesis in certain strains of rodents (Miller et al., 1963; Nishizuka et al., 1965; Balner and Dersjant, 1966), or inhibits it in others (Stutman, 1982). The effect of neonatal splenectomy on the development of host immune surveillance mechanism, however, is not clear (Kalpaktsoglou et al., 1967; Kubai and Auerbach, 1968; Moody and Reed, 1968). In adult animals, neither thymectomy nor splenectomy seems to cause any clinically recognizable immunodepression, although the former has been reported to produce diminished in vitro blastogenic response to phytohemagglutinin and concanavalin A by the host spleen cells (D. M. Jacobs and Byrd, 1975). The host antitumor surveillance is now believed to be mediated by the natural killer cell (NK) system, and its activity to be inversely correlated with tumor incidence, particularly in mice (Roder and Haliotis, 1980; Herberman and Ortaldo, 1981; Stutman, 1982).

2.6.1. Pathogenesis of Metastasizing Tumors

Naturally metastasizing solid tumors are rare in laboratory animals and, when occasionally encountered, they tend to grow expansively and metastasize only to the lung in the form of tumor cell emboli via the venous return, as most human sarcomas do. However, using the chemical carcinogens MCA and DMBA, mammary tumors can be induced in W/Fu female rats (Kim, 1970, 1977) (Table I) that metastasize spontaneously by invading the surrounding soft tissue stroma, spreading to the regional lymph node, and disseminating widely to distant organs, including the bone, lung, and liver, mimicking human breast cancer. The behavior of these chemically induced tumors varies according to the type and dosage of the inducing carcinogen, as well as to the immunological and endocrinological state of the host during tumor development and growth.

2.6.1a. Optimum Dosage of MCA in Immune-Deficient Hosts. The standard dose of MCA that produces mammary tumors in 100% of young-adult (50–55 days old) female rats (200 mg divided in ten equal doses over a 5-week period) was fed to rats that had previously been rendered partially "immune deficient" by thymectomy, splenectomy, or a combination of both 1 week prior to the first carcinogen feeding. The surgical immunosuppression caused 20, 31, and 45% increase in the incidence of mammary carcinomas, respectively, over the intact control rats during an 18-month period. When such animals in a paired experiment were immunostimulated with nonspecific immunoadjuvants, e.g., sheep red blood cells, dinitrophenol sulfonate-

TABLE I

Spontaneously Metastasizing Mammary Carcinomas Induced in W/Fu
Rats and Their Characteristics

Tumor strain	Degree of differentiation[a]	Metastasizing capacity[b]	Metastasizing routes and sites
TMT-50	W	0−+	Hematogenous; lung only
STMT-058	P	+−++	Hematogenous and lymphatic; lymph node and lung
MT-449	M	++	Hematogenous and lymphatic; lymph node and lung
SMT-077	M	++−+++	Lymphatic; lymph node, lung, and bone
DMBA-4	M	+++	Lymphatic and hematogenous; lymph node and lung
MT-450	W	+++	Hematogenous and lymphatic; lymph node and lung
SMT-2A[c]	P	++++	Lymphatic; lymph node, lung, and bone
SMT-2B	P	++++	Lymphatic; lymph node, lung, liver, bone, and spleen
TMT-081[c]	P	++++	Hematogenous and lymphatic; lymph node, lung, liver, spleen, and bone

[a]W, well differentiated; M, moderately differentiated; P, poorly differentiated.
[b]+, Slight; ++, moderate; +++, marked; ++++, extensive.
[c]Carried also in ascites form and in tissue culture lines.

conjugated bovine serum albumin, or Freund's complete adjuvant, prior to the development of tumors, the incidence decreased by 30–40% (Kim, 1970, 1977). It is evident, therefore, that surgical "immunomodulation" or suppression enhances the tumor incidence, while nonspecific immunostimulation during carcinogenesis reduces it. The growth characteristics of the developing tumors in the original hosts and those implanted in syngeneic rats were analyzed and five distinct patterns were observed: (1) tumors that regressed spontaneously in their autochthonous hosts before reaching 5 mm in average diameter, due probably to the incompatibility of their antigenic makeup with the host or to their strong immunogenicity; (2) tumors as large as 12 mm that regressed completely after an earlier, putatively more immunogenic tumor in the same host was excised, suggesting that the surgical removal evoked a "specific" antitumor immune response; (3) progressively growing tumors, larger than 15 mm, that were rejected by normal syngeneic rats upon transplantation, indicating that their antigenicity was tolerated by the immunologically attenuated autochthonous hosts, but not by normal rats; (4) tumors that grew progressively and were readily accepted by normal syngeneic hosts (the majority of the induced tumors), most of which had tumor-specific transplantation antigens (TSTA); and (5) nonimmunogenic tumors without TSTA, having the inherent capacity to metastasize to distant sites in normal rats upon transplantation.

2.6.1b. High Dosage of DMBA in Normal Hosts. A single 20-mg dose of DMBA in young-adult female rats usually produces well-differentiated, non-metastasizing mammary adenocarcinomas in 100% of the animals within 60 days, 60–70% of them being hormone dependent. Twice that amount was fed to rats over a 4-week period in doses of 10 mg/week, the intent being to produce rapidly growing, poorly differentiated, hormone-independent tumors with metastasizing potential, under the assumption that the greater the mutagenic force of the carcinogen, the faster the developing tumor cells would depart from the normal physiological control of the host, deviating from the usual evolutionary sequence of tumor progression from hormone dependence to autonomy. The dosage was found to be too toxic and about 65% of the rats died before any tumors developed. Among the surviving ones, however, one gave rise to a metastasizing tumor (DMBA-4), after the excision of another tumor that had appeared earlier, approximately 30 days after the last DMBA feeding. Although there was hardly enough time for the new tumor to go through the usual postmastectomy immunoselection process, it metastasized in normal syngeneic rats upon transplantation. Nevertheless, in its earlier transplant generations it was a fairly well-differentiated adenocarcinoma and seemed to be quite immunogenic, for it often underwent spontaneous necrosis, followed by complete regression. Eventually, however, it became poorly differentiated, grew progressively, and metastasized consistently. Being the only metastasizing tumor induced in this manner, it is surmised that it came about accidentally by an unknown pathogenic pathway, or that the tumor cells possibly went through an abbreviated immunoselection.

2.6.1c. Isolation of Dormant Metastatic Clones from an Estrogen-Dependent Mammary Tumor. In the course of studying the evolutionary pattern of a prolactin-dependent mammary tumor (MT-W9) induced by a subthreshold dose of MCA (10 mg), combined with sustained stimulation of the mammary gland by a prolactin-secreting pituitary tumor, we learned that the progression from hormone dependence to autonomy is achieved over a long period of time by sequential selection of preexisting tumor cell clones (Kim and Depowski, 1975), as will be discussed later. As it progressed, the tumor sublines were found to be less and less differentiated with respect to gland formation and their growth rate became much faster. However, such an increased virulence was not accompanied by the acquisition of metastatic potential. Interestingly enough, two naturally metastasizing tumors (MT-449 and MT-450) emerged from the estrogen-dependent MT-W9A, the first subline of MT-W9, each about 5 years apart, after a long period of consecutive passages. MT-W9A is an extremely slow-growing tumor, taking 2–3 months after transplantation to become palpable. Thus, the emergence of the metastatic clones may have been the result of a prolonged selection process. The study also suggested that the evolutionary pathway of hormone dependence to autonomy is independent of that from nonmetastatic to metastatic property.

2.6.2. Spontaneous Tumors

Some mammary carcinomas that occasionally develop in old, retired breeding female mice and rats metastasize naturally (Hewitt and Blake, 1975; Hewit et al., 1976; Willmott et al., 1979). Although little is known of the etiology and pathogenesis of these tumors, there seem to be some similarities in their host factors with those of chemically induced tumors; e.g., the hormonally stimulated mutliparous mammary gland and the prolonged latency period of the aging animals, which may provide the tumor cells with ample time to undergo immunoselection.

2.6.3. MMTV-Induced Mammary Tumors

Squartini and Bostocchi (1977) and Bostocchi et al. (1977) described mammary tumors induced in BALB/c mice with two different MMTVs, one from C3H and the other from RIII mice, which metastasized to the lung in 63 and 17% of the hosts, respectively. These tumors also had long latency periods, averaging 496 days in the former and 517 in the latter.

Thus, the tumor–host interaction during the development of naturally metastasizing mammary tumors in laboratory animals may be perceived as a continuous selection process applied to the cells by the host immune surveillance mechanism, be it T cell mediated (Thomas, 1959; Burnet, 1970) or NK regulated (Roder and Haliotis, 1980; Herberman and Ortaldo, 1981), in the following sequence: (1) tumor cells with antigen incompatible with the host are rapidly eliminated, while those with less potent antigen may be able to grow until the host immune defense mechanism is stimulated by specific or nonspecific extraneous factors, at which time they are also destroyed; (2) cells with a distinct antigen property (TSTA), which can establish an immunological equilibrium with the host and grow progressively, but are incapable of invading or metastasizing (most chemical- or virus-induced mammary tumors belong to this category); and (3) when the cells are repeatedly subjected to these immunological selective pressures, those surviving will ultimately be non- or weakly immunogenic, emerging as new clones with metastatic potential.

2.6.4. Characteristics of Metastasizing Mammary Tumors

The single most outstanding characteristic of rat mammary carcinomas which metastasize via the lymphatics, beginning with the regional lymph node and then disseminating to distant organs as most human breast cancers do, is the structural instability of their plasma membranes caused by the accelerated shedding of cell surface antigen and their renewal by actively proliferating tumor cells, apart from the exfoliation of dead or living whole cells from the primary tumor mass (Kim et al., 1975; Kim, 1983). This property seems to confer most of the phenotypic characteristics associated with metastasizing tumor cells, probably by initially helping them to detach themselves individually from the cohesive bond of organoid tumors. This loss of adhesiveness is readily observed in two established tumor cell lines in vitro, the metastasizing TMT-081-MS, which tends to grow singly or in small clusters, and the nonmetastasizing MT-100-TC, which forms large, dense cellular aggregates (Ghosh et al., 1983). These in vitro characteristics may be attributed, at least in part, to the difference in the electrostatic charge on their cell surface. The metastasizing cells migrate electrophoretically 40–50% farther than the nonmetastasizing ones in a given time period (Park et al., 1982), due perhaps to the increased net negative charge on the former that may also help to repel, or prevent the dissociated cells from sticking to each other. The elevated negative charge, on the other hand, may propel the tumor cells to the nearest vascular wall, for endothelial cells also have negative surface charge (Fishman, 1982). Needless to say, however, the migration of detached tumor cells in the subepithelial stroma is involved in more complex mechanism than just electrostatic charge-assisted passive locomotion. The possible increase in membrane fluidity, dynamic state of cyttoskeletal contractile proteins, enzymatic breaching of stromal barriers, as well as various chemotactic factors may be associated with it.

The electrostatic charge on the cell surface is considered to be an important property that probably plays a role in cell function, particularly in cell-to-cell interaction. The biochemical rationale for such physical property is based on the fact that sialic acid is one of the major negatively charged membrane-bound molecules and its levels have been found to be elevated in tumor cells (Abercrombie and Ambrose, 1962; Yogeeswaaran and Salk, 1981). Our analysis of the sialic acid content and sialyltransferase activity in metastasizing and nonmetastasizing rat mammary carcinoma cells has indeed confirmed and extended those views by finding their levels to directly correlate with the metastatic capacity (Bernacki and Kim, 1977) as well as with the electrophoretic mobility of the cells. Furthermore, the increased glycosyltransferase activity in the former is reflected in the accelerated turnover and shedding of the cell surface antigen (Bernacki and Kim, 1977; Chatterjee and Kim, 1977, 1978).

The continuous shedding of surface glycoconjugates seems to render the tumor cells non- or weakly immunogenic (Kim, 1970) and the systemic circulation of the hosts becomes progressively burdened with these molecules in the form of tumor-associated antigens (Kim et al., 1975; Ghosh et al., 1979), and perhaps with immune complexes (Yoo et al., 1983). The elevated levels of these enzymes may help to prolong the half-life of glycoprotein and glycolipid antigens by hyperglycosylating them and compounding the state of antigen excess. They may also affect T lymphocytes directly by modifying their major histocompatibility complex (MHC)-restricted recognition mechanism (Parish et al., 1981). Although excess free antigens and immune complexes are believed to stimulate suppressor T-cell activity, direct evidence to support such assumption is still lacking, and the question of immune complexes being associated with human cancer patients, as well as of their possible role in metastasis, is controversial (Yoo et al., 1983).

2.6.5. Tumor-Associated Antigens

The individuality of polymorphic TSTA in the chemically induced tumors (Prehn and Main, 1957) is evident among the MCA-induced, nonmetastasizing rat mammary carcinomas, while in the metastasizing ones it is replaced by a common, mammary gland-specific glycoprotein antigen with a molecular weight of 68,000 daltons in its native form and 28,000 upon papain digestion (Ghosh et al., 1983). This organ-specific antigen is phenotypically stable over many transplant generations and cross-reacts with all lymphogenously metastasizing mammary tumors and, less strongly, with normal rat mammary glands, but only negligibly or not at all with the non-metastasizing tumors. This situation is similar to the current characterization of human tumor-associated antigens, some of which are found at high levels in tumors but also in adjacent normal tissue at lower levels, others are the onco-fetal type, and occasionally an antigen immunologically related to MMTV is identified (see Edgington and Nakamura, 1982). this had led many investigators to doubt the existence of cancer-specific antigens in man. Perhaps the property itself of cross-reactivity with normal organotypic and developmental antigens represents the inherent status of all malignant neoplasms, i.e., invasive and metastasizing capacity, with the qualitative and quantitative difference of that property corresponding to the mode and rate of metastatic potential. Recently, Wang et al. (1982) reported the isolation of three clones of tumor cells from an MCA-induced mouse fibrosarcoma with a common, cross-reacting antigen and the capacity to metastasize to the lung. Such antigenic conversion was attributed to the modulation in the expression of MHC products in tumor cells during the immunoselection process (De Baetselier et al., 1980), associated with NK resisting capacity (Hanna, 1980). It seems as though the acquisition of metastatic potential by tumor cells is preceded by the development of new cross-reacting antigens.

3. EVOLUTION OF NEOPLASTIC STATE

Rous and colleagues (1935, 1941) first introduced the concept of cancer progressing from "bad to worse" through their observations of rabbit skin tumors, and Foulds (1949) and Furth (1953) confirmed it with mouse mammary and pituitary tumors, respectively, by correlating their progression with the gradual loss of functional capacity by neoplastic cells. Subsequently, Furth (1953) and Furth and Clifton (1966) discovered that the loss of secretory activity in the multifunctional pituitary tumors, having a combination of prolactin, growth hormone, and ACTH activities, came about one at a time in an orderly manner, relating for the first time the concept of such progression with that of heterogeneity. Since then, it has been generally accepted that tumor progression is achieved by unfolding genetically altered, preexisting phenotypic variants one by one. It may be timely, however, to reexamine these concepts by analyzing the evolution, both in vivo and in vitro, of the hormone dependence and metastatic potential of the rat mammary tumors developed in our laboratory.

Natural History of Mammary Tumors

The progression of mammary tumors from hormone dependence to autonomy may be short or long, depending upon the balance of forces between the oncogenic (mutagenic) and promoting (hormonal) factors at the time of initiation. When the tumor is induced with an optimal dose of chemical carcinogen in a physiologically prime hormonal environment for mammary gland development, the hormone dependence of the induced tumors begins at the normal ovarian and/or pituitary function, and it progresses rapidly to autonomy. In viral mammary tumorigenesis, the embryologically primitive state of the mammary cells in newborn mice seems to be one of the essential ingredients in the integration of the MMTV genome into the cellular DNA, augmented by transient stimulation of the cell by the maternal prolactin. Due probably to the undifferentiated state of the mammary gland, the tumors are hormone indifferent or autonomous from the beginning. For unknown reasons, the tumors induced by an optimal dose of ionizing radiation, either in newborn or young-adult animals, are usually hormone independent. On the other hand, when they result from a subthreshold dose of chemical carcinogen and are assisted by extraneous prolactin stimulation, their progression spans the entire range of evolution, beginning with prolactin superdependence (MT-W9), to estrogen or ovarian dependence (MT-W9A), to hormone independence (MT-W9B), to androgen or testicular dependence (MT-W9C), and finally to autonomy (MT-W9D) (Figure 1). Karyotypic analysis indicates that the progression is achieved by a sequential selection of preexisting tumor cell clones (Kim and Depowski, 1975). The five clones involved are characterized and maintained vertically in syngeneic W/Fu rats by successive transplantations. The estrogen- and androgen-dependence of MT-W9A and MT-W9C, respectively, are the most unstable characteristics to maintain, for they repeatedly disappear after several passages and the tumors become autonomous. It is not clear whether such loss of hormone sensitivity is simply caused by the shifting of stem cell populations or by other mechanisms. However, that of estrogen senstivity does not seem to affect ER levels, for in the autonomous MT-W9B they remain as high as in the parent tumor. ER is not completely lost until the tumor progresses to MT-W9D (Bronn et al., 1978; Ip et al., 1979). With the progressive loss of hormone dependence, the growth of the tumors becomes increasingly faster and structurally less differentiated, but none acquires metastasizing capacity.

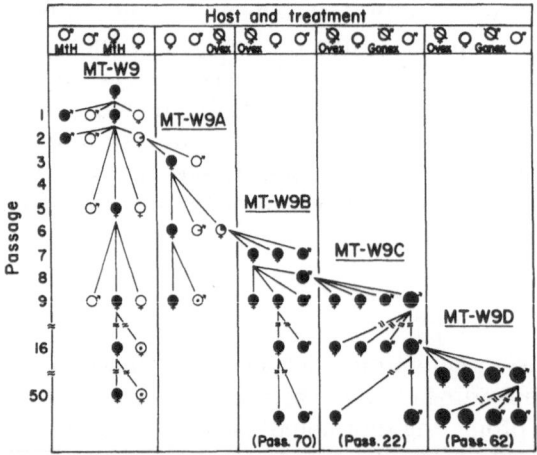

FIGURE 1. Composite pedigree of a rat mammary adenocarcinoma progressing from mammotropin dependence to full autonomy. Shaded areas in the circle indicates percentage of take; size of circle signifies relative tumor size; dot in circle denotes occasional take. MtH, mammotropin (prolactin); Ovex, oophorectomy; Gonex, orchiectomy; Pass., passage (transplant generation).

Morphological Diversity

The basic components of the mammary gland are alveolar and ductal epithelia and myoepithelium, while those of mammary tumors in rodents are roughly alveolar, ductal, epidermoid, and sarcomatoid. MMTV-induced tumors tend to be of alveolar type, chemically induced ones alveolar and ductal, and radiation-induced ones often ductal and/or sarcomatoid. However, a perfect mrophological homogeneitty is seldom seen in animal tumors. Each is more often composed of subunits that evolve independently according to the fluctuating hormonal milieu of the host.

The histological pattern of the five rat mammary tumor clones under discussion generally reflects the degree of their hormone-dependence and gland-forming capacity. The hormone-dependent MT-W9 and MT-W9A are well-differentiated adenocarcinomas, the hormone-independent MT-W9B and the androgen-dependent MT-W9C moderately to poorly differentiated, and the fully autonomous MT-W9D usually undifferentiated. However, it is difficult to distinguish these tumors by their histological pattern alone, without knowing their biological characteristics.

In human breast cancer, the degree of glandular differentiation seems to be directly correlated with ER levels in postmenopausal women (Fisher et al., 1980), and inversely with drug sensitivity (Fisher et al., 1983). Its morphological versatility is much greater than that of animal tumors, being classified into 20–30 morphologically distinct types, depending on the pathologist (World Health Organization, 1981). In addition to the most common invasive ductal carcinomas, there are prognostically more favorable types, e.g., adenocystic, tubular, juvenile secretory, medullary carcinoma with lymphoid stroma, and so on, and more unfavorable ones, e.g., inflammatory carcinomas and those with sarcomatous metaplasia, each having a predictably different biological behavior pattern (Gallager, 1984). However, these special types constitute only a small part of all human breast cancer and, as seen in animal tumors, a combination of a few histologically different ones is often observed in any given tumor, again indicating that complex inter-dependent factors may be responsible for the generation of such morpho-logical diversity.

Acquisition of Metastatic Potential

Unlike human cancers, most solid tumors in animals grow expansively at the site of origin without infiltrating the surrounding stroma or metas-tasizing to distant organs, even when they become very large. This funda-mental difference may lie in their pathogenic pathway. Most investigators tend to favor fast-growing animal tumor models that have been induced with potent oncogenic agents, selecting those with a short latency. Such tumors are usually highly immunogenic, due probably to the lack of time to undergo host immunoselective processes. In contrast, human cancers, except for those that are the sequelae of occupational or industrial hazards, usually occur late in life, with their longer latency due perhaps to a more subtle exposure to oncogens, developing through various routine immunological and en-docrinological selective forces generated by the host and thus becoming less immunogenic. This assumption was verified by the development of the me-tastasizing rat mammary carcinomas discussed previously. Nevertheless, there are still a number of lingering questions about the process by which tumor cells acquire or lose their metastatic phenotype.

Hormonal versus Immunological Selection. In addition to the devel-opment of metastasizing mammary tumors in immunologically compromised rats, the fact that the naturally metastasizing MT-449 and MT-450 tumors could be isolated from a hormone-dependent tumor in its early phase of tumor progression, rather than from its autonomous sublines, is noteworthy. When coupled with the fact that more than half of the metastatic breast cancers in postmenopausal women contain ER-positive cells, the experi-mental evidence suggests that the hormonal environment may not only be an essential factor only in mammary tumor development, but also in main-taining the metastatic potential of the transformed cells during the early stages of carcinogenesis, perhaps with the two traits encoded in gene loci close to each other. An anlogous situation was recently observed in a breast cancer patient at our Institute (RPMI Case No. 157810). After an 18-year disease-free interval following radical mastectomy for a localized breast can-cer (Stage I), the ER-positive tumor recurred in the same chest wall, dissem-inated widely, and the patient succumbed to the disease within a year. A prolonged immunological selection pressure seems to be needed to trigger the latent metastatic trait.

Lung Colonizing versus Lung Metastasizing Capacity. Fidler (1973) popularized and stimulated the research on metastasis by the introduction of a rapid method to isolate highly metastatic tumor cells from the lungs of mice repeatedly injected i.v. with B16 melanoma cells. However, Stackpole

(1981) found that a number of these lines, including the F10 of Fidler, produced numerous lung colonies only when injected i.v., rarely metastasizing from s.c. or i.m. implantation. Conversely, other lines that metastasized to the lung spontaneously produced few lung colonies after i.v. injection. He concluded that organ colonization after the cells are injected directly into the bloodstream is not necessarily predictive of metastatic potential. Indeed, the lung colonizing capacity seems to be more closely related to nonmetastatic phenotype, even in the rat mammary tumor system, for nonmetastasizing cells injected i.v. produce numerous lung nodules in the recipient rats, but the lymphogenously metastasizing ones colonize massively the peribronchial and mediastinal lymph nodes and other organs, before forming lung nodules in the animals (Kim, unpublished data).

Loss of Metastatic Potential

Although more than 30% of the mammary tumors induced with MCA in immuno-compromised rats had the capacity to metastasize in their first transplantation generation, only about a third of them retained this property, while the rest lost it after a few subpasses (Kim, 1977). The tumor strains listed in Table I have been stable for more than 8 years, some of them with occasional fluctuations in their metastasizing capacity from one transplantation generation to the next (Figure 2) (Kim et al., 1975). It was postulated at the time that such instability is probably caused by a varying ratio of metastasizing to nonmetastasizing cells in each passage. However, whether the stability of metastatic phenotype can be explained solely by the popu-

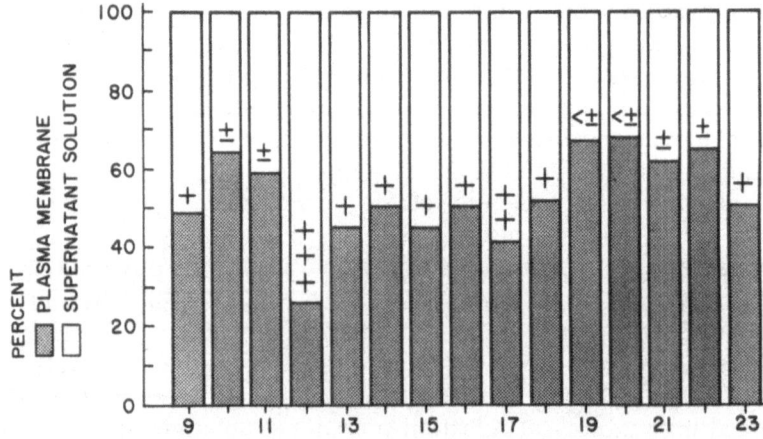

FIGURE 2. Fluctuation of metastasizing capacity in the rat mammary carcinoma TMT-50 from passage to passage, correlated with the level of the plasma membrane-associated marker enzyme 5'-nucleotidase solubilized in the supernatant of plasma membrane fractions. + + +, Highly metastasizing; + +, moderately; +, weakly; ±, occasionally; < ±, occasionally, microscopical (from Kim et al., 1975).

lation dynamics of constituent cell plurality has not been established. This metastatic instability can also be observed in the in vitro line of the TMT-081-MS tumor (Ghosh et al., 1983), which, unless cloned (Dunnington et al., 1984), becomes weakly metastatic after continuous cultivation, perhaps as a consequence of karyotypic drift of stem cells (Yoshida et al., unpublished data). Further analyses are needed to determine the significance of chromosomal changes, for this cell line frequently also contains anomalies common to rodent tumor cells grown in vitro for a long period of time. Neri and Nicolson (1981) and Ossowski and Reich (1980) observed a similar progressive loss of metastatic potential in rat mammary tumor cells and in human epidermoid carcinoma in vitro, respectively. Schirmacher (1980) proposed that a preformed genetic program can be activated by environmental signals, leading to diverse changes in genetic expression and to the generation of heterogeneity and phenotypic instability. However, the metastatic-to-non-metastatic phenotypic conversion probably does not occur in cancer patients, at least not sufficiently to cause tumors to be irreversibly localized and surgically eradicable.

Modulation of Tumor Cell Surface Antigens

It is possible to compel the putative MCA-transformed cells in laboratory animals to express native organ-specific or onco-fetal antigens, instead of TSTA, by subjecting them to sustained immunological selective pressures, as is the case in the prolactin-dependent mammary tumors induced with a subthreshold dose of carcinogen under intense hormonal stimulation. This antigenic modulation usually appears to be accompanied by other cellular changes, e.g., accelerated shedding and renewal of surface glycoconjugates, loss of immunogenicity and receptors for various biological response modifiers, increased plasma membrane fluidity or malleability, and elevated net negative electrostatic surface charge, resulting in metastatic potential. Even after the tumor becomes established, it may be amenable to further modifications by various iatrogenic environmental factors, such as treatment with hormones, drugs, vaccines, radiation, or hyperthermia, due probably to the genetic instability inherent in transformed cells. This adaptability of tumor cells to their environment seems comparable to the immune escape mechanism of protozoan parasites that have been found to evade the host immune response by the adoption of host antigens as a "disguise," continuously altering their antigenic makeup and interfering with the host defense mechanism by shedding immunosuppressive substances (Cox, 1984; Parsons et al., 1984). Thus, the antigenic modulating capacity of tumor cells places a major constraint on the development of effective anticancer measures.

4. CONCLUDING REMARKS

The phenotypic diversity or heterogeneity of tumor cells, as shown in laboratory animals, can be generated by oncogenic agents interacting with endogenous host factors and innumerable exogenous environmental influences on the target cell at the initiating phase of tumorigenesis, as well as during the evolution of the neoplastic state. The question is whether the heterogeneity is created by specific environmental signals to activate a preformed genetic program, by the application of host pressures that cause the selection of preexisting cell clones according to a predetermined sequence, or by the process of accelerated mutation and selection due possibly to the easy mutability of tumor cells with an unstable genome and their adaptability to the environment. Perhaps it would be more pertinent to ask whether (1) the conversion of metastasizing to nonmetastasizing cells in an experimental setting is a real phenomenon that can also occur in human cancers; (2) the acquisition of new characteristics by the cells during tumor progression can be reversed with appropriate biological response modifiers or drugs; or (3) there are more specific markers to identify common denominators useful for the control of tumor growth and dissemination.

REFERENCES

Aamdal, S., Børmer, O., Jørgensen, O., Høst, H., Eliassen, G., Kaalhus, O., and Pihl, A., 1984, Estrogen receptors and long-term prognosis in breast cancer, *Cancer* 53:2525–2529.

Abercrombie, A., and Ambrose, E. J., 1962, The surface properties of cancer cells: A review, *Cancer Res.* 22:525–548.

Anderson, D. E., 1973, A high risk group for breast cancer, *Cancer Bull.* 2:23–25.

Arafah, B. M., Finegan, H. M., Roe, J., Manni, A., and Pearson, O. H., 1982, Hormone dependency in N-nitrosomethylurea-induced rat mammary tumors, *Endocrinology* 111:584–588.

Armstrong, B., and Doll, R., 1975, Environmental factors and cancer incidence and mortality in different countries, with special reference to dietary practices, *Int. J. Cancer* 15:617–631.

Armstrong, B., Stevens, N., and Doll, R., 1974, Retrospective study of the association between use of rauwolfia derivatives and breast cancer in English women, *Lancet* 2:672–675.

Balner, H., and Dersjant, H., 1966, Neonatal thymectomy and tumor induction with methylcholanthrene in mice, *J. Natl. Cancer Inst.* 36:513–521.

Beatson, G. T., 1896, On the treatment of inoperable cases of carcinoma of the mamma: Suggestion for a new method of treatment with illustrative cases, *Lancet* 2:104–162.

Bentvelzen, P., and Hilgers, J., 1980, Murine mammary tumor virus, in: *Viral Oncology* (G. Klein, ed.), Raven Press, New York, pp. 311–355.

Bern, H. A., and Nandi, S., 1961, Recent studies of the hormonal influence in mammary tumorigenesis, *Prog. Exp. Tumor Res.* 2:90–144.

Bernacki, R., and Kim, U., 1977, Concomitant elevation in sialyltransferase activity and sialic acid content in rats with metastasizing mammary tumors, *Science* 195:577–580.

Bibbo, M., Haenzel, W. M., Wied, G. L., Hubby, M., and Herbst, A. L., 1978, A twenty-five year follow-up study of women exposed to diethylstilbestrol during pregnancy, *N. Engl. J. Med.* 298:763–767.

Bittner, J. J., 1940, Further studies on active milk influence in breast cancer production in mice, *Proc. Soc. Exp. Biol. Med.* 45:805–810.

Bittner, J. J., 1942, Possible relationship of the estrogenic hormones, genetic susceptibility, and milk influence in the production of mammary cancer in mice, *Cancer Res.* 2:710–721.

Bittner, J. J., 1947, Mammary tumor milk agent, *Ann. N. Y. Acad. Sci.* 49:69–73.

Bittner, J. J., 1962, Biological assay and serial passage of the mouse mammary tumors from mothers and their inbred progeny, in: *A Ciba Foundation Symposium on Tumour Viruses of Murine Origin* (G. E. W. Wolstenholme and M. O'Connor, eds.), Little, Brown, Boston, pp. 56–71.

Bjelke, E., 1975, Dietary Vitamin A and human lung cancer, *Int. J. Cancer* **15**:561–565.

Bland, K. I., Fuchs, A., and Wittliff, J. L., 1981, Menopausal status as a factor in the distribution of estrogen and progestin receptors in breast cancer, *Surg. Forum* **32**:410–412.

Bollag, W., 1972, Prophylaxis of chronically induced benign and malignant epithelial tumors by vitamin A acid (retinoic acid), *Eur. J. Cancer* **8**:689–693.

Boot, L. M., Mühlbock, O., Ropcke, G., and Van Ebbenhorts Tangbergen, W., 1962, Further investigations on induction of mammary cancer in mice by isografts of hypophyseal tissue, *Cancer Res.* **22**:713–727.

Bostocchi, M., Nuti, M., and Squartini, F., 1977, Quantitative comparison on milk-release C3H and RIII mammary tumor viruses in infected BALB/ch hosts, *Tumori* **63**:535–542.

Bowers, C. Y., Friesen, H. G., Hwang, P., Guyda, H. J., and Folkers, K., 1971, Prolactin and thyrotropin release in man by synthetic pyroglutamyl-histidyl-prolinamide, *Biochem. Biophys. Res. Commun.* **45**:1033–1041.

Brock, D. J. H., and Sutcliffe, R. G., 1972, Alfa-fetoprotein in the antenatal diagnosis of anencephaly and spina bifida, *Lancet* **2**:197.

Bronn, D. G., Webster, D. J. T., and Minton, J. P., 1978, Estrogen receptor levels in hormonally progressive mammary tumors, *Surg. Forum* **29**:174–176.

Bruni, J. E., and Montemurro, D. G., 1971, Effect of hypothalamic lesions on the genesis of spontaneous mammary tumors in the mouse, *Cancer Res.* **31**:854–863.

Bulbrook, R. D., Hayward, J. L., and Spencer, C. C., 1971, Relation between urinary androgen and corticoid excretion and subsequent breast cancer, *Lancet* **2**: 395–398.

Burnet, F. M., 1970, *Immunological Surveillance*, Pergamon Press, Elmsford, N.Y.

Burrows, H., and Horning, E. S., 1952, *Oestrogens and Neoplasia*, Blackwell, Oxford.

Cancer Research Supplement, 1983, Workshop conference on nutrition in cancer causation and prevention, *Cancer Res. Suppl.* **43**:2385s–2519s.

Cardiff, R. D., and Young, J. T., 1980, Mouse mammary tumor biology: A new synthesis, in: *Viruses in Naturally Occurring Cancers* (M. Essex, G. Todaro, and H. zur Hausen, eds.), Cold Spring Harbor Laboratory, Cold Spring Harbor, N.Y., pp. 1105–1114.

Carroll, K. K., 1973, Experimental evidence of dietary factors and hormone dependent cancers, *Cancer Res.* **33**:3374–3383.

Carroll, K. K., and Khor, H. T., 1970, Effects of dietary fat and dose level on 7,12-dimethylbenz(a)anthracene on mammary tumor incidence in rats, *Cancer Res.* **30**:2260–2264.

Cave, W. T., Jr., Dunn, J. T., and MacLeod, R. M., 1979, Effects of iodine deficiency and high-fat diet on N-nitrosomethylurea-induced mammary cancer in rats, *Cancer Res.* **39**:729–734.

Chan, P.-C., Didato, F., and Cohen, L. A., 1975, High dietary fat, elevation of rat serum prolactin, and mammary tumors, *Proc. Soc. Exp. Biol. Med.* **149**:132–135.

Chatterjee, S. K., and Kim, U., 1977, Galactosyltransferase activity in metastasizing and nonmetastasizing rat mammary carcinomas and its possible relationship with tumor cell surface antigen shedding, *J. Natl. Cancer Inst.* **58**:273–280.

Chatterjee, S. K., and Kim, U., 1978, Fucosyltransferase activity in metastasizing and nonmetastasizing rat mammary carcinomas, *J. Natl. Cancer inst.* **61**:151–162.

Chopra, I. J., Hershman, J. M., and Hornabrook, R. W., 1976, Serum thyroid hormone and thyrotropin levels in subjects from endemic goiter regions of New Guinea, *J. Clin. Endocrinol. Metab.* **40**:326–333.

Cohen, J. C., Shank, P. R., Morris, V. L., Cardiff, R., and Varmus, H. E., 1979, Integration of the DNA of mouse mammary tumor virus in virus-infected normal and neoplastic tissue of the mouse, *Cell* **16**:333–345.

Cohen, S. M., Wittenberg, J. F., and Bryan, G. T., 1976, Effect of avitaminosis A and hypervitaminosis A on urinary bladder carcinogenicity of N-[4-(5-nitro-2-furyl)-2-thiazolyl]-formamide, *Cancer Res.* **36**:2334–2339.

Cooper, G. M., 1982, Cellular transforming genes, *Science* **217**:801–806.

Costlow, M. E., Buschow, R. A., Richert, N. J., and McGuire, W. L., 1975, Prolactin and estrogen binding in transplantable hormone-dependent and autonomous mammary carcinoma, *Cancer Res.* **35**:970–974.

Cowan, L. D., Gordis, L., Tonascia, J. A., and Jones, G. S., 1981, Breast cancer incidence in women with a history of progesterone deficiency, Am. J. Epidemiol. 114:209–217.

Cox, F. E. G., 1984, How parasites evade the immune response, Immunol. Today 1984:29–33.

Cronkite, E. P., Shellabarger, C. J., Bond, V. P., and Lippincott, S. W., 1957, Studies of the mechanism of induction of radiation-induced tumors of the breast in the rat, Radiat. Res. 7:311.

Cutts, J. H., 1969, Unusual response to androgen of estrogen dependent mammary tumors, J. Natl. Cancer Inst. 42:485–488.

Cutts, J. H., and Noble, R. L., 1964, Estrogen-induced mammary tumors in the rat. I. Induction and behavior of tumors, Cancer Res. 24:1116–1123.

Dao, T. L., Bock, F. G., and Greiner, M. J., 1960, Mammary carcinogenesis by 3-methylcholanthrene. II. Inhibitory effect of pregnancy and lactation on tumor induction, J. Natl. Cancer Inst. 25:991–1003.

De Baetselier, P., Katzav, S., Gorelik, E., Feldman, M., and Segal, S., 1980, Differential expression of H-2 gene products in tumour cells is associated with their metastatogenic properties, Nature 288:179–181.

De la Monte, S. M., Hutchins, G. M., and Moore, G. W., 1984, Estrogen and progesterone receptors in prediction of metastatic behavior of breast carcinoma, Am. J. Med. 76:11–17.

Drasar, B. S., and Irving, D., 1975, Environmental factors and cancers of the colon and breast, Br. J. Cancer 27:167–172.

Dunnington, D. J., Kim, U., Hughes, C. M., Monaghan, P., and Rudland, P. S., 1984, Lack of production of myoepithelial variants by cloned epithelial cell lines derived from the TMT-081 metastasizing rat mammary tumor, Cancer Res. 44:5338–5346.

Edgington, T. S., and Nakamura, R. M., 1982, Tumor associated and tumor specific markers of human mammary cancer, in: Serono Symposium No. 46, Markers for Diagnosis and Monitoring Human Cancer (M. I. Colnaghi, G. L. Buraggi, and M. Ghione, eds.), Academic Press, New York, pp. 51–74.

Erickson, K. L., McNeill, C. J., Gershwin, M. E., and Ossmann, J. B., 1980, Influence of dietary fat concentration and saturation on immune ontogeny in mice, J. Nutr. 110:1555–1572.

Eskin, B. A., 1970, Iodine metabolism and breast cancer, Trans. N. Y. Acad. Sci. 32:911–947.

Faulkin, L. J., 1966, Hyperplastic lesions of mouse mammary glands after treatment with 3-methylcholanthrene, J. Natl. Cancer Inst. 36:289–298.

Fidler, I. J., 1973, Selection of successive lines of metastasis, Nature New Biol. 242:148–149.

Fisher, E. R., Redmond, C. K., Liu, H., Rockette, H., and Fisher, B., 1980, Correlation of estrogen receptor and pathologic characteristics of invasive breast cancer, Cancer 45:349–353.

Fisher, E. R., Redmond, C., Fisher, B., and participating NSABP investigators, 1983, Pathologic findings from the National Surpical Adjuvant Breast Project. VIII. Relationship of chemotherapeutic responsiveness to tumor differentiation, Cancer 51:181–191.

Fishman, A. P., 1982, Endothelium: A distributed organ of diverse capacity, Ann. N.Y. Acad. Sci. 401:1–8.

Fishman, J., Fukushima, D. K., O'Conner, J., and Lynch, H. T., 1979, Low urinary estrogen glucuronides in women at risk for familial breast cancer, Science 204:1089–1091.

Foulds, L., 1949, Mammary tumours in hybrid mice: Growth and progression of spontaneous tumours, Br. J. Cancer 3:345–375.

Furth, J., 1953, Conditioned and autonomous neoplasms. A review, Cancer Res. 13:477–492.

Furth, J., 1959, A meeting of ways in cancer research: Thoughts on the evolution and nature of neoplasms, Cancer Res. 19:241–258.

Furth, J., 1973, The role of prolactin in mammary carcinogenesis, in: Human Prolactin (J. L. Pasteels and C. Robyn, eds.), Exerpta Medica, Amsterdam, pp. 232–248.

Furth, J., and Clifton, K. H., 1966, Experimental pituitary tumors, in: The Pituitary Gland (G. W. Harris and B. T. Donovan, eds.) Butterworths, London, pp. 460–497.

Furth, J., and Furth, O., 1936, Neoplastic diseases produced by general irradiation with X-rays. I. Incidence and type of neoplasms, Am. J. Cancer 28:54–65.

Gallager, S., 1984, Pathologic types of breast cancer: Their prognoses, Cancer 53:623–629.

Ganther, H. E., Hafeman, D. G., Lawrence, R. A., Serfass, R. E., and Hoekstra, W. G., 1976,

Selenium and glutathione peroxidase in health and disease—A review, in: *Trace Elements in Human Health and Diseases* (A. S. Presa, ed.), Academic Press, New York, pp. 165–234.

Gardner, W. U., 1957, Hormones and carcinogenesis, *Proc. Can. Cancer Res. Conf.* **2**:207–241.

Ghosh, S. K., Grossberg, S., Kim, U., and Pressman, D., 1979, A tumor-associated organ-specific antigen characteristic of spontaneously metastatic rat mammary carcinoma, *J. Natl. Cancer Inst.* **62**:1229–1233.

Ghosh, S. K., Roholt, O. A., and Kim, U., 1983, Antigenic characteristics of metastasizing and nonmetastasizing mammary adenocarcinoma of rat, in: *Non-HLA Antigens in Health, Aging and Malignancy* (E. Cohen, J. Fitzpatrick, and G. P. Murphy, eds.), Liss, New York, pp. 227–233.

Gorski, J., Toft, D., Shyamala, G., Smith, D., and Notides, A., 1968, Hormone receptor studies on the interaction of estrogen with the uterus, *Recent Prog. Horm. Res.* **24**:45–80.

Gray, G. E., Pike, M. C., and Henderson, B. E., 1979, Breast cancer incidence and mortality rates in different countries in relation to known risk factors and dietary practices, *Br. J. Cancer* **39**:1–9.

Gridley, D. S., Kettering, J. D., Garaza, C. D., Andres, M. L., Slater, J. M., and Nutter, R. L., 1982, Modification of herpes 2-transformed cell-induced tumors in mice fed different source of protein, fat, and carbohydrate, *Cancer Lett.* **17**:161–173.

Gridley, D. S., Kettering, J. D., Slater, J. M., and Nutter, R. L., 1983, Modification of spontaneous mammary tumors in mice fed different sources of protein, fat and carbohydrate, *Cancer Lett.* **19**:133–146.

Gruenstein, M., Meranze, D. R., and Acuff, M., 1968, The role of thyroid in hydrocarbon-induced mammary carcinogenesis in rats, *Cancer Res.* **28**:471–474.

Guffy, M. M., Rosenberger, J. A., Simon, I., and Burns, C. P., 1982, Effect of cellular fatty acid alteration on hyperthermic sensitivity in cultured L1210 murine leukemia cells, *Cancer Res.* **42**:3625–3630.

Guffy, M. M., North, J. A., and Burns, C. P., 1984, Effect of cellular fatty acid alteration on adriamycin sensitivity in cultured L1210 murine leukemia cells, *Cancer Res.* **44**:1863–1866.

Guillemin, R., Yamazaki, E., Gard, D. A., Jutisz, M., and Sakiz, E., 1963, In vitro secretion of thyrotropin (TSH): Stimulation by a hypothalamic peptide (TRF), *Endocrinology* **73**:564–572.

Gullino, P. M., Pettigrew, H. M., and Grantham, F. H., 1975, N-nitrosomethylurea as mammary gland carcinogen in rats, *J. Natl. Cancer Inst.* **54**:401–409.

Hanna, N., 1980, Expression of metastatic potential of tumor cells in young nude mice is correlated with low levels of natural killer cell-mediated cytotoxicity, *Int. J. Cancer* **26**:675–680.

Harr, J. R., Exon, J. H., Weswig, P. H., and Whanger, P. D., 1973, Relationship of dietary selenium concentration, chemical cancer induction and tissue concentration of selenium in rats, *Clin. Toxicol.* **6**:287–293.

Haughton, G., and Whitmore, A. C., 1976, Genetics, the immune response and oncogenesis, *Transplant. Rev.* **28**:75–97.

Henderson, B. E., Powell, D., Rosario, I., Keys, C., Hanisch, R., Young, M., Casagrande, J., Gerkins, V., and Pike, M. C., 1974, An epidemiologic study of breast cancer, *J. Natl. Cancer Inst.* **53**:609–614.

Henderson, B. E., Gerkins, V., Rosario, I., Casagrande, J., and Pike, M. C., 1975, Elevated serum levels of estrogen and prolactin in daughters of patients with breast cancer, *N. Engl. J. Med.* **292**:790–795.

Heppner, G. H., 1984, Tumor heterogeneity, *Cancer Res.* **44**:2259–2265.

Herberman, R. B., and Ortaldo, J. R., 1981, Natural killer cells: Their role in defenses against disease, *Science* **214**:24–30.

Heuson, J. C., and Legros, N., 1970, Influence of insulin and of aloxan diabetes on growth of the rat mammary carcinoma in vivo, *Eur. J. Cancer* **6**:349–351.

Heuson, J. C., Legros, N., and Heimann, R., 1972, Influence of insulin administration on growth of the 7,12-dimethylbenz(a)anthracene-induced mammary carcinoma in intact, oophorectomized and hypophysectomized rats, *Cancer Res.* **32**:233–238.

Hewitt, H. B., and Blake, E. R., 1975, Quantitative studies of translymphnodal passage of tumor cells naturally disseminated from a nonimmunogenic murine squamous carcinoma, *Br. J. Cancer* **31**:25–35.

Hewitt, H. B., Blake, E. R., and Walder, A. S., 1976, A critique of the evidence for active host defense against cancer, based on personal studies of 27 murine tumors of spontaneous origin, *Br. J. Cancer* **33**:241–259.

Hilf, R., Hissin, P. J., and Shafie, S. M., 1978, Regulatory interrelationships for insulin and estrogen action in mammary tumors, *Cancer Res.* **38**:4075–4085.

Hirayama, T., 1978, Epidemiology of breast cancer with special reference to the role of diet, *Prev. Med.* **7**:173–195.

Horwitz, K. B., and McGuire, W. L., 1975, Specific progesterone receptors in human breast cancer, *Steroids* **25**:497–505.

Howard, D. K., Schlom, J., and Fisher, P. B., 1983, Chemical carcinogen–mouse mammary tumor virus interactions in cell transformation, *In Vitro* **19**:58–66.

Huggins, C., and Fukunishi, R., 1963, Cancer in the rat after single exposure to irradiation or hydrocarbons. Age and strain factors. Hormone dependence of the mammary cancers, *Radiat. Res.* **20**:493–503.

Huggins, C., Briziarelli, G., and Suton, H., 1959, Rapid induction of mammary carcinoma in the rat and the influence of hormones on the tumors, *J. Exp. Med.* **109**:25–42.

Huggins, C., Grand, L. C., and Brillantes, F., 1961, Mammary cancer induced by a single feeding of polynuclear hydrocarbon and its suppression, *Nature* **189**:204–207.

Huggins, C., Moon, R. C., and Morii, S., 1962, Extinction of experimental mammary cancer. I. Estradiol-17β and progesterone, *Proc. Natl. Acad. Sci. USA* **48**:379–386.

Hwang, P., Guyda, H., and Friesen, H., 1971, A radioimmunoassay for human prolactin, *Proc. Natl. Acad. Sci. USA* **68**:1902–1906.

Ichinose, R. R., and Nandi, S., 1966, Influence of hormones on lobulo-alveolar differentiation of mouse mammary gland in vitro, *J. Endocrinol.* **35**:331–340.

Ip, C., 1981, Factors influencing the anticarcinogenic efficacy of selenium on dimethylbenz(a)anthracene-induced mammary tumorigenesis in rats, *Cancer Res.* **41**:2683–2686.

Ip, C., and Ip, M. M., 1981, Serum estrogen and estrogen responsiveness in 7,12-dimethylbenz(a)anthracene-induced mammary tumors as influenced by dietary fat, *J. Natl. Cancer Inst.* **66**:291–295.

Ip, C., and Sinha, D. K., 1981, Enhancement of mammary tumorigenesis by dietary selenium deficiency in rats with a high polyunsaturated fat intake, *Cancer Res.* **41**:31–34.

Ip, C., Yip, P., and Bernardis, L. L., 1980, The role of prolactin in the promotion of dimethylbenz(a)anthracene-induced mammary tumors by dietary fat, *Cancer Res.* **40**:374–378.

Ip, M. M., Milholland, R. J., Kim, U., and Rosen, F., 1978, Characterization of androgen receptors in 7,12-dimethylbenz(a)anthracene-induced and transplantable rat mammary tumors, *Cancer Res.* **38**:2879–2885.

Ip, M., Milholland, R. J., Rosen, F., and Kim, U., 1979, Mammary cancer: Selective action of the estrogen receptor complex, *Science* **203**:361–363.

Itoh, K., and Maruchi, N., 1975, Breast cancer in patients with Hashimoto's thyroiditis, *Lancet* **2**:1119–1121.

Jacobs, M. M., 1980, Effects of selenium on chemical carcinogenesis, *Prev. Med.* **9**:362–367.

Jacobs, D. M., and Byrd, W., 1975, Addult thymectomy results in loss of T-dependent mitogen response in mouse spleen cells, *Nature* **255**:153–155.

Jensen, E. V., Suzuku, T., Kawashima, T., Stumpf, W. E., Jungblut, P. W., and DeSombre, E. R., 1968, A two-step mechanism for the interaction of estradiol with rat uterus, *Proc. Natl. Acad. Sci. USA* **59**:632–639.

Jensen, E. V., Block, G. E., Smith, S., Keyser, K., and DeSombre, E. R., 1971, Estrogen receptors and breast cancer response to adrenalectomy, *Natl. Cancer Inst. Monogr.* **34**:55–79.

Jull, J. W., 1958, Hormonal mechanisms in mammary carcinogenesis, in: *Endocrine Aspects of Breast Cancer* (A. R. Currie and C. F. W. Illingworth, eds.), Livingstone, Edinburgh, pp. 305–317.

Kalpaktsoglou, P. K., Yunis, E. J., and Good, R. A., 1967, Early splenectomy and survival of inbred mice, *Nature* **215**:633–634.

Kapdi, C. C., and Wolf, J. N., 1976, Breast cancer—Relationship to thyroid supplements for hypothyroidism, *J. Am. Med. Assoc.* **23:**1124–1127.

Katz, L., Steinitz, R., and Sela, T., 1981, Epidemiological review of breast cancer in Israel, *Isr. J. Med. Sci.* **17:**810–815.

Kellen, J. A., 1972, Effect of hypothyroidism on induction of mammary tumors in rats by 7,12-dimethylbenz(a)anthracene, *J. Natl. Cancer Inst.* **48:**1901–1904.

Keydar, I., Selzer, G., Chaitchik, S., Horeuveni, M., Karby, S., and Hizi, A., 1982, A viral antigen as a marker for the prognosis of human breast cancer, *Eur. J. Cancer Clin. Oncol.* **18:**1321–1328.

Kiang, D. T., and Kennedy, B. J., 1977, Factors affecting estrogen receptors in breast cancer, *Cancer* **40:**1571–1576.

Kim, U., 1970, Metastasizing mammary carcinomas in rats: Induction and study of their immunogenicity, *Science* **167:**72–74.

Kim, U., 1977, Pathogenesis of spontaneously metastasizing mammary carcinomas in rats, *Gann Monogr.* **20:**73–81.

Kim, U., 1983, On the characteristics of tumor cells and host responses associated with metastatic potential, in: *13th International Cancer Congress, Part C, Biology of Cancer* (E. Mihich and E. Mirand, eds.), Liss, New York, pp. 45–50.

Kim, U., and Depowski, M., 1975, Progression from hormone dependence to autonomy in mammary tumors as an *in vitro* manifestation of sequential clonal selection, *Cancer Res.* **35:**2068–2077.

Kim, U., and Furth, J., 1960a, Relation of mammary tumors to mammotropes. I. Induction of mammary tumors in rats, *Proc. Soc. Exp. Biol. Med.* **103:**640–642.

Kim, U., and Furth, J., 1960b, Relation of mammary tumors to mammotropes. II. Hormone responsiveness of 3-methylcholanthrene induced mammary carcinomas, *Proc. Soc. Exp. Biol. Med.* **103:**643–645.

Kim, U., and Furth, J., 1961, Relation of mammary tumors to mammotropes. IV. Development of highly hormone-dependent mammary tumors. *Proc. Soc. Exp. Biol. Med.* **105:**490–492.

Kim, U., and Furth, J., 1976, The role of prolactin in carcinogenesis, *Vitam. Horm. (N.Y.)* **34:**107–136.

Kim, U., Furth, J., and Yannopoulos, K., 1963, Observations on hormonal control of mammary cancer. I. Estrogen and mammotropes, *J. Natl. Cancer Inst.* **31;**233–259.

Kim, U., Baumler, A., Carruthers, C., and Bielat, K., 1975, Immunological escape mechanism in spontaneously metastasizing mammary tumors, *Proc. Natl. Acad. Sci. USA* **72:**1012–1016.

Klug, H. L., Moxon, A. L., Petersen, D. F., and Painter, E. P., 1953, Inhibition of rat liver succinic dehydrogenase by selenium compounds, *J. Pharmacol. Exp. Ther.* **108:**437–441.

Kollmorgen, G. M., Sansing, W. A., Lehman, A. A., Fischer, G., Longley, R. E., Alexander, S. S., Jr., King, M. M., and McCoy, P. B., 1979, Inhibition of lymphocyte function in rats fed high-fat diets, *Cancer Res.* **39:**3458–3462.

Kubai, L., and Auerbach, R., 1968, Neonatal splenectomy: Absence of runting in mice, *Nature* **217:**460.

Kwa, H. G., DeJong-Bekker, M., Engelsman, E., and Cleton, F. J., 1974, Plasma-prolactin in human breast cancer, *Lancet* **1:**433–434.

Lacassagne, A., and Duplan, J. F., 1959, Le mécanisme de la cancérisation de la mamelle chez la Souris, considéré d'apre les résultats d'expériences au moyen de la réserpine, *C. R. Acad. Sci.* **249:**810–812.

Lewko, W. M., and McConnell, W. P., 1982, Biphasic influence of selenium on cell growth and the synthesis of collagen in cultured mammary tumor cells, *Fed. Proc.* **41:**623.

Lo, L. W., Koropatnick, J., and Stitch, H. F., 1978, The mutagenicity and cytotoxicity of selenite, "activated" selenite and selenate for normal and DNA repair-deficient human fibroblasts, *Mutat. Res.* **49:**305–312.

Loeb, L., and Kirtz, M. M., 1939, The effects of transplants of anterior lobes of the hypophysis on the growth of the mammary gland and on the development of mammary gland carcinoma in various strains of mice, *Am. J. Cancer* **36:**56–82.

Lorber, J., Stewart, C. R., and Ward, A. M., 1973, Alfa-fetoprotein in antenatal diagnosis of anencephaly and spina bifida, *Lancet* **1:**1187.

Lynch, H. T., Albano, W. A., Danes, B. S., Layton, M. A., Kimberling, W. J., Cheng, S. C., Costello, K. A., Mulcahy, G. M., Wagner, C. A., and Tindall, S. L., 1984, Genetic predisposition to breast cancer, *Cancer* **53**:612–622.

Lyons, W. R., Li, C. H., and Johnson, R. E., 1958, The hormonal control of mammary growth and lactation, *Recent Prog. Horm. Res.* **14**:219–248.

McKeehan, W. L., Hamilton, W. G., and Ham, R. G., 1976, Selenium is an essential trace element for growth of W-38 diploid human fibroblasts, *Proc. Natl. Acad. Sci. USA* **73**:2023–2027.

MacMahon, B., Cole, P., and Brown, J., 1973, Etiology of human breast cancer: A review, *J. Natl. Cancer Inst.* **50**:21–42.

Maiorana, A., and Gullino, P. M., 1980, Effect of retinyl acetate on the incidence of mammary carcinomas and hepatomas in mice, *J. Natl. Cancer Inst.* **64**:655–663.

Medina, D., and Shepherd, F., 1980, Selenium-mediated inhibition of mammary tumorigenesis, *Cancer Lett.* **8**:241–245.

Medina, D., and Shepherd, F., 1981, Selenium-mediated inhibition of 7,12-dimethyl-benz(a)anthracene-induced mouse mammary tumorigenesis, *Carcinogenesis* **2**:451–455.

Medina, D., De Ome, K. B., and Young, L., 1970, Tumor producing capabilities of hyperplastic alveolar nodules in virgin and hormone-stimulated BALB/c C3H and C3Hf mice, *J. Natl. Cancer Inst.* **44**:167–174.

Mehta, R. G., McCormick, D. L., Cerny, W., and Moon, R. C., 1982, Correlation between retinoid inhibition of N-methyl-N-nitrosourea-induced mammary carcinogenesis and levels of retinoic acid binding proteins, *Carcinogenesis* **3**:89–91.

Mettlin, C., Graham, S., Priore, R., Marshall, J., and Swanson, M., 1981, Diet and cancer of the esophagus, *Nutr. Cancer* **2**:143–147.

Miller, J. F. A. P., Grant, G. A., and Roe, F. J. C., 1963, Effect of thymectomy on the induction of skin tumours by 3,4-benzpyrene, *Nature* **199**:920–922.

Mittra, I., and Haywood, J. L., 1977, The hypothalamic–pituitary–thyroid axis in breast cancer, *Lancet* **1**:885–889.

Moody, J. K., and Reed, N. D., 1968, Neonatal splenectomy and survival of mice, *Nature* **218**:1056–1057.

Moon, R. C., 1962, Influence of graded thyroxine levels on mammary gland, *Am. J. Physiol.* **203**:942–946.

Moon, R. C., and Mehta, R. G., 1982, Retinoid binding in normal and neoplastic mammary tissue, in: *Hormones and Cancer* (W. W. Leavit, ed.), Plenum Press, New York, pp. 231–249.

Moon, R. C., Grubbs, C. J., and Sporn, M. B., 1976, Inhibition of 7,12-dimethylbenz(a)anthracene-induced mammary carcinogenesis by retinyl acetate, *Cancer Res.* **36**:2626–2630.

Moon, R. C., Grubbs, C. J., Sporn, M. B., and Goodman, D. G., 1977, Retinyl acetate inhibits mammary carcinogenesis induced by N-methyl-N-nitrosourea, *Nature* **267**:620–621.

Moon, R. C., McCormick, D. L., and Mehta, R. G., 1983, Inhibition of carcinogenesis by retinoid, *Cancer Res. (Suppl.)* **43**:2469–2475.

Moore, D. H., Charney, J., and Pullinger, B. D., 1970, Mouse mammary tumor virus infectivity as a function of age at inoculation, breeding, and total lapsed time, *J. Natl. Cancer Inst.* **45**:561–565.

Mori, S., 1922, The changes in the para-ocular glands which follow the administration of diets low in fat-soluble A; with notes of the effects of the same diets on the salivary glands and the mucosa of the larynx and trachea, *Johns Hopkins Hosp. Bull.* **33**:357–359.

Mühlbock, O., and Boot, L. M., 1959, Induction of mammary cancer in mice without the mammary tumor agent by isograft of hypophyses, *Cancer Res.* **19**:402–412.

Nagataki, S., Shizume, K., and Nakao, K., 1967, Thyroid function in chronic excess iodine ingestion: Comparison of thyroidal absolute iodine uptake and degradation of thyroxine in euthyroid Japanese subjects, *J. Clin. Endocrinol. Metab.* **27**:638–647.

Nandi, S. J., 1958, Endocrine control of mammary gland development in the C3H/He Crgl mouse, *J. Natl. Cancer Inst.* **21**:1039–1055.

Nandi, S., and Bern, H. A., 1960, Relation between mammary-gland responses to lactogenic hormone combinations and tumor susceptibility in various strains of mice, *J. Natl. Cancer Inst.* **24**:907–931.

Neri, A., and Nicolson, G. L., 1981, Phenotypic drift of metastatic and cell-surface properties of mammary adenocarcinoma cell clones during growth in vitro, Int. J. Cancer 28:731–738.

Nishizuka, Y., Nakakuki, K., and Usui, M., 1965, Enhancing effect of thymectomy on hepato-tumorigenesis in Swiss mice following neonatal injection of 20-methylcholanthrene, Nature 205:1236–1238.

Noble, R. L., and Collip, J. B., 1941, Regression of estrogen-induced mammary tumors in female rats following removing of the stimulus, Can. Med. Assoc. J. 44:1–5.

Nusse, R., and Varmus, H. E., 1982, Many tumors induced by the mouse mammary tumor virus contain a provirus integrated in the same region of the host genome, Cell 31:99–109.

Ossowski, L., and Reich, E., 1980, Experimental model for quantitative study of metastasis, Cancer Res. 40:2300–2309.

Parish, C. R., O'Neill, H. C., and Higgins, T. J., 1981, Glycosyltransferases and T-cell recognition, Immunol. Today 2:98–102.

Park, B. H., Fike, R. M., and Kim, U., 1982, Increased electrophoretic mobility of rat mammary tumor cells: A positive correlation with metastatic potential, IRCS Med. Sci. 10:96–97.

Parsons, M., Nelson, R. G., and Agabian, N., 1984, Antigenic variation in African trypanosomes: DNA rearrangements program immune evasion, Immunol. Today 5:43–50.

Peters, G., Brookes, S., Smith, R., and Dickson, C., 1983, Tumorigenesis by mouse mammary tumor virus: Evidence for a common region for provirus integration in mammary tumors, Cell 33:369–377.

Pingitore, R., and Squartini, F., 1982, Relationship between morphology and viral etiology in mammary tumors of BALB/cf C3H and BALB/cf RIII mice, Tumori 68:199–203.

Prehn, R. T., and Main, J. M., 1957, Immunity to methylcholanthrene-induced sarcomas, J. Natl. Cancer Inst. 18:769–778.

Rao, B. R., and Meyer, J. S., 1977, Estrogen and progestin receptors in normal and cancer tissue, in: Progesterone Receptors in Normal and Neoplastic Tissues (W. L. McGuire, J. P. Raynaud, and E. E. Baulieu, eds.), Raven Press, New York, pp. 155–169.

Rao, G. A., and Abraham, S., 1975, Enhanced growth rate of transplanted mammmary adeno-carcinomas induced in C3H mice by dietary linoleate, J. Natl. Cancer Inst. 54:401–414.

Rhomberg, W., 1975, Metastasierendes Mammakarzinom and diabetes mellitus—Eine prog-nostisch günstige krankheitskombination, Dtsch. Med. Wochenschr. 100:2422–2427.

Ringold, G. M., Dobson, D. E., Grove, J. R., Hall, C. V., Lee, F., and Vannice, J. L., 1983, Glucocorticoid regulation of gene expression: Mouse mammary tumor virus as a model system, Recent Prog. Horm. Res. 39:387–424.

Rivera, E. M., 1966, Strain differences in mouse mammary tissue sensitivity to prolactin and somatotrophin in organ culture, Nature 209:1151–1152.

Roder, J. C., and Haliotis, T., 1980, Do NK cells play a role in anti-tumor surveillance? Immunol. Today 1:96–100.

Rogers, A. E., Herndon, B. J., and Newberne, P. M., 1973, Induction by dimethylhydrazine of intestinal carcinoma in normal rats and rats fed high and low levels of vitamin A, Cancer Res. 33:1003–1009.

Ross, R. K., Paganini-Hill, A., Gerkins, V. R., Mack, T. M., Pfeffer, R., Arthur, M., and Henderson, B. E., 1980, A case-control study of menopausal estrogen therapy and breast cancer, J. Am. Med. Assoc. 243:1635–1639.

Rous, P., and Beard, J. W., 1935, The progression to carcinoma of virus-induced rabbit papilloma (Shope), J. Exp. Med. 62:523–548.

Rous, P., and Kidd, J. G., 1941, Conditional neoplasms and subthreshold neoplastic states: A study of tar tumors of rabbits, J. Exp. Med. 73:365–389.

Rudland, P. S., Bennett, D. C., and Warburton, M. J., 1979, Hormonal control of growth and differentiation of cultured rat mammary gland epithelial cells, in: Hormones and Cell Culture, Cold Spring Harbor Laboratory, Cold Spring Harbor, N.Y., pp. 677–699.

Schally, A. V., and Bowers, C. Y., 1963, The nature of thyrotropin-releasing hormone (TRH), Proc. 6th Midwest. Conf. Thyroid Endocrinol. pp. 25–63.

Schirmacher, V., 1980, Shift in tumor cell phenotypes induced by signals from the microen-vironment: Relevance for the immunobiology of cancer metastasis, Immunobiology 157:89–98.

Severi, L., Biancifiori, C., Olivi, M., and Squartini, F., 1958, On hormone dependence in the transmission of mammary tumour agent from males, in: *Endocrine Aspects of Breast Cancer* (A. R. Currie and C. F. W. Illingworth, eds.), Livingston, Edinburgh, pp. 283–290.

Shamberger, G. N., White, D. A., and Schneider, C. J., 1978, Selenium and cancer: Effects of selenium and of the diet on the genesis of spontaneous mammary tumors in virgin inbred female C3H/St. mice, *Bioinorg. Chem.* **8**:387–396.

Shellabarger, C. J., Bond, V. P., and Cronkite, E. P., 1960, Studies on radiation-induced mammary gland neoplasia in the rat. IV. The response of females to a single dose of sublethal total-body gamma radiation as studied until first appearance of breast neoplasia to death of the animals, *Radiat. Res.* **13**:242–249.

Silverstone, H., and Tannenbaum, A., 1950, The effect of the proportion of dietary fat on the rate of formation of mammary carcinoma in mice, *Cancer Res.* **10**:448–453.

Singh, D. V., De Ome, K. B., and Bern, H. A., 1970, Strain differences in response of the mouse mammary gland to hormones *in vitro*, *J. Natl. Cancer Inst.* **45**:657–675.

Sinha, Y. N., Selby, F. W., and Vanderlaan, W. P., 1974, The natural history of prolactin and GH secretion in mice with high and low incidence of mammary tumors, *Endocrinology* **94**:757–764.

Skipper, H. E., 1983, Stepwise progress in the treatment of disseminated cancers, *Cancer* **51**:1773–1776.

Smithline, F., Sherman, L., and Kolodny, H. D., 1975, Prolactin and breast carcinoma, *N. Engl. J. Med.* **292**:784–792.

Spiegelman, S., 1974, Molecular evidence for viral agents in human cancer and its chemotherapeutic consequences, *Cancer Chemother. Rep.* **58**:595–613.

Spiegelman, S., Mesa-Tejada, R., Ohno, T., Ramanarayanan, M., Nayak, R., Bausch, J., and Fenoglio, C., 1980, The presence and clinical implications of a virus-related protein in human breast cancer, *Cold Spring Harbor Conf. Cell Prolif.* **7**:1149–1167.

Sporn, M. B., Squire, R. A., Brown, C. C., Smith, J. M., Wenk, M. L., and Springer, S., 1977, 13-cis-retinoic acid: Inhibition of bladder carcinogenesis in the rat, *Science* **195**:487–489.

Squartini, F., and Bostocchi, M., 1977, Bioreactivity of C3H and RIII mammary tumor viruses in virgin female BALB/cf mice: Brief communication, *J. Natl. Cancer Inst.* **58**:1845–1847.

Stackpole, C. W., 1981, Distinct lung-colonizing and lung-metastasizing cell populations in B16 mouse melanoma, *Nature* **289**:798–800.

Stutman, O., 1982, Natural and induced immunity to mouse mammary tumors and the mammary tumor virus (MuMTV), in: *Springer Seminars in Immunopathology*, Springer-Verlag, Berlin, pp. 333–372.

Talwalker, P. K., and Meites, J., 1961, Mammary lobulo-alveolar growth induced by anterior pituitary hormones in adreno-ovariectomized and adreno-ovariectomized-hypophysectomized rats, *Proc. Soc. Exp. Biol. Med.* **107**:880–883.

Tashjian, A. H., Jr., Barosky, N. J., and Jensen, D. K., 1971, Thyrotropin-releasing hormone: Direct evidence for stimulation of prolactin production by pituitary cells in culture, *Biochem. Biophys. Res. Commun.* **43**:516–523.

Thomas, D. B., 1980, Epidemiologic and related studies of breast cancer etiology, in: *Reviews in Cancer Epidemiology*, Volume 1 (A. M. Lilienfeld, ed.), Elsevier/North-Holland, Amsterdam, pp. 153–217.

Thomas, L., 1959, Discussion in: *Cellular and Humoral Aspects of Hypersensitive States* (H. S. Lawrence, ed.), Cassell, London, p. 529.

Thompson, H. J., and Becci, P. J., 1980, Selenium inhibition of N-methyl-N-nitrosourea-induced mammary carcinogenesis in the rat, *J. Natl. Cancer Inst.* **65**:1299–1301.

Thompson, H. J., Becci, P. J., Brown, C. C., and Moon, R. C., 1979, Effect of retinyl acetate feeding on inhibition of 1-methyl-1-nitrosourea-induced mammary carcinogenesis in the rat, *Cancer Res.* **39**:3977–3980.

Tonelli, Q. J., and Sorof, S., 1980, Epidermal growth factor requirement for development of cultured mammary glands, *Nature* **285**:250–252.

Tonelli, Q. J., and Sorof, S., 1981, Expression of a phenotype of normal differentiation in cultured mammary glands is promoted by epidermal growth factor and blocked by cyclic adenine nucleotide and prostaglandins, *Differentiation* **20**:253–259.

Topper, Y. J., and Oka, T., 1974, Some aspects of mammary gland development in mature mouse, in: *Lactation: A Comprehensive Treatise*, Volume 1 (G. L. Larson and V. R. Smith, eds.), Academic Press, New York, pp. 327–348.

Vagenakis, A. G., Koutras, D. A., Burger, A., Malamos, B., Ingbar, S. H., and Braverman, L. E., 1973, Studies on serum triiodothyronine, thyroxine and thyrotropin concentrations in endemic goiter in Greece, *J. Clin. Endocrinol. Metab.* **37**:485–488.

Varmus, H., Bishop, J. M., Nowinski, R., and Sarkar, N., 1972, Mammary tumour virus specific nucleotide sequences in mouse DNA, *Nature New Biol.* **238**:189–191.

Wagner, D. A., Naylor, P. H., Kim, U., Shea, W., Ip, C., and Ip, M. M., 1982, Interaction of dietary fat and the thymus in the induction of mammary tumors by 7,12-dimethylbenz(a)anthracene, *Cancer Res.* **42**:1266–1273.

Wang, N., Yu, S. H., Leiner, I. E., Hebbel, R. P., Easton, J. W., and McKhann, C. F., 1982, Characterization of high- and low-metastatic clones derived from a methylcholanthrene-induced murine fibrosarcoma, *Cancer Res.* **42**:1046–1051.

Weinberg, R. A., 1981, Use of transfection to analyze genetic information and malignant transformation, *Biochim. Biophys. Acta* **651**:25–35.

Weinstein, I. B., 1981, Current concepts and controversies in chemical carcinogenesis, *J. Supramol. Struct. Cell. Biochem.* **17**:99–120.

Weinstein, I. B., Gattoni-Celli, S., Kirschmeier, P., Hsiao, W., Horowitz, A., and Jeffrey, A., 1984, Cellular target and host genes in multistage carcinogenesis, *Fed. Proc.* **43**:2287–2294.

Welsch, C. W., and Meites, J., 1969, Effects of a norethynodrel–mestranol combination (enovid) on development and growth of carcinogen-induced mammary tumors in female rats, *Cancer* **23**:601–607.

Welsch, C. W., and Nagasawa, H., 1977, Prolactin and murine mammary tumorigenesis: A review, *Cancer Res.* **37**:951–963.

Welsch, C. W., Nagasawa, H., and Meites, J., 1970, Increased incidence of spontaneous mammary tumors in female rats with induced hypothalamic lesions, *Cancer Res.* **30**:2310–2313.

Welsch, C. W., Bron, C. K., Goodrich-Smith, M., Chuisano, J., and Moon, R. C., 1980, Synergistic effect of chronic prolactin suppression and retinoid treatment in the prophylaxis of N-methyl-N-nitrosourea-induced mammary tumorigenesis in female Sprague–Dawley rats, *Cancer Res.* **40**:3095–3098.

Willmott, N., Austin, E. B., and Baldwin, R. W., 1979, Comparative studies of the metastasizing potential of three transplantable rat mammary carcinomas of spontaneous origin, *Br. J. Exp. Pathol.* **60**:499–506.

Wittliff, J. L., 1979, The steroid receptors of experimental mammary tumors, and their relationship to those of human-breast carcinoma, *Mol. Aspects Med.* **2**:395–437.

Wittliff, J. L., 1984, Steroid-hormone receptors in breast cancer, *Cancer* **53**:630–643.

Wolbach, S. D., and Howe, P. R., 1925, Tissue changes following deprivation of fat-soluble A vitamin, *J. Exp. Med.* **42**:753–777.

Wood, B. G., Washburn, L. L., Mukerjee, A. S., and Banerjee, M. R., 1975, Hormonal regulation of lobulo-alveolar growth, functional differentiation and regression of whole mouse mammary gland in organ culture, *J. Endocrinol.* **65**:1–6.

World Health Organization, 1981, Histological classification of tumours, No. 2, Histological typing of breast tumours, World Health Organization, 2nd ed., Geneva.

Wynder, E. L., Bross, I. J., and Hirayama, T., 1960, A study of the epidemiology of cancer of the breast, *Cancer* **13**:559–601.

Yanai, R., and Nagasawa, H., 1970, Effects of ergocornine and 2-Br-alpha-ergokryptin (CB-154) on the formation of mammary hyperplastic alveolar nodules and the pituitary prolactin levels in mice, *Experientia* **26**:645–650.

Yang, N. C., Castro, A. J., Lewis, M., and Wong, T. W., 1961, Polynuclear aromatic hydrocarbons, steroids and carcinogens, *Science* **134**:386–387.

Yogeeswaaran, G., and Salk, P., 1981, Metastatic potential is positively correlated with cell surface sialylation of cultured murine tumor cell lines, *Science* **212**:1514–1516.

Yokoro, K., and Furth, J., 1962, Determining role of "mammotropin" in induction of mammary tumors in mice by virus, *J. Natl. Cancer Inst.* **29:**887–909.

Yokoro, K., Furth, J., and Haran-Ghera, N., 1961, Induction of mammotropic pituitary tumors by X-rays in rats and mice: The role of mammotropes in development of mammary tumors, *Cancer Res.* **21:**178–186.

Yoo, T. J., Balint, J. P., Jr., Whiteaker, R. S., Floyd, R. A., and Kim, U., 1983, Circulating immune complexes in rats with metastasizing and nonmetastasizing mammary tumor, *Int. Arch. Allergy Appl. Immunol.* **71:**224–227.

CHAPTER 6

THE MAMMARY GLAND
A Model for Hormonal Control of
Differentiation and Preneoplasia

BARBARA K. VONDERHAAR and
MAITREYI BHATTACHARJEE

1. INTRODUCTION

In order to achieve full functional differentiation, i.e., copious synthesis and secretion of milk, the mammary gland undergoes a dramatic series of changes in morphology, size, composition, and activity throughout the life cycle of the animal. These changes begin in fetal life, continue throughout puberty and the attainment of sexual maturity, and are very pronounced during pregnancy and lactation. Development occurs in discrete stages throughout ontogency and is marked by changes in sensitivity of the glandular components to multiple hormones and growth factors. In addition, in several species, there exists in the otherwise dormant, mature glands morphologically discrete, pregnancylike structures (hyperplastic nodules) that have a high rate of developing into overt neoplasms. Because many of the morphogenetic and differentiative events that occur *in vivo* can be mimicked in various culture systems under controlled conditions, especially with murine tissue, the mouse mammary gland has proven to be an excellent model system for studying hormonal control of differentiation and preneoplasia.

BARBARA K. VONDERHAAR and MAITREYI BHATTACHARJEE • Laboratory of Pathophysiology, National Cancer Institute, National Institutes of Health, Bethesda, Maryland 20205. This paper is dedicated to Sr. Marguerite Neumann, Ph.D., Professor of Chemistry, Clarke College, mentor and friend, on the occasion of her retirement from active teaching.

2. MORPHOLOGICAL DEVELOPMENT

2.1. The Fetal and Neonatal Mammary Gland

Early in embryonic life (about the 11th day of gestation in the mouse), the mammary crest begins to appear on either side of the trunk as a zone of raised epiderm (Propper, 1978). Mitosis occurs in the mammary rudiment at a lower rate than in the surrounding epidermis, indicating that early fetal development is achieved by morphogenic movement of epidermal cells and displacement of neighboring ectodermal cells (Balinsky, 1950a). The fully formed mammary bud then goes into a brief (1- to 3-day) resting phase after which epithelial proliferation accelerates and sprout formation begins. Secondary sprout formation ensues so that by late gestation (day 19 in the mouse) the primitive ductal gland, present at birth, has been established (Figure 1) (Balinsky, 1950b).

Sexual dimorphism and hormonal control of mammary gland development are apparent early in fetal life. This is most obvious as an inhibition of growth of the epithelium and nipple attachment in the male (Raynaud *et al.*, 1970), which occurs between days 13 and 15 in the mouse and coincides with the emergence of androgens from the fetal testes. Under the influence of the male sex hormones, the mesenchyme condenses around the mammary bud ultimately leading to the isolation and partial destruction of the mammary bud. Development of the bud in the male mouse ceases (Raynaud and Raynaud, 1953; Colard and Gomot, 1975). Destruction of the embryonic mouse testes by X-radiation on day 13 prevents the condensation of mesenchyme around the mammary bud and subsequently the partial destruction of the mammary epithelium (Raynaud and Frilley, 1947; Raynaud, 1961). Destruction of the ovaries by X-radiation on day 13 does not alter mammary development in the female mouse (Raynaud, 1950), pointing out the dominance of the female phenotype. Destruction of the pituitary in 13-day mouse embryos does not affect normal morphogenesis of the mammary glands in either sex (Raynaud, 1971).

The destruction of the mammary rudiment in the male mouse is a precisely timed biological event that can be mimicked in explant culture *in vitro*. Kratochwil (1971, 1977) showed that mammary rudiments of both male and female embryos acquire androgen sensitivity on day 13 of fetal life and lose it during day 15. Development of the 14- and 15-day rudiments from either sex ceases when 10^{-9} M testosterone is added to the explanted tissues. The target tissue for the androgen is the mesenchyme (Kratochwil and Schwartz, 1976; Drews and Drews, 1977). Recombinants of mammary epithelium and mesenchyme from normal males and androgen-insensitive Tfm mutant embryos cultured in the presence of testosterone show that the mutant epithelium developed as a normal male gland when combined with normal mesenchyme whereas normal epithelium combined with Tfm mesenchyme gave a normal female type of mammary development. Autoradiography of [^{3}H]testosterone has localized the hormone binding sites to those mesen-

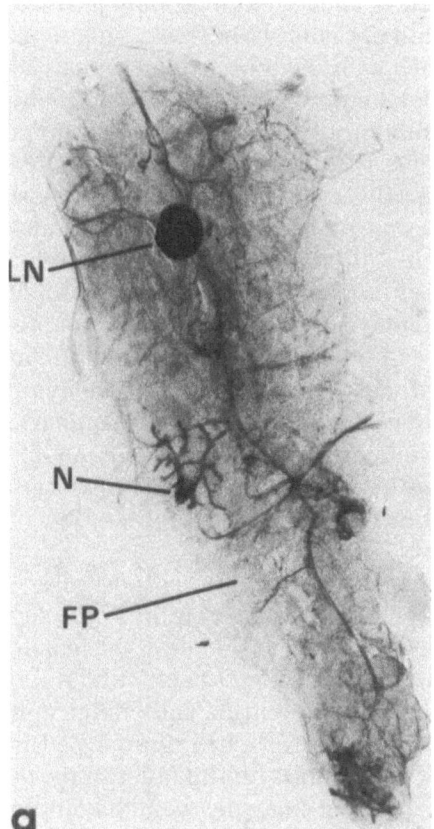
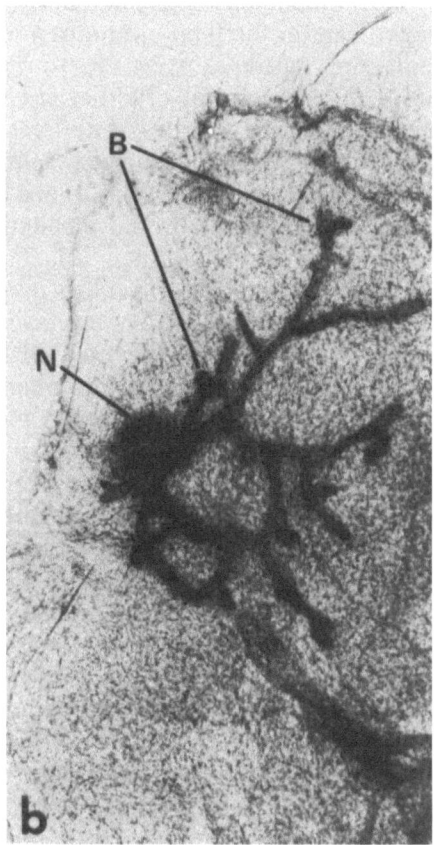

FIGURE 1. Whole mount preparation (a) of a #4 abdominal mammary gland from a 2-day-old female mouse (C3H/HeN MMTV$^+$). Panel b is a 6× enlargement of the nipple and epithelium of a similar gland. LN, lymph node; FP, fat pad; N, nipple; B, end bud. Glands were stained with hematoxylin (Vonderhaar and Greco, 1979).

chymal cells closest to the epithelial mammary bud (Heuberger et al., 1982). These receptors in mesenchyme are induced by the adjacent epithelium. The high-affinity androgen binding sites are present in mesenchyme at very low levels on day 12 but increase at least 20-fold by day 14 of fetal life. This high level is maintained until birth (Wasner et al., 1983). Thus, while acquisition of androgen sensitivity can be correlated with induction of receptors, loss of androgen responsiveness on day 15 is not assocaited with either a change in the number of binding sites or their affinity for the male sex hormones.

Estrogen receptors are also present in the mesenchyme but not the epithelium of 16-day female embryonic mammary gland (Narbaitz et al., 1980). Differentiation of the nipple accompanied by extensive proliferation of the surrounding mesenchyme can be induced by estrogen (Raynaud, 1955).

The mammary mesenchyme profoundly affects the morphological development of the fetal epithelium but does not alter its intrinsic functional potential. Sakakura et al. (1976) combined salivary mesenchyme obtained from 14-day embryos of either sex with mammary epithelium from 16-day female embryos in vitro. After transplantation of the recombinants under the kidney capsule of syngeneic female mice, the mammary grafts developed the typical histological appearance of the salivary gland. But when the host mice became pregnant and lactated, the transplants became secretory and synthesized the milk protein α-lactalbumin. The ability of fetal mesenchyme to affect morphogenesis persists even in adult mammary tissue (Sakakura et al., 1979). Embryonic mammary mesenchyme transplanted into intact glands of adult female mice promoted local areas of typical mammary gland ductal branching whereas similarly transplanted embryonic salivary mesenchyme promoted local areas of salivary gland-like growth of the adult mammary epithelium. More recently (Taga et al., 1983), embryonic mesenchyme has been shown to elaborate an epidermal growth factor (EGF)-like growth activity that blocks functional differentiation and promotes proliferation of adult mammary epithelial cells in primary culture.

A differentiative product of the mesenchyme, i.e., the adipose tissue that forms the mammary fat pad (Sakakura et al., 1982), continues to play an important role in mammary development throughout the life of the female animal. The mammary epithelium cannot grow or differentiate without the fat pad. It is the medium through which the ducts elongate and branch and in which the lobulo-alveolar structures propagate. At birth, the fat pad is small and well vascularized (Figure 1a). The mammary epithelium in the 1- to 5-day-old female consists of a primary duct that emanates from the nipple and short secondary and tertiary ducts. At the ends of the tertiary ducts are small dense end buds (Figure 1b).

Little change is observed in the gross morphology of the mammary gland during the first 3 weeks of life. The epithelial component slowly increases in size through elongation of the ducts. The growing end-buds are not as dense as during the first week. The fat pad increases in size and is not as well vascularized as in 1-day-old females (Figure 2a,b).

2.2. Attaining Sexual Maturity

At the beginning of the fourth week of life, puberty begins in the mouse. During the next several weeks, the fat pad and epithelium grow with the latter increasing in both size and degree of branching. Dense terminal end buds are still evident on the ends of the growing branched ducts. The growth of the epithelium occurs in an ordered fashion and is restricted by the dimensions of the fat pad. There is an inhibitory zone of unoccupied fat between each duct into which other ducts normally do not penetrate (Faulkin and DeOme, 1960) so that by week 8–10, the epithelial component has filled the entire fat pad with a network of highly branched ducts with many growing ends. Occasionally alveolar buds can be seen.

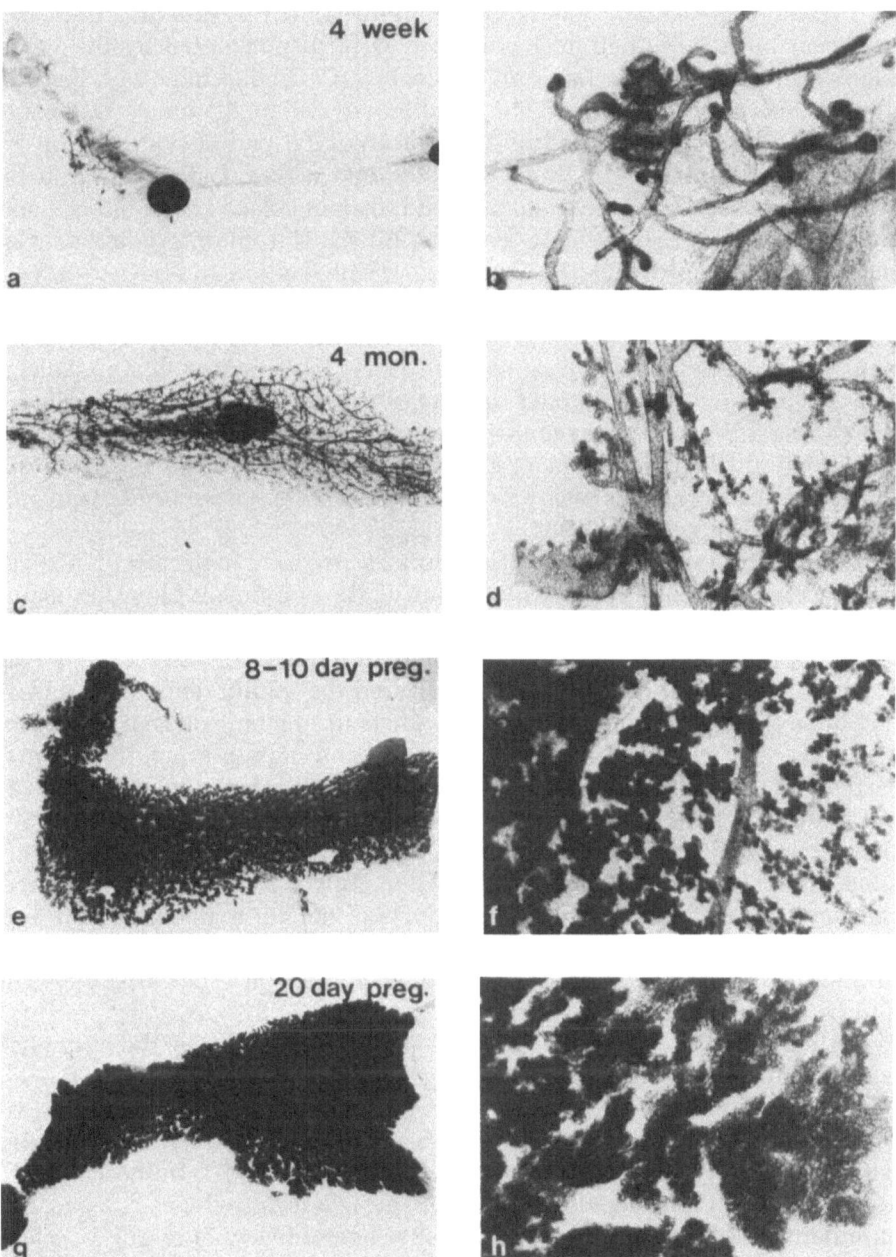

FIGURE 2. Whole mount preparations of #4 abdominal mammary glands from 4-week-old (a, b), 4-month-old sexually mature (c, d), 8- to 10-day pregnant (e, f), and 20-day pregnant (g, h) female mice (C3H/HeN MMTV⁺). Panels b, d, f, and h are 6× enlargements of the epithelial region of the glands shown in panels a, c, e, and g, respectively. Glands were stained with hematoxylin (Vonderhaar and Greco, 1979).

The importance of the fatty matrix in directing this ordered outgrowth of the mammary epithelium has been clearly demonstrated by the transplantation studies of DeOme and colleagues (DeOme et al., 1959; Faulkin and DeOme, 1960), Hoshino (1962), and Slavin (1966). Mammary fragments transplanted into the epithelium-free "cleared" fat pad of nonpregnant female mice grew out to the limits of the fat pad with a characteristic ductal pattern. However, similarly transplanted fragments placed in an intact gland were inhibited in their outgrowth by the interductal inhibitory fat zones of the endogenous epithelium (DeOme et al., 1959; Faulkin and DeOme, 1960). Transplants of mammary fragments successfully grew out only in the white fatty tissue of the mammary fat pad and transiently in the parametrial fat pad. No other tissue including spleen, ovary, liver, uterus, brain, skeletal muscle, or brown fat promoted mammary growth (Hoshino, 1962; Slavin, 1966). The difference in the ability of these tissues (especially white versus brown fat) to promote mammary growth is believed to be due in part to the quality of the fatty acids of the tissues' membrane phospholipids (Kidwell et al., 1982; Young et al., 1984).

Multiple hormones and growth factors are involved in the morphological development of the mammary gland during the attainment of sexual maturity. In an attempt to ascertain precisely which of these are involved in morphogenesis and which in functional differentiation, Nandi and colleagues (Richards et al., 1982, 1983) cultured the undifferentiated terminal end buds of immature mouse mammary ducts in a rat tail collagen gel matrix supplemented with various sera, hormones, and growth-promoting agents. Media containing horse and porcine serum and cholera toxin promoted growth but not functional differentiation of the epithelial cells. The presence of 5% porcine serum, insulin, cholera toxin, estradiol, progesterone, hydrocortisone, and prolactin in the media stimulated growth maximally and induced the synthesis of the differentiated products of the adult gland, caseins and thioesterase as well as a secretory ultrastructure. The nature of the growth-promoting factors in the sera remains to be defined, but this culture system affords an excellent method to do so.

After full sexual maturity is reached (3–4 months of age), the epithelial component that fills the fat pad undergoes cyclic variations during the estrous cycle. Epithelial DNA synthesis is highest during proestrus, the estrogenic phase of the cycle (Sutton and Suhribier, 1967). Mitosis occurs during late estrus and metestrus (Grahame and Bertalanffy, 1972; Dulbecco et al., 1982). Although only small increments of growth occur with each cycle, the cumulative effect is extensive ductal side branching (Figure 2c). In some strains, especially those containing the mammary tumor virus (Squartini et al., 1983), isolated alveolar structures can be seen (Figure 2d).

2.3. Pregnancy and Lactation

Full functional differentiation of the mammary gland is dependent upon the number of cells in the gland producing the milk as well as the amount synthesized per cell. To achieve this end, the gland goes through marked changes during pregnancy exemplified by controlled cellular proliferation. This results in enlargement of the lobulo-alveolar structures in preparation for the synthetic and secretory activity that occurs during lactation.

Proliferation of the epithelial cells occurs at the expense of the fat cells of the gland and within 3 days after coitus, increased ductal branching and extensive alveolar formation has already occurred. Alveolar buds begin to form along the lateral walls of the mammary ducts and their numerous side branches. By day 6–8 of gestation, the alveoli begin to cluster to form true lobulo-alveolar structures (Figure 2e,f). Small lumina can occasionally be seen in histological sections. Toward the end of the second week of pregnancy, lobulo-alveolar formation begins to slow and these structures predominate in the gland. Histological sections show lobules that are now well formed and composed of many alveoli.

After the middle of pregnancy, cellular synthesis of the secretory products is initiated. A marked increase in the size of individual epithelial cells results from accumulation of the secretion products (Foster, 1977). As a result, alveoli expand and unfold so that by day 20 of gestation the thickness of the gland has increased considerably. The highly vascularized gland of late pregnancy is dominated by the alveoli (Figure 2g) so that the ductal elements are not visible in whole mount preparations. This predominance of alveoli (Figure 2h) continues throughout active lactation.

The size of the secretory cell population increases drmatically during gestation with an estimated 78% of mammary cell growth in the mouse taking place during this period (Brookreson and Turner, 1959). There is also a transient surge of cell proliferation between days 3 and 5 postpartum in the mouse (Traurig, 1967a,b; Knight and Peaker, 1982a). Within 3 days of parturition the alveoli are highly distended and the gland becomes engorged with milk. This appearance of the gland remains virtually unchanged throughout the 21–22 days of lactation in the mouse.

Following lactation, or premature separation of the nursing young from the dam, the alveolar components begin to involute. Within 5 days, milk accumulation has completely ceased and extensive cellular debris is present in the lumen. By day 10 of involution, the lobules and alveoli have significantly decreased in number. The gland eventually regresses until only a highly branched ductal system with a few alveoli remains. This gland is similar in appearance to the gland of a sexually mature virgin animal (Figure 2c).

Many hormones are necessary for the cellular replication during pregnancy that leads to the appearance of the lobulo-alveolar structures. Delineation of the hormones involved, their individual functions and their multiple interactions has been examined in vivo by several laboratories using hormonal ablation or hormone treatment or a combination of both. The work of Turner and Gomez (1934) and Nandi and colleagues (Nandi, 1958, 1959; Nandi and Bern, 1961) established that maintenance of alveoli in mice requires intact ovaries and pituitary. In ovariectomized, hypophysectomized animals, estrogen and progesterone or estrogen and growth hormone can maintain alveoli. Thyroid hormones, in concert with prolactin (Vonderhaar, 1982), stimulate the formation of alveoli in the mouse (Mixner and Turner, 1942; Dubnik et al., 1950; Vonderhaar and Greco, 1979). Adrenalectomy has little effect on maintenance of alveoli (Turner and Gomez, 1934; Nandi, 1958); however, adrenal steroids are important in development of lobules (Banerjee, 1976). Development of lobulo-alveolar structures in triply operated (ovariectomy, hypophysectomy, adrenalectomy) mice requires prolonged treatment with estrogen, progesterone, deoxycorticosterone acetate, and prolactin and/or growth hormone (Nandi, 1958; Nandi and Bern, 1960).

The natural cycles of growth, lobulo-alveolar development, and loss of alveoli during glandular involution can be sequentially mimicked in vitro using a whole organ culture technique first described by Ichinose and Nandi (1964, 1966) and refined by Banerjee and co-workers (Banerjee et al., 1973; Banerjee, 1976) and by Tonelli and Sorof (1980). Full lobulo-alveolar development is achieved in culture using the entire second thoracic gland from 3- to 4-week-old female BALB/c mice primed by daily injections of estradiol-17β (1 μg) and progesterone (1 mg) or s.c. insertion of a slow-release cholesterol-based pellet containing the two steroids (Vonderhaar, 1984) for 9 days, cultivated in chemically defined hormonally supplemented medium. The length of the estrogen–progesterone priming required to allow for a full response in vitro varies among strains of mice (Singh et al., 1970) and is dependent on the hormones and growth factors in the medium (Vonderhaar, 1984). Initially, this culture method yielded only a single round of development by the glands of mice primed for 9 days and cultured at least 5 or 6 days under the influence of the minimum hormonal combination of insulin, prolactin, aldosterone and hydrocortisone (Table I and Figure 3b). The estrogen–progesterone priming process itself is insufficient to initiate lobulo-

TABLE I

Hormone Priming Required in Vivo for Responsiveness of
Tissue in Vitro[a]

Priming conditions		Hormones in culture		
Hormones	Days	IPrlAH	IPrlAH + EGF	IPrlAH + E + P
None	None	0/15	0/15	0/9
E	9	0/9	—	—
P	9	0/9	—	—
E/P	3	0/15	0/15	—
E/P	6	1/15	14/15	—
E/P	9	15/15	15/15	—

[a]Four-week-old female BALB/c mice were primed with s.c. cholesterol-based pellets containing estradiol-17β (E) or progesterone (P) or both E/P as described by Vonderhaar (1984). The second thoracic glands were then cultured in serum-free medium containing insulin, prolactin, aldosterone, and hydrocortisone (IPrlAH); or ECF (10^{-9} M) or estradiol 17β (10^{-9} M) and progesterone (10^{-7} M). After 9 days in culture, glands were removed, fixed, and stained with hematoxylin (Vonderhaar and Greco, 1979).

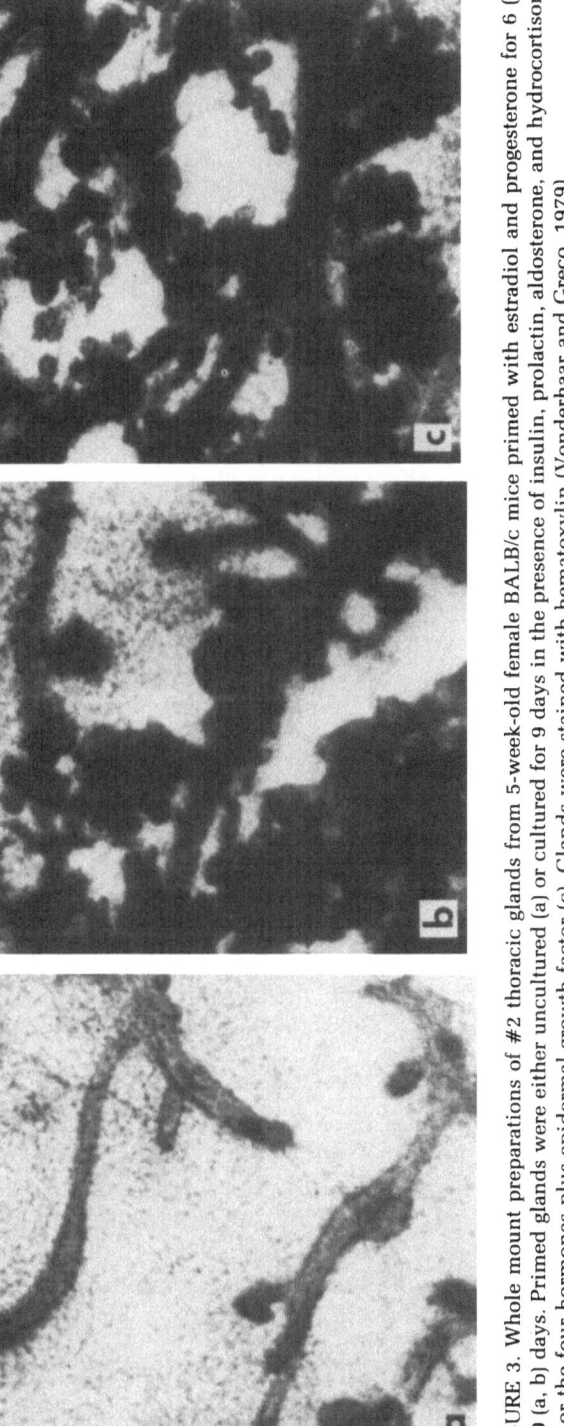

FIGURE 3. Whole mount preparations of #2 thoracic glands from 5-week-old female BALB/c mice primed with estradiol and progesterone for 6 (c) or 9 (a, b) days. Primed glands were either uncultured (a) or cultured for 9 days in the presence of insulin, prolactin, aldosterone, and hydrocortisone (b) or the four hormones plus epidermal growth factor (c). Glands were stained with hematoxylin (Vonderhaar and Greco, 1979).

alveolar growth *in vivo* (Figure 3a), but is an absolute requirement for response *in vitro* (Ichinose and Nandi, 1966; Vonderhaar, 1984). Neither estrogen nor progesterone alone is sufficient during the priming period to prepare the gland to respond to the four hormones *in vitro* to initiate lobulo-alveolar development (Table I).

Addition of thyroid hormones, which are essential for alveolar formation in mice *in vivo* (Vonderhaar and Greco, 1979), is not required *in vitro*. This is presumably due to the presence of endogenous hormone carried into the medium by the tissue (Vonderhaar, 1982) since it is the ratio of prolactin to thyroid hormones in the system that greatly affects the degree of lobulo-alveolar development observed. Using the whole organ culture system, Singh and Bern (1969) showed that addition of T_4 (0.01–5 μg/ml) to the medium altered the responsiveness of the tissue to prolactin. Both positive and negative effects of the thyroid hormone were demonstrated. In the presence of optimal concentrations of insulin, glucocorticoids, and prolactin, low concentrations of T_4 had no effect on lobulo-alveolar development whereas high concentrations of T_4 were inhibitory. In cultures maintained with suboptimal amounts of prolactin, low levels of T_4 enhanced lobulo-alveolar development whereas higher concentrations of T_4 were inhibitory. In the absence of prolactin, thyroxine cannot promote lobulo-alveolar development *in vitro* (Warner, 1978).

Addition of estrogen and progesterone to the medium is not essential even though these ovarian steroids are required for alveolar formation *in vivo* in the sexually mature female. It has been suggested that the lack of a requirement for estradiol and progesterone may reflect either residual steroids from the priming process that are carried into culture or the persistence *in vitro* of their biological effects initiated *in vivo* (Topper and Freeman, 1980). That the former possibility is not the sole answer is clear in that addition of estradiol and progesterone to medium containing insulin, prolactin, aldosterone, and hydrocortisone is not sufficient to initiate lobulo-alveolar development *in vitro* in glands from unprimed mice (Table I). That the latter possibility is more likely the case is supported by recent work from the laboratories of Banerjee, Sorof, and ourselves.

Viability of the ductal elements of the glands from estrogen–progesterone-primed mice requires only the presence of insulin in the culture medium (Mehta and Banerjee, 1975). Following lobulo-alveolar development *in vitro* under the influence of the four-hormone mammogenic combination, withdrawing all of the hormones except insulin for 9 days results in full alveolar regression (involution), leaving only the ductal structures intact (Wood *et al.*, 1975). The regressed epithelial components resemble the postlactational involuted mammary gland, thus completing *in vitro* the natural developmental cycle of the gland *in vivo*.

A second round of development *in vitro*, following complete regression, can only be initiated if EGF or EGF-like growth factors are added to the medium with insulin, prolactin, aldosterone, and hydrocortisone (Tonelli and Sorof, 1980, 1981). This second round of development can only be achieved if the mice are primed with estradiol and progesterone for a minimum of 9 days prior to the onset of culture. The lack of a requirement for EGF in the initial round of development after 9 days of priming is believed to reflect the presence of EGF and/or EGF-like growth factors supplied to the cultures by the primed tissue. When glands from the mice are cultured after only 6 days of priming, full lobulo-alveolar development is achieved only if EGF or a mammary gland-derived EGF-like growth factor is added to the four-hormone mammogenic combination (Figure 3c, Table I). Glands from unprimed animals or animals primed for only 3 days are unable to develop even in the presence of EGF (Table I). This requirement for EGF cannot be met by platelet-derived growth factor or fibroblast growth factor (Vonderhaar, 1984).

The estrogen–progesterone priming process increases submaxillary gland EGF synthesis. However, extracts of glands of mice primed by the steroids for 9 days do not contain EGF at levels detectable by radioimmunoassay (Vonderhaar, 1984). These same extracts, however, do contain an activity that competes for hepatic EGF receptors and when added with the four-hormone mammogenic combination to cultures of glands from animals primed with estrogen and progesterone for 6 days, promote full lobulo-alveolar development. This mammary-derived EGF-like growth factor is extracted from the epithelium-rich region of the mammary glands and is more effective than EGF since levels as low as 0.3 ng EGF equivalents/ml (based on binding competition) are equivalent in activity to 30–60 ng EGF/ml in vitro (Vonderhaar, 1984). Thus, it appears that estrogen–progesterone priming may induce an EGF-like factor in the mammary glands of the mice. The site of synthesis of this factor, its molecular nature, and which hormone (estradiol or progesterone) induces it are yet to be elucidated. However, the whole organ mammary culture system affords an excellent model for unraveling these events in vitro and shedding light on the sequence of events involved in the natural development and involution of the mammary gland in vivo.

2.4. Preneoplastic Hyperplastic Nodules

The whole organ culture system has also proven effective in studies designed to define the sequence of events occurring during neoplastic transformation of the mammary gland and the genesis of overt mammary tumors. This is a complex, multistep process (Nandi and McGrath, 1973; Medina, 1978; Cairns and Logan, 1983) characterized in the early stages in several species by the appearance of morphologically distinct preneoplastic lesions. Preneoplastic elements are demonstrable in carcinogen-treated rat mammary glands (Dao et al., 1975; Sinha and Dao, 1977; Rivera et al., 1981) and in human breast samples (Jensen et al., 1976; King et al., 1983). In the human breast, dysplasias such as carcinoma in situ and precancerous cystic hyperplasia are considered as high-risk lesions more likely to produce overt tumors (Black and Chabon, 1969; Wellings et al., 1975). Although ductal dysplasias of the mammary gland have been described (Ethier and Ullrich, 1982), the

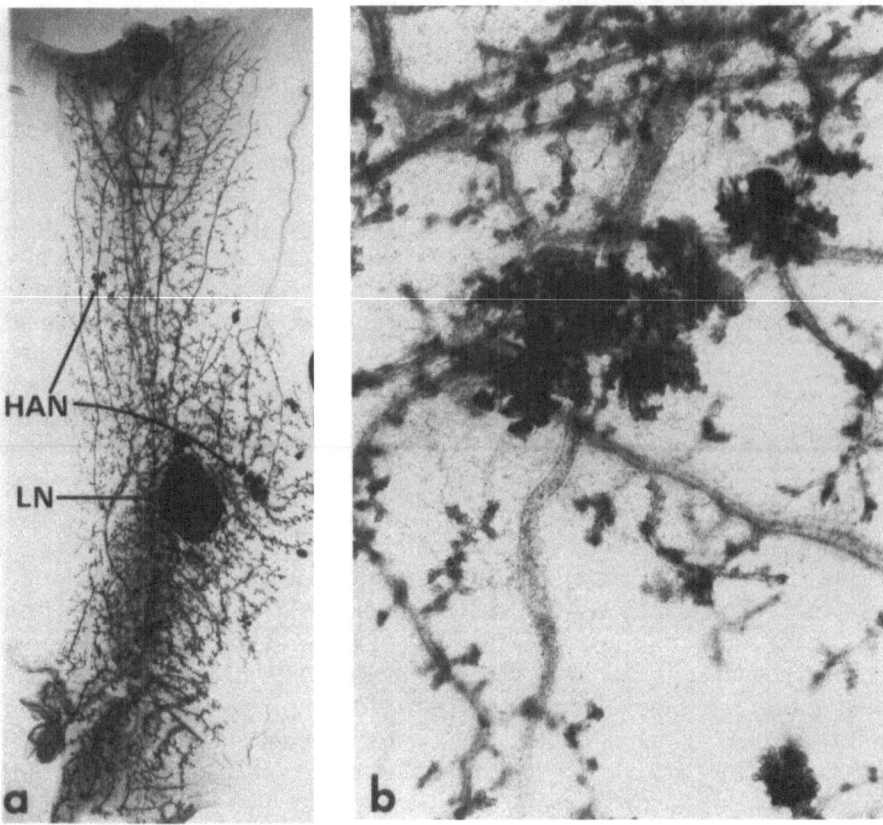

FIGURE 4. Whole mount preparation (a) of a #4 abdominal mammary gland of an 8-month-old virgin female mouse (C3H/HeN MMTV[+]) containing numerous hyperplastic alveolar nodules (HAN). Panel b is a 6× enlargement of a region of the gland containing overt HAN. Panel

principal preneoplastic lesion in the mouse is the hyperplastic alveolar nodule (HAN), which appears as a distinct concentration of dense hyperplastic lobulo-alveolar development in an area containing predominantly nonstimulated ductal epithelium with occasional small clusters of alveoli (Figure 4a,b). The HAN can be induced in mice by hormones, the murine mammary tumor virus (MMTV), or chemical carcinogens (Faulkin, 1966; Medina and DeOme, 1968, 1970b). The HAN may exist in the mouse either as a primary lesion or it can be transplanted as an outgrowth within the epithelium-free, "cleared" mammary fat pad of a syngeneic host (DeOme et al., 1959; Medina and DeOme, 1970a,b; Ashley et al., 1980). Primary HAN arise in MMTV-bearing virgin animals any time after 6 months of age. In involuted postlactational glands of parous animals, the lesions are more numerous and may appear earlier. In histological sections the HAN appear to be composed of many alveoli with large lumina frequently containing secretory material. Lining the alveolus is a single layer of highly vacuolated columnar cells

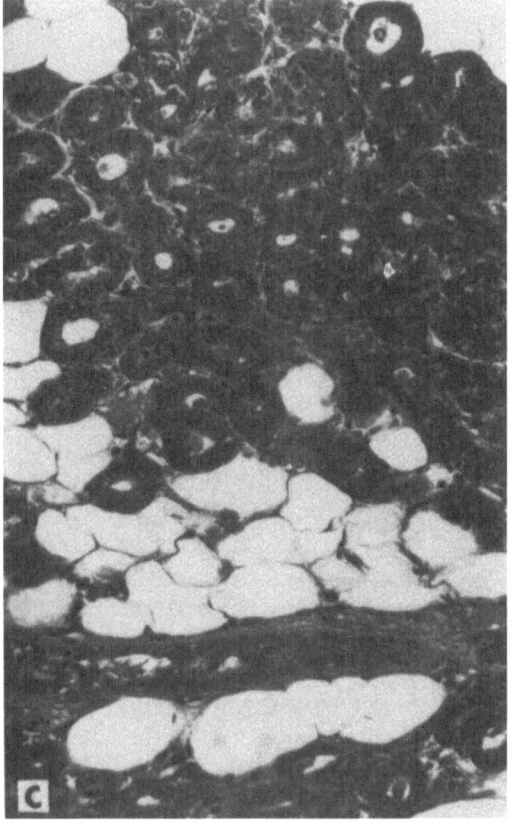

c is a histological section through the pregnancylike HAN. Whole mounts were stained with hematoxylin (Vonderhaar and Greco, 1979); histological section was stained with hematoxylin and eosin. LN, lymph node.

surrounded by a thin layer of connective tissue. Typical HAN are histologically and cytochemically indistinguishable from normal prelactational lobules at approximately day 14 of gestation (Figure 4c).

The preneoplastic nature of the murine HAN was first demonstrated by DeOme et al. (1959) by transplantation of selected foci into the epithelium-free fat pad. Normal tissue grew out into the pad with characteristic ductal outgrowths while preneoplastic tissue filled the fat pads with hyperplastic alveolar tissue. This latter tissue outgrowth produced overt mammary tumors sooner and with greater frequency than did the normal outgrowth in the contralateral fat pads. The cells of the HAN outgrowths are stably hyperplastic and outgrowth lines have been established from these lesions. These are used to examine the characteristics that account for their preneoplastic condition and the various factors that may affect their development (Medina, 1973). In general, the characteristics of the HAN are similar whether they result from chemical, viral, or hormonal transformation.

The number of HAN and appearance of overt tumors are enhanced in MMTV-bearing mice by a single pregnancy (Riley, 1975; B. K. Vonderhaar, unpublished observations). Ovariectomy and hypophysectomy, but not adrenalectomy, inhibit the growth of several nodule lines (Medina, 1973). This suggests that HAN induction, as well as maintenance, may be under hormonal control. *In vivo* studies have suggested that estrogen plus progesterone or glucocorticoids plus growth hormone or prolactin are necessary for noduligenesis (Nandi *et al.*, 1960; Nandi, 1963). The same hormones, except for estrogen, are necessary for maintenace of the HAN *in vivo* (Nandi, 1961). The hormonal requirements for nodule induction and maintenance are the same as those for mammogenesis. In part this is due to the hormonally induced increase in proliferative activity in the mammary epithelial cells. Increased levels of DNA synthesis in the tissue at the time of carcinogen treatment result in increased noduligenesis and tumorigenesis (Adamson *et al.*, 1971) presumably by an increase in the susceptibility of the mitotic mammary tissue to the transforming action of the oncogenic agents. How this occurs and the role of hormones and growth-modifying factors in this event have been the subject of investigations in several laboratories using the *in vitro* serum-free conditions of the whole organ culture model.

Initially, Banerjee *et al.* (1974) showed that the mammary glands of estrogen–progesterone-primed C3HfC57BL mice, treated with either 7,12-dimethylbenz(a)anthracene (DMBA) or 3-methylcholanthrene (MCA) for 24 hr *in vitro* during the first wave of hormonally induced DNA synthesis, followed by carcinogen-free periods of growth and regression, resulted in the presence of isolated microscopic areas of lobulo-alveolar structures in 26% of the regressed glands. Nonregressed alveolar areas were absent in control glands treated only with the solvents for the carcinogens. Histologically, these nonregressed lobulo-alveolar structures resembled primary HAN found in mice, but they failed to produce HAN-like hyperplastic outgrowths or overt tumors when transplanted into the cleared fat pads of syngeneic virgin hosts. Similar results were subsequently reported by Sorof and coworkers using glands from estrogen–progesterone-primed BALB/c mice and either DMBA or 2-acetylaminofluorene (FAA) and derivatives as the carcinogens *in vitro* (Tonelli *et al.*, 1979; Schaefer *et al.*, 1983). The appearance *in vitro* of the transformed foci induced by procarcinogens, but not by many activated carcinogens, can be prevented by the simultaneous addition to the culture medium of retinoids, the natural and synthetic analogues of vitamin A (Dickens *et al.*, 1979; Dickens and Sorof, 1981; Mehta *et al.*, 1983; Banerjee, 1985).

The inability of the nodulelike alveolar lesions (NLAL) to produce hyperplastic outgrowths and overt tumors was overcome by Banerjee and coworkers by modifications of the original experimental design. The hormonal combination used for morphogenesis was reduced to insulin, prolactin, aldosterone, and hydrocortisone to give maximum lobulo-alveolar development and limited functional differentiation. Under the influence of these four hormones, two waves of DNA synthesis are observed during the initial round of development. The first wave, which primarily represents those cells (35–40% of the epithelial cells) that entered the S phase of the cell cycle in vivo as a result of the estrogen–progesterone priming of the mice, reaches a peak at 48 hr of culture in the presence of the hormones. This is followed by a second wave of DNA synthesis between days 3 and 4 of culture and involves about 10% of the epithelial cells (Lin et al., 1976). The cytotoxicity of the carcinogen (i.e., DMBA) was examined in detail to allow for maximal retention of cell proliferation and normal lobulo-alveolar development after carcinogen treatment. Treatment of the glands with the carcinogen even at reduced dosage, during the first wave of DNA synthesis, results in some cytotoxic effects (Banerjee, 1984). Consequently, a sublethal dose of DMBA was chosen for treatment of the cultures during the second wave of DNA synthesis, thus allowing for enhanced transformation of the mammary gland in vitro followed by near-normal hormonally supported development of the glands subseqeunt to carcinogen treatment. Under this schedulee, glands cultured in the presence of insulin, prolactin, aldosterone, and hydrocortisone and treated with DMBA between day 3 and 4 of culture show NLAL in 79% of the glands (Telang et al., 1979; Iyer and Banerjee, 1981). MCA treatment under similar conditions in vitro produced NLAL transformed foci in 40% of the glands (Lin et al., 1976).

The importance of all four hormones, and the adrenal steroids in particular, during the transformation process is clear in that a greatly reduced (35%) incidence of NLAL formation was obtained when hydrocortisone was omitted from the culture medium and no NLAL were obtained when aldosterone was omitted during the carcinogen treatment (Banerjee, 1985). Since the hormone combinations of insulin, prolactin, aldosterone, and hydrocortisone or insulin, prolactin, and aldosterone are virtually identical in this culture system for promoting morphogenesis (Banerjee et al., 1976), it would appear that hydrocortisone plays some role in transformation of the epithelial cells at a level other than stimulation of cell proliferation.

That the NLAL thus induced are truly transformed "preneoplastic" structures requires that they display true stable outgrowth characteristics and tumorigenicity upon transplantation into cleared fat pads of syngeneic mice. To establish this relationship, Banerjee and co-workers (Telang et al., 1979; Iyer and Banerjee, 1981) transplanted a single piece of the tissue from the DMBA-treated glands into one cleared fat pad and a piece of control (solvent treated) tissue into the contralateral cleared fat pad of virgin mice. These host mice were then given a pituitary isograft under the kidney capsule for 6 weeks to provide for continual prolactin stimulation of the mammary cells (Welsch and Nagasawa, 1977). The graft and resulting prolactin stimulus was removed and 10 to 12 weeks later the glands whole mounted and examined for hyperplastic outgrowths. Such hyperplasias were apparent in 46% of the outgrowths from DMBA-treated tissue, whereas control tissue produced only normal ductal outgrowth patterns. Mammary carcinomas were obtained from 13% of the implants carried into another transplant generation in syngeneic virgin mice carrying no pituitary isograft. The tumorigenicity of the in vitro DMBA-induced outgrowth can be enhanced by using colla-genase-digested cells obtained from first-generation outgrowths. In this case, 56% of the implants gave hyperplastic outgrowths with a 31% tumor inci-dence. One of these hyperplastic outgrowths subsequently produced 80% mammary tumors in the third generation (Banerjee, 1985).

Thus, like the hyperplastic outgrowths from primary in vivo MMTV- or DMBA-induced HAN (Medina, 1973; DeOme et al., 1978), implants of in vitro DMBA-induced NLAL produce stable, morphologically similar hyper-plastic outgrowths and can result in overt mammary tumors in syngeneic mice. This in vitro whole organ culture system, which can now give two complete rounds of hormone- and growth factor-induced development (To-nelli and Sorof, 1980; Vonderhaar, 1984), can be used to systematically define those hormonal conditions that influence the various steps in transformation of the normal mammary epithelium to the preneoplastic state by oncogenic agents. The hormones and growth factors involved in maintenance and prop-agation of the preneoplastic condition can be clearly defined. In addition, the mechanism of carcinogenesis by several chemicals may be clarified under the controlled conditions that this model system provides.

3. FUNCTIONAL DIFFERENTIATION

3.1. Lactogenesis

It is during lactation that the total synthetic and secretory capabilities of the mammary epithelial cells are displayed, resulting in production of all components of milk necessary to sustain the life of the nursing young. Milk yield increases gradually for the first 7 days of lactation in the mouse (Knight and Peaker, 1982a), reaching a peak at day 10. Since cell proliferation has ceased in the mouse by day 5 postpartum (Traurig, 1967a,b; Knight and Peaker, 1982a), the final increase in milk production is due to enhanced, hormonally induced synthesis and secretion of the various components of milk. The individual epithelial cells of a given alveolus differentiate in an all-or-none fashion (Keenan et al., 1970) while adjacent alveoli, in histolog-ical section, can range from nearly undifferentiated in appearance to fully differentiated milk-filled secretory structures (Nolin, 1979; Smith and Von-derhaar, 1981).

Milk is a complex biological fluid composed of many proteins, hor-mones, growth factors, vitamins, cellular metabolites, minerals, immuno-globulins, sugars, and lipids (Kuhn, 1977; Cowie et al., 1980; Tucker, 1981). The synthesis, secretion, and transport of these components by and through the mammary gland have been the subject of extensive research in many laboratories. Although other factors such as nutrition, environment, and neurological agents can affect lactogenesis (Knight and Peaker, 1982b), the mammary gland has proven most useful in examining the role of hormones and growth factors in differentiation. These studies have been greatly aided by culture systems (primary epithelial cells, explant and whole organ) that use chemically defined, serum-free medium.

3.2. Milk-Protein Synthesis and Secretion

Several useful markers of the fully differentiated mammary epithelial cells are the characteristic milk proteins, the caseins, α-lactalbumin, and whey acid protein. The maximum hormonally induced synthesis and secretion of these proteins by the mouse mammary gland in vitro requires that the epithelial cells in culture first elaborate the synthetic machinery or rough endoplasmic reticulum (RER). Using explants of glands from midpregnancy primiparous mice and the culture system first defined by Elias (1957), Topper and co-workers attempted to define the hormonal requirements for production of stable RER and secretory Golgi apparatus. Explants cultured for 96 hr in the presence of insulin and hydrocortisone contain cells with abundant RER that is mostly undilated and is randomly distributed in the cytoplasm. The Golgi are fairly well developed but are lateral to the nucleus and virtually devoid of granules (Mills and Topper, 1970). Between 48 and 96 hr after addition of prolactin to this culture medium, nearly all of the epithelial cells take on an ultrastructure similar to that of cells from lactating tissue with highly polarized organelles. The RER and nucleus are in the basal cytoplasm and the highly developed Golgi are in the apical cytoplasm. Nucleoli are enlarged and mitochondrial abundant; secretory protein granules and abundant lipid droplets are present in the apical cytoplasm.

If the initial incubation of the explants is with insulin only, no RER develop until 48 hr after subsequent addition of hydrocortisone and prolactin. By 96 hr of culture in the presence of all three hormones, the fully secretory appearance is attained (Mills and Topper, 1970). Oka and Topper (1971) found that a transient formation of RER occurs when prolactin alone is added to explants previously cultured in the presence of insulin alone. Production of RER under the influence of insulin and glucocorticoids appears to be through association of previously free ribosomes with newly synthesized membranes without a net increase in total ribosomes. In a similar study, using explants of mammary glands from virgin mice, the essential role of insulin and hydrocortisone in establishing a secretory ultrastructure and the role of prolactin in maintaining it were confirmed (Vonderhaar and Smith, 1982).

The characteristic secretory proteins of the mammary gland are synthesized on the RER. The hormonal requirements for RER formation, accumulation of the milk-protein mRNA, and synthesis of the secretory products are very similar. For expression of casein genes in mouse mammary tissue in vitro, which may result from changes in DNA methylation patterns (Razin and Riggs, 1980; Bolander, 1983), a minimum of four hormones (insulin, glucocorticoid, prolactin, and estrogen) is required. Insulin is specifically required for the accumulation of casein mRNAs and synthesis of the four major casein species by explants of mammary glands from midpregnancy mice. After 4 hr of culture in the presence of cortisol and prolactin, only 20% of the casein mRNA initially present in the tissue remains (Bolander et al., 1981). When insulin is included in the medium, however, a 14-fold increase in the accumulation of casein mRNas is observed. Neither EGF nor somatomedin C can substitute for insulin (Topper et al., 1984). The level of insulin that supports casein synthesis in the presence of cortisol and pro- lactin is in the physiological range (Bolander et al., 1981), and can be replaced by antiinsulin receptor serum (Nicholas and Topper, 1983).

The essential role of the glucocorticoid, which was demonstrated in vivo (Ganguly et al., 1979), was confirmed in vitro using the whole organ culture system described previously. Casein mRNA levels increase 134-fold when morphologically developed glands previously cultured in corticoste- roid-free growth-promoting medium are transferred to medium containing the lactogenic combination of insulin, prolactin, and cortisol. After 6 days in this lactogenic medium, abundant milklike secretory material is found in the alveolar lumina of the cultured tissue. Omission of either cortisol or prolactin from the latter incubation results in no increase in casein mRNAs or peptide synthesis (Terry et al., 1977; Mehta et al., 1980). Although this requirement for glucocorticoid may not be absolute, the presence of the steroid is essential for maximal accumulation of the casein mRNAs induced by prolactin (Nagaiah et al., 1981).

The requirement for estrogen is not as readily demonstrated since this hormone is frequently carried into the culture medium by the mammary tissue from the adult or estrogen–progesterone-primed immature mice. How- ever, using ovariectomized mice, Bolander and Topper (1980b) demonstrated that the mammary tissue from these mice does not synthesize casein in vitro in response to insulin, cortisol, and prolactin. Neither does this cultured tissue accumulate casein mRNA (Bolander and Topper, 1981b). Respon- siveness of the tissue in vitro is restored by estrogen replacement therapy in vivo (Bolander and Topper, 1980b). An estrogen effect on functional dif- ferentiation in vitro using tissue from intact adult, midpregnancy mice could only be demonstrated in the presence of suboptimal concentrations of pro- lactin (Bolander and Topper, 1980a).

Similar hormonal requirements for casein gene expression in vitro have been reported for primary MMTV-induced HAN, transplanted hyperplastic outgrowth lines (Smith et al., 1984), and in vitro DMBA-induced NLAL (Ganguly et al., 1982; Banerjee et al., 1983).

Whey acidic protein (WAP) has only recently been identified as a major secretory product of the mouse mammary gland. This protein is distinct from α-lactalbumin, although both of these milk proteins have molecular weights of 14,000 (Piletz et al., 1981; Hennighausen and Sippel, 1982a,b; Bhatta- charjee and Vonderhaar, 1983). Using a cDNA probe synthesized from an mRNA fraction highly enriched for WAP sequences (Henninghausen and Sippel, 1982a; Motojima and Oka, 1983), Banerjee and colleagues have investigated the hormonal requirements for WAP gene expression using the two-step whole organ culture system and glands from estrogen–

progesterone-primed mice (Banerjee *et al.*, 1983). They report that WAP mRNA is virtually undetectable in the morphologically developed glands after 6 days of culture in the corticosteroid-free medium. After 3 days of culture in the lactogenic medium containing insulin, prolactin, and cortisol, WAP mRNA is induced to a level of 0.015% of the total RNA of the gland. Neither prolactin nor cortisol alone was stimulatory even in the presence of insulin. Although a role for estrogens in WAP gene expression has yet to be demonstrated, it currently appears that the accumulation of WAP mRNA in the mouse mammary gland *in vitro* is under similar hormonal control as is casein.

Another major milk protein used as a marker for functional differentiation of the mammary gland is α-lactalbumin. This protein modifies the specificity of galactosyltransferase so that glucose becomes a physiologically significant substrate for the enzyme system and lactose is produced during lactation (Ebner *et al.*, 1966; Brodbeck *et al.*, 1967). The α-lactalbumin purified from mouse milk (Zamierowski and Ebner, 1980) and lactating mammary glands (Bhattacharjee and Vonderhaar, 1983) has an apparent molecular weight of 14,000. The α-lactalbumin purified from the lactating gland exists as two charged forms with pIs of 6.2 and 5.8 (Bhattacharjee and Vonderhaar, 1983) and is distinct from WAP, which has a pI of 4.7 (Piletz *et al.*, 1981). Accumulation of the α-lactalbumin mRNA and synthesis of the secretory protein *in vitro* has the same minimal hormonal requirement of insulin (Nicholas and Topper, 1983; Topper *et al.*, 1984), prolactin (Vonderhaar *et al.*, 1973; Perry and Oka, 1984), glucocorticoid (Ono and Oka, 1980a,b; Nagamatsu and Oka, 1983; Terada *et al.*, 1983), and estrogen (Bolander and Topper, 1980a,b, 1981b). However, in order to more accurately mimic *in vitro* the physiological conditions for α-lactalbumin synthesis and secretion, both quantitatively and qualitatively, addition of thyroid hormone to the culture medium is also required (Vonderhaar, 1975, 1979; Bhattacharjee and Vonderhaar, 1984). An increase in α-lactalbumin activity is achieved at physiological concentrations of L-T_3 (3,5,3'-triiodothyronine). Neither D-T_3 nor monoiodothyronine nor diiodotyrosine is effective and L-T_4 (3,5,3'5'-tetraiodothyronine or thyroxine) requires as much as a 100-fold greater concentration in the medium to achieve the same maximal effect as L-T_3 (Table II). This effect of L-T_3 is selective for α-lactalbumin since neither [^{3}H]thymidine incorporation into DNA, nor casein synthesis, nor the activities of galactosyltransferase, glucose-6-phosphate dehydrogenase, and gluconate-6-phosphate dehydrogenase were increased by the addition of L-T_3 to the cultures (Vonderhaar, 1975). L-T_3 does not substitute for any of the other hormones in the culture, including prolactin (Vonderhaar, 1977). However, it does increase the sensitivity of the mammary gland to the action of prolactin both *in vivo* and *in vitro* (Vonderhaar, 1977; Bhattacharya and Vonderhaar, 1979a). Mammary glands from virgin mice cultured in the presence of insulin, hydrocortisone, and prolactin in the presence or absence of L-T_3 showed a differential sensitivity to prolactin for induction of lactose synthetase activity depending on the thyroid status of the animal. Figure 5

TABLE II

Effect of Various Concentrations of Thyroid Hormones and Derivatives on Lactose Synthetase Activity in Cultured Midpregnancy Mammary Tissue[a]

Hormones in culture	Molar conc. of thyroid hormone:	Lactose synthetase activity (pmoles lactose formed/mg tissue per 30 min)							
		0	10^{-12}	10^{-11}	10^{-10}	10^{-9}	10^{-8}	10^{-7}	10^{-6}
Expt. A IFPrl		103							
+ L-T$_3$			159	270	266	242	266		
+ L-T$_4$			—	—	—	265	287	206	200
+ D-T$_3$			—	81	110	122	119		
Expt. B IFPrl		50							
+ L-T$_4$						313			
+ I-thyronine						49			
+ I$_2$-tyrosine						58			

[a]Midpregnancy mammary glands were cultured for 48 hr in the presence of insulin (I: 5 μg/ml), hydrocortisone (F: 1 μg/ml), and prolactin (Prl: 5 μg/ml) plus either L-T$_3$, L-thyroxine (L-T4), D-T$_3$, or monoiodo-L-thyronine or diiodotyrosine at the indicated concentrations. Lactose synthetase activity was measured in the presence of endogenous galactosyltransferase (Vonderhaar et al., 1973).

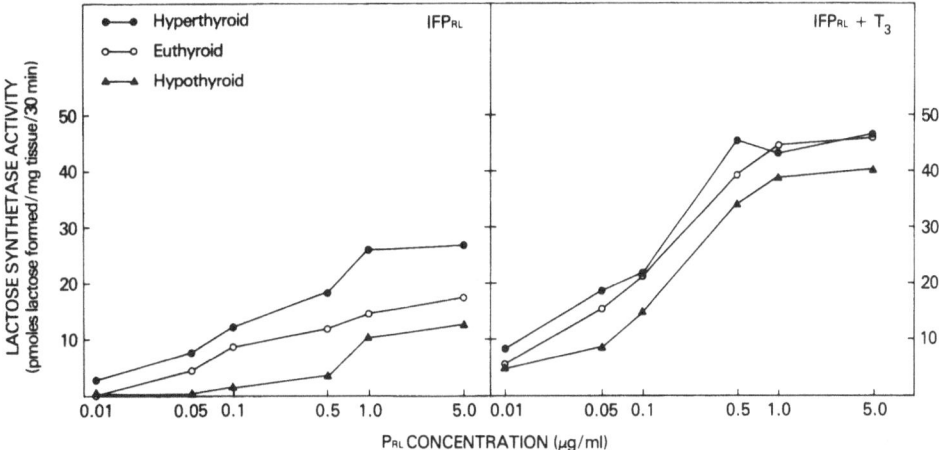

FIGURE 5. Induction of lactose synthetase activity in mammary explants from virgin mice in various thyroid states. Explants from virgin mice (4 months old) were cultured in serum-free medium for 72 to 96 hr in the presence of insulin (I; 5 μg/ml) and hydrocortisone (F; 1 μg/ml) or insulin, hydrocortisone, and 10^{-9} M L-T_3 and various concentrations of prolactin (Prl). Lactose synthetase activity was determined in the presence of endogenous galactosyltransferase (Vonderhaar et al., 1973).

shows that in the absence of exogenous L-T_3, lactose synthetase activity in tissue from hyperthyroid animals is induced at a prolactin concentration as low as 0.01 μg/ml (4.5×10^{-10} M). Euthyroid tissue requires at least 0.05 μg/ml (2.25×10^{-9} M), whereas induced lactose synthetase activity is not observed in hypothyroid tissue until prolactin concentrations are at least 0.1 μg/ml (4.5×10^{-9} M) with a consistent result being obtained at 0.5 μg/ml (2.25×10^{-8} M). In the presence of 10^{-9} M L-T_3, all tissues are able to respond to prolactin concentrations as low as 0.01 μg/ml (4.5×10^{-10} M). Similar results were obtained when glands from euthyroid midpregnancy mice were cultured in the presence of the same hormone combinations (Vonderhaar, 1977). In the absence of exogenous L-T_3, 1×10^{-3} μg prolactin/ml (4.5×10^{-11} M) is required to observed an effect on induction of lactose synthetase activity. In the presence of L-T_3 (10^{-9} M), effects are consistently seen at a prolactin concentration of 1×10^{-4} μg/ml (4.5×10^{-12} M). Thus, it appears that addition of thyroid hormone to culture medium decreases the minimal effective concentration of prolactin necessary for induced α-lactalbumin activity by 10- to 20-fold depending on the developmental state and thyroid status of the animal.

The effect of thyroid hormones is not just on the activity of α-lactalbumin in the lactose synthetase system, but also on the production of the milk sugar lactose (Bolander and Topper, 1981a; Bhattacharjee and Vonderhaar, 1984) and the synthesis and secretion of α-lactalbumin itself and of its mRNA (Terada and Oka, 1982; M. Bhattacharjee and B. K. Vonderhaar, unpublished observations). The increase in total α-lactalbumin synthesis by midpregnancy tissue in the presence of L-T_3 ranged from 40 to 100%. A significant portion of the newly synthesized milk proteins is found in the medium in explant cultures (Ono and Oka, 1980b). Table III shows that relatively low levels of newly synthesized caseins are found in the medium in the presence or absence of L-T_3 and no selective effect of this hormone on secretion can be demonstrated. However, significantly more α-lactalbumin is found in the medium in the presence of L-T_3 (i.e., two- to fivefold for a given experiment). The level of α-lactalbumin found in the medium in the presence of L-T_3 can be as high as 37% of the total and is independent of the assay used (Bhattacharjee and Vonderhaar, 1984). Thus, it appears that this hormone, in addition to oxytocin *in vivo* (Soloff *et al.*, 1979), plays an important role in the secretion of the milk protein α-lactalbumin.

The presence of L-T_3 in the culture medium is essential for secretion of the milk proteins in the presence of hydrocortisone. This steroid hormone is a prerequisite for the formation of RER (Oka and Topper, 1971) but the concentration present in the culture medium is critical and can differentially affect the synthesis of the caseins and α-lactalbumin (Ono and Oka, 1980a,b; Bolander and Topper, 1981a). At high concentrations of hydrocortisone (>0.1 μg/ml), the α-lactalbumin present in the tissue, as determined by its activity in the lactose synthetase system, is inhibited (Ono and Oka, 1980a,b). This effect is partially overcome by addition of L-T_3 to the medium (Bolander and Topper, 1981a) or by substituting corticosterone and aldosterone for hydrocortisone in the medium (Bhattacharjee and Vonderhaar, 1985). The addition of high concentrations of hydrocortisone to the medium, in addition to its effects on tissue content of the milk proteins, inhibits the secretion of caseins and α-lactalbumin into the medium (Figure 6). Addition of L-T_3 to the medium selectively overcomes this inhibition and actually stimulates secretion only of α-lactalbumin.

In addition to these quantitative differences in α-lactalbumin synthesis and secretion by midpregnancy mammary gland explants in the presence of

TABLE III
Effect of L-T_3 on the Synthesis and Secretion of Milk Proteins[a]

Milk protein			cpm $\times$ 10^{-3}/mg tissue		
			IFPrl	IFPrl + T_3	IFPrl + T_3/IFPrl
Expt. 1	Casein	Tissue	45.6 ± 1.6	48.0 ± 1.0	1.05
		Media	23.2 ± 1.4	25.5 ± 0.9	1.10
	α-Lactalbumin	Tissue	38.6 ± 0.6	53.9 ± 1.0	1.39
		Media	18.9 ± 0.8	37.7 ± 0.6	2.00
Expt. 2	α-Lactalbumin	Tissue	85.4 ± 1.8	145.7 ± 0.6	1.70
		Media	18.8 ± 1.1	95.5 ± 0.8	5.10

[a]Midpregnancy mammary gland explants were cultured as described in Table II. ^{3}H-labeled amino acids were present throughout the 48-hr culture period after which the tissue and media were collected and assayed individually for casein and α-lactalbumin by specific immunoprecipitation (Bhattacharjee and Vonderhaar, 1984).

FIGURE 6. The Effect of hydro-cortisone and L-T₃ on milk-protein secretion. Explants from midpregnancy mammary glands were cultured and labeled for 48 hr as described in Tables II and III. Tissue and media were collected and assayed for the presence of newly synthesized caseins or α-lactalbumin using specific immunoprecipitation. The percent of milk protein secreted into the media was then calculated as (media/total) × 100 and the data expressed as milk protein secreted into the media at a given concentration of hydrocortisone (F) relative to that secreted in the absence of the steroid (designated as 1.0). Casein secreted in the absence (●---●) or presence (▲---▲) of L-T₃; α-lactalbumin secreted in the absence (●—●) or presence (▲—▲) of L-T₃ (Bhattacharjee and Vonderhaar, 1984).

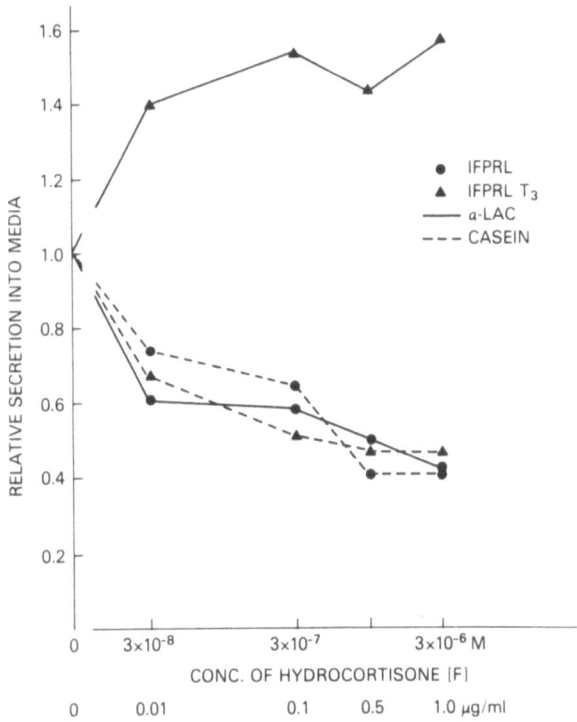

L-T₃, qualitative differences also occur. Figure 7 shows that tissue cultured in the presence of insulin, hydrocortisone, and prolactin synthesizes α-lactalbumin that is seen on SDS–polyacrylamide gels, after precipitation with an α-lactalbumin-specific antibody, as predominantly a broad single peak. When L-T₃ is included in the culture medium, two distinct forms of α-lactalbumin are detected in the tissue extracts. Although these two forms are synthesized in the presence of the thyroid hormone, only one, as seen as a single broad peak on the SDS–polyacrylamide gels (Figure 8), is secreted in the presence or absence of L-T₃. No differences in the patterns of caseins synthesized or secreted are seen whether or not L-T₃ is present in the culture medium (Bhattacharjee and Vonderhaar, 1984). By coelectrophoresis of the immunoprecipitated α-lactalbumins from tissue and medium labeled with [14]C- or ^{3}H-amino acids, it is clear that the slower-migrating peak represents the form of α-lactalbumin that is secreted in the presence of L-T₃ and that this is the same as the form that is synthesized and secreted in the absence of the thyroid hormone. The two forms of α-lactalbumin synthesized in the presence of L-T₃ are distinct from WAP (Bhattacharjee and Vonderhaar, 1984) and differ from each other only in their carbohydrate content (M. Bhattacharjee and B. U. Vonderhaar, unpublished). Synthesis of two forms of α-lactalbumin in the presence of L-T₃, but secretion of primarily one form, is consistent with the results obtained on purification of this milk protein.

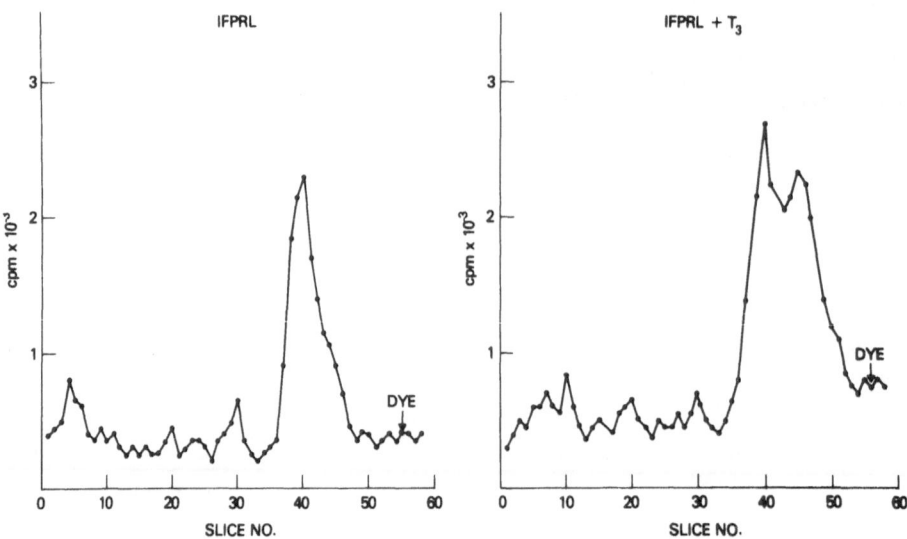

FIGURE 7. SDS–polyacrylamide gel electrophoresis of α-lactalbumin in tissue after 48 hr of culture in the presence or absence of L-T$_3$. Immunoprecipitated α-lactalbumin was prepared from midpregnancy mammary tissue cultured and labeled as described in Tables II and III (Bhattacharjee and Vonderhaar, 1984).

Only one major form of α-lactalbumin is purified from mouse milk (Zamierowski and Ebner, 1980; Nagamatsu and Oka, 1980) whereas two forms differing in their pIs are purified from lactating mouse mammary glands (Bhattacharjee and Vonderhaar, 1983). These results illustrate the physiological importance of L-T$_3$ in lactogenesis and suggest that all four hormones (insulin, glucocorticoid, prolactin, and thyroid hormone) should be used in explant cultures to achieve qualitatively as well as quantitatively meaningful results. In the presence of such a hormonal combination, the in vitro mouse mammary gland can be used as an effective model to acquire greater insights into the complex series of regulatory events during functional differentiation.

3.3. Receptor Regulation during Development and Functional Differentiation

The action of any given hormone or growth factor is believed to be mediated through its initial interaction with specific cellular receptors. The requisite receptors for the various hormones and growth factors that are involved in development and differentiation of the mouse mammary gland have been described. These include the receptors for insulin (O'Keefe and Cuatrecasas, 1974; Apostolova et al., 1976), glucocorticoids (Terada and Oka, 1983; Banerjee et al., 1983), prolactin (Bhattacharya and Vonderhaar, 1979a), estrogen and progesterone (Puca and Bresciani, 1969; Richards et al., 1974; Auricchio et al., 1976; Haslam and Shyamala, 1981), thyroid hormones (Bhat-

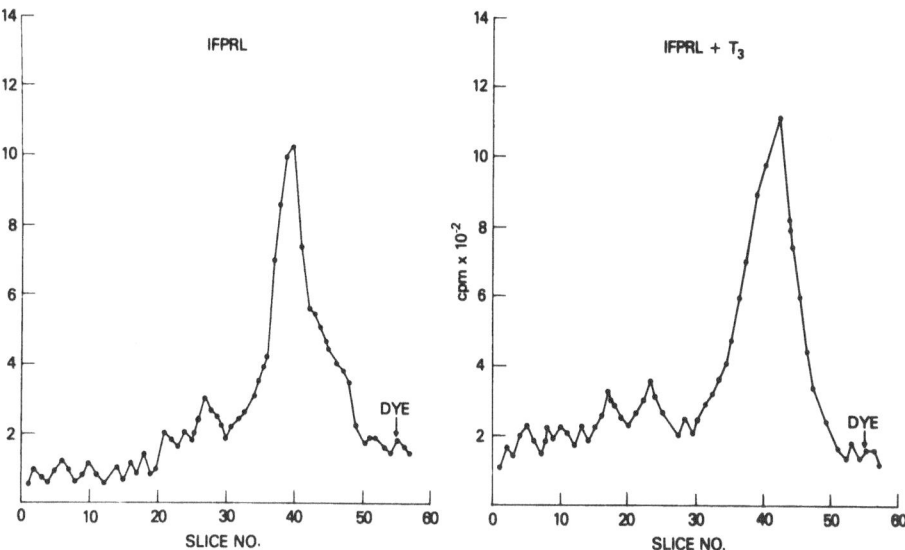

FIGURE 8. SDS–polyacrylamide gel electrophoresis of α-lactalbumin in the media after 48 hr of culture in the presence or absence of L-T$_3$. Immunoprecipitated α-lactalbumin was prepared from the media in which midpregnancy mammary explants were cultured and labeled as described in Tables II and III (Bhattacharjee and Vonderhaar, 1984).

tacharya and Vonderhaar, 1977), testosterone (Heuberger et al., 1982), oxytocin (Soloff et al., 1979), and EGF (Taketani and Oka, 1983a; Vonderhaar, 1984). But the mere presence of a receptor in the target tissue is not sufficient to explain a hormone or growth factor's biological action. Modulation of the receptors of one hormone by another is an important regulatory mechanism in many systems (Toft and O'Malley, 1972; Gelato et al., 1975; Vignon and Rochefort, 1976; Madsen and Sonne, 1976; Ciaraldi and Marinetti, 1977; Williams et al., 1977; Knazek et al., 1978; Taketani and Oka, 1983a,b). The mammary gland, because of its multiple hormonal and growth factor requirements during development and differentiation, provides an excellent model for studying how receptor regulation influences various biological events.

Estrogen and progesterone act in concert during mammary gland morphogenesis (Nandi, 1958). Progesterone, even in the presence of estrogen, exerts negative effects on functional differentiation of the mammary gland. Before parturition, progesterone prevents the initiation of lactation (Kuhn, 1969; Denamur and DeLouis, 1972; Vonderhaar, 1977; Rosen et al., 1978; Banerjee et al., 1983). Once lactation is established, it can proceed normally, even in the absence of ovaries (Cowie and Tindall, 1971). Regulation of the progesterone receptor is under estrogenic control (Leavitt et al., 1977; Haslam and Shyamala, 1979b). The concentration of the progesterone receptor per cell in the mammary gland varies with the developmental state of the animal: it is present in virgin tissue, decreases during pregnancy, is undetectable during lactation, and reappears during involution (Haslam and Shyamala, 1979a). In the virgin mouse, the level of mammary gland progesterone receptor is augmented by estrogen administration (Haslam and Shyamala, 1979b). However, not only is the receptor for progesterone absent during lactation (Shyamala and McBlain, 1979), but estrogen administration to either intact or ovariectomized lactating mice fails to induce the receptor in the epithelial cells (Haslam and Shyamala, 1979b). Thus, even though estrogen receptors are present in lactating mammary tissue (Richards et al., 1974; Auricchio et al., 1976), the gland develops an insensitivity to the action of estradiol in terms of progesterone receptor induction and thus becomes refractory to progesterone inhibition of lactogenesis (Haslam and Shyamala, 1980).

Examination of the regulation of the prolactin receptor by thyroid hormones has proven useful in understanding the mechanism by which L-T_3 increases the sensitivity of the mammary gland to this peptide hormone. Initially, prolactin binding activity was evaluated in membranes prepared from mammary tissue (Bhattacharya and Vonderhaar, 1979a) and on isolated mammary epithelial cells from mice in various thyroid states. As seen in Table IV, there is no specific binding of prolactin to epithelial cells derived from mammary glands of hypothyroid virgin mice whereas cells from glands of hyperthyroid animals show binding that is double that of cells from euthyroid animals. Similar results were found with membranes prepared from the whole mammary glands of virgin and primiparous mice in various thyroid states (Bhattacharya and Vonderhaar, 1979a). Using the explant culture system of midpregnancy tissue in which the L-T_3-induced altered sensitivity of mammary glands to prolactin was originally demonstrated (Vonderhaar, 1977), it is possible to explore the ability of thyroid hormones to induce prolactin binding activity in vitro. As shown in Table V, prolactin binding to membranes prepared from explants cultured overnight in the presence of

TABLE IV
The Effect of Thyroid Status on Prolactin
Binding to Epithelial Cells from Virgin
Mouse Mammary Glands[a]

Thyroid status	[^{125}I]oPrl bound specifically (cpm/mg DNA)	Relative binding
Euthyroid	$45,510 \pm 13,090$	1.0
Hyperthyroid	$94,160 \pm 20,710$	2.04
Hypothyroid	Not detectable	—

[a]Virgin mice were made mildly hyperthyroid by ingestion of L-T_4 and mildly hypothyroid by ingestion of 2-thiouracil in the drinking water (Vonderhaar and Greco, 1979). Mammary epithelial cells were prepared by collagenase digestion of the glands (Topper et al., 1975). Specific binding of ^{125}I-labeled ovine prolactin (oPrl) to the cells were determined by incubation at 37°C for 3 hr in the presence and absence of excess unlabeled oPrl.

TABLE V
Effect of L-T$_3$ on Prolactin Binding to
Membranes Prepared from Cultured
Midpregnancy Mammary Glands[a]

Culture conditions		[^{125}I]oPrl bound specifically (cpm/mg protein)	
		Expt. A	Expt. B
Uncultured		2074 ± 1269	—
16 hr	IF	2731 ± 723	3305 ± 297
	IF + T$_3$	4886 ± 318	5020 ± 449

[a]Explants from mammary glands from midpregnancy mice were cultured in the presence of insulin and hydrocortisone (IF) in the absence or presence of 10^{-9} M L-T$_3$ as described in Table II. Specific binding to membranes prepared from the tissue was according to the method of Shiu et al. (1973) as modified (Bhattacharya and Vonderhaar, 1979a) using excess unlabeled ovine prolactin (oPrl) to determine nonspecific binding.

insulin, hydrocortisone, and L-T$_3$ is more than double the level of binding to membranes from uncultured tissue and nearly double that of tissue cultured in the absence of L-T$_3$. No significant difference in the binding is seen between uncultured tissue and tissue cultured in the presence of insulin and hydrocortisone, suggesting that there is no loss of prolactin receptor during the culture period and thyroid hormones are not selectively stabilizing prolactin receptors in vitro. The induction of prolactin binding capacity by L-T$_3$ in short-term culture does not require protein synthesis (Bhattacharya and Vonderhaar, 1979a), thus suggesting that thyroid hormones increase the sensitivity of mammary epithelial cells to prolactin at least in part by unmasking cryptic receptor sites (Bhattacharya and Vonderharr, 1979b).

4. CONCLUSION

The mammary gland goes through multiple discrete stages of morphological development and differentiation under the influence of several hormones and growth factors. Many of the events involved in these processes in vivo can be mimicked in vitro in the presence of serum-free, hormonally supplemented media, thus making the mammary gland an excellent model system for examining differentiation, preneoplasia, hormone action, and receptor regulation.

REFERENCES

Adamson, R. D., Banerjee, M. R., and Medina, D., 1971, Susceptibility of mammary tumor virus-free BALB/c mice in DNA synthesis to 3-methylcholanthrene tumorigenesis, J. Natl. Cancer Inst. **46:**899–907.

Apostolova, J., Sirakov, L. M., and Barth, T., 1976, Insulin receptors in lactating mouse mammary gland, *Collect. Czech. Chem. Commun.* **41**:3830–3836.

Ashley, R. L., Cardiff, R. D., Mitchell, D. J., Faulkin, L. J., and Lund, J. K., 1980, Development and characterization of mouse hyperplastic mammary outgrowth lines from BALB/cfC3H hyperplastic alveolar nodules, *Cancer Res.* **40**:4232–4242.

Auricchio, F., Rotondi, A., and Bresciani, F., 1976, Oestrogen receptor in mammary gland cytosol of virgin, pregnant and lactating mice, *Mol. Cell. Endocrinol.* **4**:55–60.

Balinsky, B. I., 1950a, On the pre-natal growth of the mammary gland rudiment in the mouse, *J. Anat.* **84**:227–235.

Balinsky, B. I., 1950b, On the developmental processes in mammary glands and other epidermal structures, *Trans. R. Soc. Edinburgh* **62**:1–32.

Banerjee, M. R., 1976, Responses of mammary cells to hormones, *Int. Rev. Cytol.* **46**:1–97.

Banerjee, M. R., 1985, An in vitro model for neoplastic transformation of epithelial cells in a whole mammary organ in the mouse, in: *In Vitro Models for Cancer Research* (M. Weber and L. Sekely, eds.), CRC Press, Boca Raton, Fla. (in press).

Banerjee, M. R., Wood, B. G., and Kinder, D. L., 1973, Whole mammary gland organ culture: Selection of appropriate gland, *In Vitro* **9**:129–133.

Banerjee, M. R., Wood, B. G., and Washburn, L. L., 1974, Chemical carcinogen-induced alveolar nodules in organ culture of mouse mammary gland, *J. Natl. Cancer Inst.* **53**:1387–1393.

Banerjee, M. R., Wood, B. G., Lin, F. K., and Crump, L. R., 1976, Organ culture of the whole mammary gland of the mouse, *Tissue Culture Assoc. Man.* **2**:457–462.

Banerjee, M. R., Antoniou, M., Joshi, J. B., and Majumder, P. K., 1983, Recent advances in hormonal regulation of milk protein gene expression, in: *Understanding Breast Cancer: Clinical and Laboratory Concepts* (M. A. Rich, J. C. Hager, and P. Furmanski, eds.), Dekker, New York, pp. 335–364.

Bhattacharjee, M., and Vonderhaar, B. K., 1983, Purification and characterization of mouse α-lactalbumin from lactating mammary glands, *Biochim. Biophys. Acta* **755**:279–286.

Bhattacharjee, M., and Vonderhaar, B. K., 1984, Thyroid hormones enhance the synthesis and secretion of α-lactalbumin by mouse mammary tissue in vitro, *Endocrinology* **115**:1070–1077.

Bhattacharya, A., and Vonderhaar, B. K., 1977, Specific binding proteins for 3,5,3'-triiodothyronine in mouse mammary epithelium, *J. Cell Biol.* **75**:47a.

Bhattacharya, A., and Vonderhaar, B. K., 1979a, Thyroid hormone regulation of prolactin binding to mouse mammary glands, *Biochem. Biophys. Res. Commun.* **88**:1405–1411.

Bhattacharya, A., and Vonderhaar, B. K., 1979b, Phospholipid methylation stimulates lactogenic binding in mouse mammary gland membranes, *Proc. Natl. Acad. Sci. USA* **76**:4489–4492.

Black, M. M., and Chabon, A. B., 1969, In situ carcinoma of the breast, *Pathol. Annu.* **4**:185–210.

Bolander, F. F., Jr., 1983, The effect of 5-azacytidine on mammary gland differentiation *in vitro*, *Biochem. Biophys. Res. Commun.* **111**:150–155.

Bolander, F. F., Jr., and Topper, Y. J., 1980a, Stimulation of lactose synthetase activity and casein synthesis in mouse mammary explants by estradiol, *Endocrinology* **106**:490–495.

Bolander, F. F., Jr., and Topper, Y. J., 1980b, Loss of differentiative potential of the mammary gland in ovariectomized mice: Prevention and reversibility of the defect, *Endocrinology* **107**:1281–1285.

Bolander, F. F., Jr., and Topper, Y. J., 1981a, The asynchronous hormonal induction of lactose synthetase components, α-lactalbumin and galactosyltransferase, in relation to lactose secretion by mouse mammary explants, *Endocrinology* **108**:1594–1596.

Bolander, F. F., Jr., and Topper, Y. J., 1981b, Loss of differentiative potential of the mammary gland in ovariectomized mice: Identification of a biochemical lesion, *Endocrinology* **108**:1649–1653.

Bolander, F. F., Jr., Nicholas, K. R., Van Wyk, J. J., and Topper, Y. J., 1981, Insulin is essential for accumulation of casein mRNA in mouse mammary epithelial cells, *Proc. Natl. Acad. Sci. USA* **78**:5862–5864.

Brodbeck, U., Denton, W. L., Tanahashi, N., and Ebner, K. E., 1967, The isolation and identification of the B protein of lactose synthetase as α-lactalbumin, *J. Biol. Chem.* **242**:1391–1397.

Brookreson, A. D., and Turner, C. W., 1959, Normal growth of mammary gland in pregnant and lactating mice, *Proc. Soc. Exp. Biol. Med.* **102**:744–745.

Cairns, J., and Logan, J., 1983, Step by step into carcinogenesis, *Nature* **304**:582–583.

Ciaraldi, T., and Marinetti, G. V., 1977, Thyroxine and propylthiouracil effects in vivo on alpha and beta adrenergic receptors in rat heart, *Biochem. Biophys. Res. Commun.* **74**:984–991.

Colard, C., and Gomot, L., 1975, Etude comparee de l'ultrastructure des bourgeons mammaries primaries d'embryons de souris males et femelles au stade de la differenciation sexuelle, *C. R. Acad. Sci. Ser. D* **280**:1821–1824.

Cowie, A. T., and Tindall, J. S., 1971, The physiology of lactation, in: *Physiology Society Monograph No. 22* (H. Davson and A. D. M. Greenfield, eds.), Arnold, London.

Cowie, A. T., Forsyth, I. A., and Hart, I. C., 1980, Hormonal control of lactation, *Monogr. Endocrinol.* **1980**:146–162.

Dao, T. L., Sinha, D., Christakos, S., and Varela, R., 1975, Biochemical characterization of carcinogen-induced mammary hyperplastic alveolar nodule and tumor in the rat, *Cancer Res.* **35**:1128–1134.

Denamur, R., and DeLouis, C., 1972, Effects of progesterone and prolactin on the secretory activity and the nucleic acid content of mammary gland of pregnant rabbits, *Acta Endocrinol.* **70**:603–617.

DeOme, K. B., Faulkin, L. J., Bern, H. A., and Blair, P. B., 1959, Development of mammary tumors from hyperplastic alveolar nodules transplanted into gland-free mammary fat pads of female C3H mice, *Cancer Res.* **19**:515–520.

DeOme, K. B., Miyamoto, M. J., Osborn, R. C., Guzman, R. C., and Lum, K., 1978, Detection of inapparent nodule-transformed cells in the mammary gland tissues of virgin female BALB/cfC3H mice, *Cancer Res.* **38**:2103–2111.

Dickens, M. S., and Sorof, S., 1981, Retinoid prevents transformation of cultured mammary glands by procarcinogens but not by many activated carcinogens, *Nature* **285**:581–584.

Dickens, M. S., Custer, R. P., and Sorof, S., 1979, Retinoid prevents mammary gland transformation by carcinogenic hydrocarbon in whole-organ culture, *Proc. Natl. Acad. Sci. USA* **76**:5891–5895.

Drews, U., and Drews, U., 1977, Regression of mouse mammary gland anlagen in recombinants of TfM and wild-type tissue: Testosterone acts via the mesenchyme, *Cell* **10**:401–404.

Dubnik, C. S., Morris, H. P., and Dalton, A. J., 1950, Inhibition of mammary-gland development and mammary-tumor formation in female C3H mice following ingestion of thiouracil, *J. Natl. Cancer Inst.* **10**:815–841.

Dulbecco, R., Henahan, M., and Armstrong, B., 1982, Cell types and morphogenesis in the mammary gland, *Proc. Natl. Acad. Sci. USA* **79**:7346–7350.

Ebner, K. E., Denton, W. L., and Brodbeck, U., 1966, The substitution of α-lactalbumin for the B protein of lactose synthetase, *Biochem. Biophys. Res. Commun.* **24**:232–236.

Elias, J. J., 1957, Cultivation of adult mouse mammary gland in hormone-enriched synthetic medium, *Science* **126**:842–843.

Ethier, S. P., and Ullrich, R. L., 1982, Detection of ductal dysplasia in mammary outgrowths derived from carcinogen-treated virgin female BALB/c mice, *Cancer Res.* **42**:1753–1760.

Faulkin, L. J., Jr., 1966, Hyperplastic lesions of mouse mammary glands after treatment with 3-methylcholanthrene, *J. Natl. Cancer Inst.* **36**:289–297.

Faulkin, L. J., Jr., and DeOme, K. B., 1960, The regulation of growth and spacing of gland elements in the mammary fat pad of the C3H mouse, *J. Natl. Cancer Inst.* **24**:953–969.

Foster, R. C., 1977, Changes in mouse mammary epithelial cell size during mammary gland development, *Cell Differ.* **6**:1–8.

Ganguly, N., Ganguly, R., Mehta, N. M., and Banerjee, M. R., 1982, Growth and differentiation of hyperplastic outgrowths derived from mouse mammary epithelial cells transformed in organ culture, *J. Natl. Cancer Inst.* **69**:453–463.

Ganguly, R., Mehta, N. M., Ganguly, N., and Banerjee, M. R., 1979, Glucocorticoid modulation of casein gene transcription in mouse mammary gland, *Proc. Natl. Acad. Sci. USA* **76**:6466–6470.

Gelato, M., Marshall, S., Boudreau, M., Bruni, J., Campbell, G. A., and Meites, J., 1975, Effects of thyroid and ovaries on prolactin binding activity in rat liver, *Endocrinology* **96:**1292–1296.

Grahame, R. E., and Bertalanffy, F. D., 1972, Cell division in normal and neoplastic mammary gland tissue in the rat, *Anat. Rec.* **174:**1–7.

Haslam, S. Z., and Shyamala, G., 1979a, Progesterone receptors in normal mammary glands of mice: Characterization and relationship to development, *Endocrinology* **105:**786–795.

Haslam, S. Z., and Shyamala, G., 1979b, Effect of oestradiol on progesterone receptors in normal mammary glands and its relationship with lactation, *Biochem. J.* **182:**127–131.

Haslam, S. Z., and Shyamala, G., 1980, Progesterone receptors in normal mammary gland: Receptor modulations in relation to differentiation, *J. Cell Biol.* **86:**730–737.

Haslam, S. Z., and Shyamala, G., 1981, Relative distribution of estrogen and progesterone receptors among the epithelial adipose and connective tissue components of the normal mammary gland, *Endocrinology* **108:**825–830.

Hennighausen, L. G., and Sippel, A. E., 1982a, Mouse whey acidic protein is a novel member of the family of four-disulfide core proteins, *Nucleic Acid Res.* **10:**2677–2684.

Hennighausen, L. G., and Sippel, A. E., 1982b, Characterization and cloning of the mRNAs specific for the lactating mouse mammary gland, *Eur. J. Biochem.* **125:**131–141.

Heuberger, B., Fitzka, I., Wasner, G., and Kratochwil, K., 1982, Induction of androgen receptor formation by epithelium–mesenchyme interaction in embryonic mouse mammary gland, *Proc. Natl. Acad. Sci. USA* **79:**2957–2961.

Hoshino, H., 1962, Morphogenesis and growth potentiality of mammary glands in mice. I. Transplantability and growth potentiality of mammary tissue in virgin mice, *J. Natl. Cancer Inst.* **29:**835–851.

Ichinose, R. R., and Nandi, S., 1964, Lobuloalveolar differentiation in mouse mammary tissue *in vitro*, *Science* **145:**496–497.

Ichinose, R. R., and Nandi, S., 1966, Influence of hormones on lobuloalveolar differentiation of mouse mammary glands *in vitro*, *J. Endocrinol.* **35:**331–340.

Iyer, A. P., and Banerjee, M. R., 1981, Sequential expression of preneoplastic and neoplastic characteristics of mouse mammary epithelial cells transformed in organ culture, *J. Natl. Cancer Inst.* **66:**893–905.

Jensen, H. M., Rice, J. R., and Wellings, S. R., 1976, Preneoplastic lesions in the human breast, *Science* **191:**295–297.

Keenan, T. W., Saacke, R. G., and Patton, S., 1970, Prolactin, the Golgi apparatus and milk secretion: Brief interpretative review, *J. Dairy Sci.* **53:**1349–1352.

Kidwell, W. R., Knazek, R. A., Vonderhaar, B. K., and Losonczy, I., 1982, Effects of unsaturated fatty acids on the development and proliferation of normal and neoplastic breast epithelium, in: *Molecular Interrelations of Nutrition and Cancer* (M. S. Arnott, J. vanEys, and Y. M. Wang, eds.), Raven Press, New York, pp. 219–236.

King, E. B., Chew, K. L., Petrakis, N. L., and Ernster, V. L., 1983, Nipple aspirate cytology for the study of breast cancer precursors, *J. Natl. Cancer Inst.* **71:**1115–1121.

Knazek, R. A., Liu, S. C., Graeter, R. L., Wright, P. C., Mayer, J. R., Lewis, R. H., Gould, E. B., and Keller, J. A., 1978, Growth hormone causes a rapid induction of lactogenic receptor activity in the Snell dwarf mouse liver, *Endocrinology* **103:**1590–1596.

Knight, C. H., and Peaker, M., 1982a, Mammary cell proliferation in mice during pregnancy and lactation in relation to milk yield, *Q. J. Exp. Physiol.* **67:**165–177.

Knight, C. H., and Peaker, M., 1982b, Development of the mammary gland, *J. Reprod. Fertil.* **65:**521–536.

Kratochwil, K., 1971, In vitro analysis of the hormonal basis for the sexual dimorphism in the embryonic development of the mouse mammary gland, *J. Embryol. Exp. Morphol.* **25:**141–153.

Kratochwil, K., 1977, Development and loss of androgen responsiveness in the embryonic rudiment of the mouse mammary gland, *Dev. Biol.* **61:**358–365.

Kratochwil, K., and Schwartz, P., 1976, Tissue interaction in androgen response of embryonic mammary rudiment of mouse: Identification of target tissue for testosterone, *Proc. Natl. Acad. Sci. USA* **73:**4041–4044.

Kuhn, N. J., 1969, Specificity of progesterone inhibition of lactogenesis, *J. Endocrinol.* **45:**615–623.

Kuhn, N. J., 1977, Lactogenesis: The search for trigger mechanisms in different species, in: *Comparative Aspects of Lactation* (M. Peaker, ed.), Academic Press, New York, pp. 165–192.

Leavitt, W. W., Chen, T. J., and Allen, T. C., 1977, Regulation of progesterone receptor formation by estrogen action, *Ann. N.Y. Acad. Sci.* **286**:210–225.

Lin, F. K., Banerjee, M. R., and Crump, L. R., 1976, Cell cycle-related hormone carcinogen interaction during chemical carcinogen induction of nodule-like mammary lesions in organ culture, *Cancer Res.* **36**:1607–1614.

Madsen, S. N., and Sonne, O., 1976, Increase of glucagon receptors in hyperthyroidism, *Nature* **262**:793–795.

Medina, D., 1973, Preneoplasia in breast cancer, in: *Breast Cancer*, Volume 2 (W. L. McGuire, ed.), Plenum Press, New York, pp. 47–102.

Medina, D., and DeOme, K. B., 1968, Influence of mammary tumor virus on the tumor-producing capabilities of nodule outgrowths free of mammary tumor virus, *J. Natl. Cancer Inst.* **40**:1303–1308.

Medina, D., and DeOme, K. B., 1970a, Carcinogen-induced mammary tumors from preneoplastic nodule outgrowths in BALB/c mice, *Cancer Res.* **30**:1055–1059.

Medina, D., and DeOme, K. B., 1970b, Effects of various oncogenic agents on tumor producing capabilities of series D BALB/c mammary nodule outgrowth lines, *J. Natl. Cancer Inst.* **45**:353–363.

Mehta, N. M., Ganguly, N., Ganguly, R., and Banerjee, M. R., 1980, Hormonal modulation of the casein gene expression in a mammogenesis–lactogenesis culture model of the whole mammary gland of the mouse, *J. Biol. Chem.* **255**:4430–4434.

Mehta, R. G., and Banerjee, M. R., 1975, Action of growth promoting hormones on macromolecular biosynthesis during lobuloalveolar development of the entire mammary gland in organ culture, *Acta Endocrinol.* **80**:501–516.

Mehta, R. G., Cerny, W. L., and Moon, R. C., 1983, Retinoids inhibit prolactin-induced development of the mammary gland *in vitro*, *Carcinogenesis* **4**:23–26.

Mills, E. S., and Topper, Y. J., 1970, Some ultrastructural effects of insulin, hydrocortisone and prolactin on mammary gland explants, *J. Cell Biol.* **44**:310–328.

Mixner, J. P., and Turner, C. W., 1942, Influence of thyroxin upon mammary lobule-alveolar growth, *Endocrinology* **31**:345–348.

Motojima, K., and Oka, T., 1983, 5′-terminal sequence of the mRNA of mouse whey acidic protein contains three possible sites of interaction with 18S rRNA, *Biochem. Biophys. Res. Commun.* **116**:167–172.

Nagaiah, K., Bolander, F. F., Jr., Nicholas, K. R., Takemoto, T., and Topper, Y. J., 1981, Prolactin-induced accumulation of casein mRNA in mouse mammary explants: A selective role of glucocorticoids, *Biochem. Biophys. Res. Commun.* **98**:380–387.

Nagamatsu, Y., and Oka, T., 1980, Purification and characterization of mouse α-lactalbumin and preparation of its antibody, *Biochem. J.* **185**:227–237.

Nagamatsu, Y., and Oka, T., 1983, The differential actions of cortisol on the synthesis and turnover of α-lactalbumin and casein and on accumulation of their mRNA in mouse mammary gland in organ culture, *Biochem. J.* **212**:507–515.

Nandi, S., 1958, Endocrine control of mammary-gland development and function in the C3H/HeCrgl mouse, *J. Natl. Cancer Inst.* **21**:1039–1063.

Nandi, S., 1959, *Hormonal Control of Mammogenesis and Lactogenesis in the C3H/HeCrgl Mouse*, Univ. Calif. Berkeley Publ. Zool. **65**:1–128.

Nandi, S., 1961, Effect of hormones on maintenance of hyperplastic alveolar nodules in mammary glands of various strains of mice, *J. Natl. Cancer Inst.* **27**:187–201.

Nandi, S., 1963, New method for detection of mouse mammary tumor virus. I. Influence of hyperplastic mammary nodules in BALB/cCrgl mice, *J. Natl. Cancer Inst.* **31**:57–73.

Nandi, S., and Bern, H. A., 1960, Relation between mammary-gland responses to lactogenic hormone combinations and tumor susceptibility in various strains of mice, *J. Natl. Cancer Inst.* **24**:907–931.

Nandi, S., and Bern, H. A., 1961, The hormones responsible for lactogenesis in BALB/cHeCrgl mouse, *Gen. Comp. Endocrinol.* **1**:195–210.

Nandi, S., and McGrath, C. M., 1973, Mammary neoplasia in mice, *Adv. Cancer Res.* **17**:353–414.

Nandi, S., Bern, H. A., and DeOme, K. B., 1960, Effect of hormones on growth and neoplastic development of transplanted hyperplastic alveolar nodules of the mammary gland of C3H/Crgl mice, *J. Natl. Cancer Inst.* **24**:883–905.

Narbaitz, R., Stumpf, W. E., and Sar, M., 1980, Estrogen receptors in mammary gland primordia of fetal mouse, *Anat. Embryol.* **158**:161–166.

Nicholas, K. R., and Topper, Y. J., 1983, Anti-insulin receptor serum mimics the developmental role of insulin in mouse mammary explants, *Biochem. Biophys. Res. Commun.* **111**:988–993.

Nolin, J. M., 1979, The prolactin incorporation cycle of the milk secretory cell, *J. Histochem. Cytochem.* **27**:1203–1204.

Oka, T., and Y. J. Topper, 1971, Hormone-dependent accumulation of rough-endoplasmic reticulum in mouse mammary epithelial cells in vitro, *J. Biol. Chem.* **246**:7701–7707.

O'Keefe, E., and Cuatrecasas, P., 1974, Insulin receptors in murine mammary cells: Comparison in pregnant and non-pregnant animals, *Biochim. Biophys. Acta* **343**:64–77.

Ono, M., and Oka, T., 1980a, α-Lactalbumin–casein induction in virgin mouse mammary explants: Dose-dependent differential action of cortisol, *Science* **207**:1367–1369.

Ono, M., and Oka, T., 1980b, The differential actions of cortisol on the accumulation of α-lactalbumin and casein in midpregant mouse mammary gland in culture, *Cell* **19**:473–480.

Perry, J. W., and Oka, T., 1984, The study of differentiative potential of the lactating mouse mammary gland in organ culture, *In Vitro* **20**:59–65.

Piletz, J. E., Heinlen, M., and Ganschow, R. E., 1981, Biochemical characterization of a novel whey protein from murine milk, *J. Biol. Chem.* **256**:11509–11516.

Propper, A. Y., 1978, Wandering epithelial cells in the rabbit embryo milk line, *Dev. Biol.* **67**:225–231.

Puca, G. A., and Bresciani, F., 1969, Interactions of 6,7-^{3}H-17β-estradiol with mammary gland and other organs of the C3H mouse in vivo, *Endocrinology* **85**:1–10.

Raynaud, A., 1950, Recherches experimentales sur le developpement de l'appareil genital et le fonctionnement des glandes endocrines des foetus de souris et de mulot, *Arch. Anat. Microsc. Morphol. Exp.* **39**:518–576.

Raynaud, A., 1955, Observations sur les modifications provoquees par les hormones oestrogenes, du mode de developpement des mamelons des foetus de souris, *C. R. Acad. Sci.* **240**:674–676.

Raynaud, A., 1961, Morphogenesis of the mammary gland, in: *Milk: The Mammary Gland and Its Secretion*, Volume 1 (S. K. Kon and A. T. Cowie, eds.), Academic Press, New York, pp. 3–46.

Raynaud, A., 1971, Foetal development of the mammary gland and hormonal effects on its morphogenesis, in: *Lactation* (I. R. Falconer, ed.), Butterworths, London, pp. 3–29.

Raynaud, A., and Frilley, M., 1947, Destruction des glands genitales, de l'embryon de souris, par une irradiation au moyen des rayons X, a l'age de treize jours, *Ann. Endocrinol.* **8**:400–419.

Raynaud, A., and Raynaud, J., 1953, Les principales etapes de la separation, d'avec l'epiderme, des ebauches mammaires des foetus male de souris; recherches sur les processus de la rupture de la tige du bourgeon mammaire, *C. R. Soc. Biol.* **147**:1872–1876.

Raynaud, A., Raynaud, J., Dobrovolskaia, N., Rudali, G., Adamoff, N., and Defoort, J., 1970, Sur l'etat de developpement des ebauches mammaires et mamelonnaires chez des souris nouveau-nees appartenant a cinq lignees selectionnees elevees a l'Institut du Radium de Paris, *Bull. Cancer* **57**:447–476.

Razin, A., and Riggs, A. D., 1980, DNA methylation and gene function, *Science* **210**:604–610.

Richards, J. E., Shyamala, G., and Nandi, S., 1974, Estrogen receptor in normal and neoplastic mouse mammary tissues, *Cancer Res.* **34**:2764–2772.

Richards, J., Guzman, R., Konrad, M., Yang, J., and Nandi, S., 1982, Growth of mouse mammary gland end buds cultured in a collagen gel matrix, *Exp. Cell Res.* **141**:433–443.

Richards, J., Hamamoto, S., Smith, S., Pasco, D., Guzman, R., and Nandi, S., 1983, Response of end bud cells from immature rat mammary gland to hormones when cultured in collagen gel, *Exp. Cell Res.* **147**:95–109.

Riley, V., 1975, Mouse mammary tumors: Alteration of incidence as apparent function of stress, *Science* **189**:465–467.

Rivera, E. M., Hill, S. D., and Taylor, M., 1981, Organ culture passage enhances the oncogenicity of carcinogen-induced hyperplastic mammary nodules, In Vitro 17:159–166.

Rosen, J. M., O'Neal, D. L., McHugh, J. E., and Comstock, J. P., 1978, Progesterone-mediated inhibition of casein mRNA and polysomal casein synthesis in the rat mammary gland during pregnancy, Biochemistry 17:290–297.

Sakakura, T., Nishizuka, Y., and Dawe, C. J., 1976, Mesenchyme-dependent morphogenesis and epithelium-specific cytodifferentiation in mouse mammary gland, Science 194:1439–1441.

Sakakura, T., Sakagami, Y., and Nishizuka, Y., 1979, Persistence of responsiveness of adult mouse mammary gland to induction by embryonic mesenchyme, Dev. Biol. 72:201–210.

Sakakura, T., Sakagami, Y., and Nishizuka, Y., 1982, Dual origin of mesenchymal tissues participating in mouse mammary gland embryogenesis, Dev. Biol. 91:202–207.

Schaefer, F. V., Tonelli, Q. J., Dickens, M. S., Custer, R. P., and Sorof, S., 1983, Nononcogenic hormone-independent alveoli produced by carcinogens in cultured mouse mammary glands, Cancer Res. 43:3310–3315.

Shiu, R. P. C., Kelly, P. A., and Friesen, H. G., 1973, Radioreceptor assay for prolactin and other lactogenic hormones, Science 180:968–971.

Shyamala, G., and McBlain, W. A., 1979, Distinction between progestin- and glucocorticoid-binding sites in mammary glands, Biochem. J. 178:345–352.

Singh, D. V., and Bern, H. A., 1969, Interaction between prolactin and thyroxine in mouse mammary gland lobulo-alveolar development in vitro, J. Endocrinol. 45:579–583.

Singh, D. V., DeOme, K. B., and Bern, H. A., 1970, Strain differences in response of the mouse mammary gland to hormones in vitro, J. Natl. Cancer Inst. 45:657–675.

Sinha, D., and Dao, T. L., 1977, Hyperplastic alveolar nodules of the rat mammary gland: Tumor producing capabilities in vivo and in vitro, Cancer Lett. 2:153–160.

Slavin, B., 1966, Growth of mammary transplants in various tissue and organ sites in the mouse, Anat. Rec. 154:423.

Smith, G. H., and Vonderhaar, B. K., 1981, Functional differentiation in mouse mammary gland epithelium is attained through DNA synthesis, inconsequent of mitosis, Dev. Biol. 88:167–179.

Smith, G. H., Vonderhaar, B. K., Graham, D. E., and Medina, D., 1984, Expression of pregnancy-specific genes in preneoplastic mouse mammary tissues from virgin mice, Cancer Res. 44:3426–3437.

Soloff, M. S., Alexandrova, M., and Fernstrom, M. J., 1979, Oxytocin receptors: Triggers for parturition and lactation?, Science 204:1313–1315.

Squartini, F., Basolo, F., and Bistocchi, M., 1983, Lobuloalveolar differentiation and tumorigenesis: Two separate activities for mouse mammary tumor virus, Cancer Res. 43:5879–5882.

Sutton, H., and Suhrbier, K., 1967, The estrous cycle and DNA synthesis in the mammary gland, Argonne Natl. Lab. U.S. Atomic Energy Commission Annual Report pp. 157–158.

Taga, M., Sakakura, T., and Oka, T., 1983, Identification and partial characterization of mesenchyme-derived growth factor that stimulates proliferation and inhibits functional differentiation of mammary epithelium in culture, J. Cell Biol. 97:317a.

Taketani, Y., and Oka, T., 1983a, Biological action of epidermal growth factor and its functional receptors in normal mammary epithelial cells, Proc. Natl. Acad. Sci. USA 80:2647–2650.

Taketani, Y., and Oka, T., 1983b, Epidermal growth factor stimulates cell proliferation and inhibits functional differentiation of mouse mammary epithelial cells in culture, Endocrinology 113:871–877.

Telang, N. T., Banerjee, M. R., Iyer, A. P., and Kundu, A. B., 1979, Neoplastic transformation of epithelial cells in whole mammary gland in vitro, Proc. Natl. Acad. Sci. USA 76:5886–5890.

Terada, N., and Oka, T., 1982, Selective stimulation of α-lactalbumin synthesis and its mRNA accumulation by thyroid hormone in the differentiation of the mouse mammary gland in vitro, FEBS Lett. 149:101–104.

Terada, N., and Oka, T., 1983, Cortisol 21-mesylate exerts glucocorticoid action on the induction of milk protein synthesis in cultured mammary gland, Horm. Metab. Res. 15:508–512.

Terada, N., Leiderman, L. J., and Oka, T., 1983, The interaction of cortisol and prostaglandins on the phenotypic expression of the α-lactalbumin gene in the mouse mammary gland in culture, Biochem. Biophys. Res. Commun. 111:1059–1065.

Terry, P. M., Banerjee, M. R., and Lui, R. M., 1977, Hormone-inducible casein messenger RNA in a serum-free organ culture of whole mammary gland, *Proc. Natl. Acad. Sci. USA* **74:**2441–2445.

Toft, D. O., and O'Malley, B. W., 1972, Target tissue receptors for progesterone: The influence of estrogen treatment, *Endocrinology* **90:**1041–1045.

Tonelli, Q. J., and Sorof, S., 1980, Epidermal growth factor requirement for development of cultured mammary gland, *Nature* **285:**250–252.

Tonelli, Q. J., and Sorof, S., 1981, Expression of a phenotype of normal differentiation in cultured mammary glands is promoted by epidermal growth factor and blocked by cyclic adenine nucleotide and prostaglandins, *Differentiation* **20:**253–259.

Tonelli, Q. J., Custer, R. P., and Sorof, S., 1979, Transformation of cultured mouse mammary glands by aromatic amines and amides and their derivatives, *Cancer Res.* **39:**1784–1792.

Topper, Y. J., and Freeman, C. S., 1980, Multiple hormone interactions in the developmental biology of the mammary gland, *Physiol. Rev.* **60:**1049–1106.

Topper, Y. J., Oka, T., and Vonderhaar, B. K., 1975, Techniques for studying development of normal mammary epithelial cells in organ culture, *Methods Enzymol.* **39:**443–454.

Topper, Y. J., Nicholas, K. R., Sankaran, L., and Kulski, J., 1984, Insulin as a developmental hormone, in: *Hormones and Cancer* (E. Gurpide, R. Calandra, C. Levy, and R. J. Soto, eds.), Liss, New York, pp. 63–77.

Traurig, H. H., 1967a, Cell proliferation in the mammary gland during late pregnancy and lactation, *Anat. Rec.* **157:**489–503.

Traurig, H. H., 1967b, A radioautographic study of cell proliferation in the mammary gland of the pregnant mouse, *Anat. Rec.* **159:**239–244.

Tucker, H. A., 1981, Physiological control of mammary growth, lactogenesis, and lactation, *J. Dairy Sci.* **64:**1403–1421.

Turner, C. W., and Gomez, E. T., 1934, The experimental development of the mammary gland. I. The male and female albino mouse, *Univ. Mo. Columbia Coll. Agric. Agric. Exp. Stn. Res. Bull.* **206:**1–16.

Vignon, F., and Rochefort, H., 1976, Regulation of estrogen receptors in ovarian-dependent rat mammary tumors. I. Effect of castration and prolactin, *Endocrinology* **98:**722–729.

Vonderhaar, B. K., 1975, A role of thyroid hormones in differentiation of mouse mammary gland in vitro, *Biochem. Biophys. Res. Commun.* **67:**1219–1225.

Vonderhaar, B. K., 1977, Studies on the mechanism by which thyroid hormones enhance α-lactalbumin activity in explants from mouse mammary glands, *Endocrinology* **100:**1423–1431.

Vonderhaar, B. K., 1979, Lactose synthetase activity in mouse mammary glands is controlled by thyroid hormones, *J. Cell Biol.* **82:**675–681.

Vonderhaar, B. K., 1982, Effect of thyroid hormones on mammary tumor induction and growth, in: *Hormonal Regulation of Experimental Mammary Tumors*, Volume II (B. S. Leung, ed.), Eden Press, Montreal, pp. 138–154.

Vonderhaar, B. K., 1984, Hormones and growth factors in mammary gland development, in: *Control of Cell Growth and Proliferation* (C. M. Veneziale, ed.), Van Nostrand–Reinhold, Princeton, N. J., pp. 11–33.

Vonderhaar, B. K., and Greco, A. E., 1979, Lobulo-alveolar development of mouse mammary glands is regulated by thyroid hormones, *Endocrinology* **104:**409–418.

Vonderhaar, B. K., and Smith, G. H., 1982, Dissociation of cytological and functional differentiation in virgin mouse mammary gland during DNA synthesis inhibition, *J. Cell Sci.* **53:**97–114.

Vonderhaar, B. K., Owens, I. S., and Topper, Y. J., 1973, An early effect of prolactin on the formation of α-lactalbumin by mouse mammary epithelial cells, *J. Biol. Chem.* **248:**467–471.

Warner, M. R., 1978, Effect of perinatal oestrogen on the pretreatment required for mouse mammary lobular formation in vitro, *J. Endocrinol.* **77:**1–10.

Wasner, G., Hennermann, I., and Kratochwil, K., 1983, Ontogeny of mesenchymal androgen receptors in the embryonic mouse mammary gland, *Endocrinology* **113:**1771–1780.

Wellings, S. R., Jensen, H. M., and Marcum, R. G., 1975, An atlas of subgross pathology of the human breast with special reference to possible precancerous lesions, *J. Natl. Cancer Inst.* **55**:231–273.

Welsch, C. W., and Nagasawa, H., 1977, Prolactin and murine mammary tumorigenesis: A review, *Cancer Res.* **37**:951–963.

Williams, L. T., Lefkowitz, R. J., Watanabe, A. M., Hathaway, D. R., and Besch, H. R., Jr., 1977, Thyroid hormone regulation of β-adrenergic receptor number, *J. Biol. Chem.* **252**:2787–2789.

Wood, B. G., Washburn, L. L., Mukherjee, A. S., and Banerjee, M. R., 1975, Hormonal regulation of lobulo-alveolar growth, functional differentiation and regression of whole mouse mammary gland in organ culture, *J. Endocrinol.* **65**:1–6.

Young, P., Arch, J. R. S., and Ashwell, M., 1984, Brown adipose tissue in the parametrial fat pad of the mouse, *FEBS Lett.* **167**:10–14.

Zamierowski, M. M., and Ebner, K. E., 1980, A radioimmunoassay for mouse α-lactalbumin, *J. Immunol. Methods* **36**:211–220.

CHAPTER 7

ROLE OF CYCLIC AMP IN MODIFYING THE GROWTH OF MAMMARY CARCINOMAS
Genomic Regulation

YOON SANG CHO-CHUNG, FREESIA L. HUANG, and C. LAL KAPOOR

1. INTRODUCTION

It has become a widely held view that cyclic adenosine $3',5'$-monophosphate (cAMP), an intracellular chemical switch, regulates cellular growth and differentiation. The precise mechanism of cAMP action is, however, unknown at present.

In eukaryotic cells, cAMP acts as the intracellular mediator for a set of nonsteroid hormones (Robison et al., 1971). The action of cAMP is then mediated through activation of protein kinases, which phosphorylates specific proteins and thereby modifies their biological activity (Kuo and Greengard, 1969). In bacteria, however, the action of cAMP has been shown to involve no protein phosphorylation (Pastan and Perlman, 1972). Upon binding to cAMP receptor protein (CRP), cAMP in E. coli induces an allosteric change in CRP and the resulting cAMP–CRP complex then interacts directly with DNA to initiate gene transcription (Pastan and Perlman, 1972). Thus, two apparently different mechanisms of cAMP action have been elucidated— one involves promotion of protein phosphorylation and the other involves induction of an allosteric change or an activation of a receptor protein.

YOON SANG CHO-CHUNG, FREESIA L. HUANG, and C. LAL KAPOOR ● Laboratory of Pathophysiology, National Cancer Institute, National Institutes of Health, Bethesda, Maryland 20205.

The mechanism of cAMP action in bacteria resembles that of steroid hormones in eukaryotes. Steroid hormones enter the cell and bind to steroid receptor proteins. The activated steroid–protein complex formed in the cytoplasm enters the nucleus where it can interact with chromatin (Jensen and DeSombre, 1972; O'Malley and Means, 1974). Although this type of mechanism has not been demonstrated for the action of cAMP in eukaryotic cells, indirect evidence from recent studies suggests (Cho-Chung, 1980b) that cAMP-binding protein in mammalian organisms might also exert an action similar to that of CRP in *E. coli* in regulating gene transcription

This chapter deals with the mechanism of cAMP action in growth control of hormone-dependent mammary tumors. The evidence presented shows that: (1) cAMP acts antagonistically with estrogen in the hormone-dependent mammary tumors and the antagonism requires the respective binding proteins to be present in the cytoplasm; (2) the counteraction between cAMP and estrogen is exerted on the endogenous nuclear protein phosphorylation and in the differential gene expression observed during growth and regression of mammary tumors; (3) cAMP suppresses the hormone-dependent expression of the cellular ras^H oncogene in mammary carcinomas *in vivo*. It is proposed tht cAMP and steroid hormones may counteract each other through their respective binding proteins in the regulation of hormone-dependent tumor growth.

2. GROWTH ARREST BY cAMP

Growth and morphology of a number of cultured cell lines have been reported to be influenced by cAMP or its derivatives. Exposure of various lines of transformed cells to cAMP or cAMP derivatives resulted in inhibition of growth rate without affecting cell viability (Pastan *et al.*, 1975; Prasad, 1975; Dubpernell and Gavurin, 1978; Puck, 1979). These actions of cAMP raise the question as to whether exogenous cAMP derivatives or agents altering intracellular cAMP levels might contribute to pharmacological control of cancer.

2.1. Mammary Tumors in Rats

Administration of cAMP derivatives, $N^6,O^{2'}$-dibutyryl cAMP (DBcAMP), 8-thiomethyl cAMP, and 8-bromo cAMP (10 mg/day per 200-g rat, s.c. or os) (Cho-Chung, 1974; Cho-Chung and Gullino, 1974a), or cholera toxin (2 μg/day per 200-g rat, s.c.) (Cho-Chung *et al.*, 1983), an agent that specifically increases intracellular cAMP levels (Holmgren, 1981), to host rats resulted in the arrest of growth of hormone-dependent tumors, primary, 7,12-dimethylbenz(α)anthracene (DMBA)-induced (Huggins *et al.*, 1961) and transplanted MTW9 (Kim and Furth, 1960). The same treatment of hormone-responsive and -independent tumors produced growth arrest in a fraction of tumors. The inhibition of growth by DBcAMP was dose-dependent and reversible, and no toxic effect of DBcAMP was observed in the animals (Cho-Chung, 1974).

Of particular importance is the synergistic growth inhibitory response elicited by DBcAMP and arginine (Cho-Chung et al., 1980). When a dose of DBcAMP (1 mg/200-g rat s.c.) that alone had no effect on tumor growth was injected into the animals along with arginine (50 mg/200-g rat s.c.), the growth inhibitory effect was enhanced. Tumors regressed rapidly and within 2 weeks the majority of tumors regressed to 15% of their initial size. The dose–response curves of DBcAMP in the absence and presence of arginine showed that arginine enhanced the growth inhibition at all doses of DBcAMP and lowered the dose of DBcAMP required for maximal growth inhibition to one-tenth of that in the absence of arginine.

Arginine alone also produced inhibition of tumor growth; at a dose of 50 mg/200-g rat per day s.c., appreciable tumor regression occurred within 2 weeks (Cho-Chung et al., 1980). The growtht inhibitory effect of arginine has been demonstrated on various experimental tumors (Levy et al., 1954; Nakanishi, 1969; Kojima et al., 1973; Takeda et al., 1975; Milner and Stepanovich, 1979), but the mechanism of its action has not been elucidated.

The synergistic effect of arginine and DBcAMP on growth arrest was not mimicked by DBcAMP and other amino acids, such as lysine or serine. Moreover, arginine enhanced both the cAMP-induced increase of the 56,000-dalton cAMP receptor protein (CR) in DMBA tumor slices in vitro and the penetration of the cAMP receptor complex into tumor nuclei in a cell-free system (Cho-Chung et al., 1979). In vivo growth arrest by arginine was accompanied by a sharp increase in cellular cAMP content, which was preceded by parallel increases in NAD-dependent ADP-ribosylation of the membrane proteins and NAD-dependent activation of adenylate cyclase (Cho-Chung et al., 1980). These results suggest a specific role for arginine in the cAMP-mediated inhibition of mammary tumors.

2.2. Human Breast Cancer Cells in Culture

Growth of human breast cancer cells (MCF-7) in culture has been arrested by DBcAMP (10^{-4} M) (Shafie and Brooks, 1977; Cho-Chung et al., 1981a) or cholera toxin (10^{-10} M) (Cho-Chung et al., 1983), and the growth arrest accompanied the morphological change of the cells (Cho-Chung et al., 1981a). Arginine also exhibited a synergistic growth inhibitory effect with DBcAMP on MCF-7 cells. When DBcAMP, at a dose (10^{-6} M) that alone had no effect on cell growth, was added to the cell culture along with a dose of arginine, the growth inhibitory effect was greatly enhanced (Cho-Chung et al., 1981a). Cell replication ceased completely within 2 days after treatment and the growth arrest was preceded by an increase in the intracellular content of cAMP and adenylate cyclase activity and by a decrease in estrogen-binding. Thus, mammary cancer cell growth is subject to cAMP-mediated regulation and arginine appears to play a specific role in this process.

3. ANTAGONISM BETWEEN cAMP AND ESTROGEN IN HORMONE-DEPENDENT MAMMARY TUMORS

The first indication that a relationship exists between estrogen and cAMP in mammary tumor regression was provided by the observation that both hormone removal (ovariectomy) and DBcAMP treatment produce new synthesis of acid RNase within a few hours after initiation of treatment (Cho-Chung and Gullino, 1973, 1974a; Cho-Chung, 1974). In regressing DMBA tumors, an increase in the cAMP level follows ovariectomy (Matusik and Hilf, 1976; Bodwin *et al.*, 1978; Cho-Chung *et al.*, 1978a), high-dose estrogen or tamoxifen administration (Bodwin *et al.*, 1981b), inhibition of prolactin secretion (Matusik and Hilf, 1976), streptozotocin-induced diabetes (Matusik and Hilf, 1976; Shafie *et al.*, 1979), and DBcAMP treatment (Bodwin *et al.*, 1978; Cho-Chung *et al.*, 1978a). In rat uterus, the cAMP level decreases when a low-dose estrogen injection is given following ovariectomy, or during proestrus when the plasma estrogen level is maximal (Kuehl *et al.*, 1974). These data indicate that cAMP levels are low in estrogen-target tissues that are under a physiological concentration of estrogen. Thus, there appears to be an antogonistic relationship between cAMP and estrogen in target tissues.

3.1. cAMP- and Estrogen-Binding Activities

How might cAMP and estrogen interact? Involvement of the specific cytoplasmic receptor proteins for cAMP and estrogen has been shown in hormone-dependent mammary tumors (Bodwin *et al.*, 1978; *Cho-Chung et al.*, 1978a; Cho-Chung, 1979b). During growth, high estrogen-binding and low cAMP-binding activities are found in DMBA-induced tumors. When DMBA tumors undergo growth arrest following either ovariectomy or DBcAMP treatment of the host, a change in the specific binding of estrogen and cAMP occurs in the tumors: cAMP binding markedly increases whereas estrogen binding sharply decreases in tthe regressing tumors. These reciprocal changes in cAMP- and estrogen-binding activities are detectable within 1 day after either ovariectomy or DBcAMP treatment, when there is no appreciable change in tumor size, indicating that the changes are early events in the regression process rather than the result of tumor regression. The changes are reversed, however, when tumor growth is resumed following either the injection of estradiol valerate or the cessation of DBcAMP treatment. The increased cAMP-binding activitty seems to be the result of new protein synthesis since the increase can be blocked by cycloheximide. The decrease of estrogen-binding activity was due to the decrease in total binding sites without any modification of either binding affinity or sedimentation characteristics.

We have observed that the inverse relationship between cAMP- and estrogen-binding activities was closely related to the hormone-dependency of tumor growth. In hormone-independent mammary tumors that continue to grow and fail to regress after hormonal deprivation, we found a wide range

of estrogen- and cAMP-binding activities that do not change after ovariectomy or DBcAMP treatment. It appears that the integrity of both cAMP-
binding protein and estrogen receptor is probably essential for the control
of hormone-dependent mammary tumor growth. Thus, cAMP and estrogen
may counteract each other through their respective binding proteins in the
regulation of hormone-dependent tumor growth (Cho-Chung, 1979b).

3.2. Nuclear Protein Phosphorylation

Nuclear proteins are a complex of many different molecules whose heterogeneity and specificity may be varied further by phosphorylative modification. There is evidence that certain steroid and thyroid hormones mediate
nuclear protein phosphorylation and regulation of DNA transcription primarily through stimulation of nuclear cAMP-independent protein kinase. In
the case of hormones and exogenous stimuli that act via cAMP, however,
nuclear protein phosphorylation and gene expression are stimulated after
the cAMP-mediated translocation of cytoplasmic cAMP-dependent protein
kinase to nuclear acceptor sites (Jungmann and Kranias, 1977). In both cases,
hormone-mediated stimulation of nuclear cAMP-dependent and -indepen-
dent protein kinases could result in phosphorylative modification of certain
nuclear proteins. Studies from our laboratory (Cho-Chung and Redler, 1977;
Cho-Chung and Doud, 1978) have shown a correlation between specific nuclear protein phosphorylation and growth arrest of hormone-dependent
mammary tumors. In growing DMBA tumor nuclei, a low-molecular-weight
basic protein species, GAP (growth-associated protein), was found to be the
major endogenous substrate for nuclear protein kinase; whereas in nuclei
from tumors regressing after ovariectomy or DBcAMP treatment, the phosphorylation of GAP decreases and a new nonhistone basic protein species
of higher molecular weight, RAP (regression-associated protein), becomes
the predominant substrate of the endogenous kinase. These changes in phosphorylation take place within 1 day after ovariectomy or DBcAMP treatment
and are reversed by injection of estradiol valerate or cessation of DBcAMP
treatment. Phosphorylation of RAP was also induced in vitro by preincu-
bation of growing DMBA tumor slices with 10^{-5} M cAMP but when 10^{-7}
M 17β-estradiol was added simultaneously with cAMP, the effect of cAMP
was inhibited. Moreover, the exogenous substrate specificity and the effect
of protein inhibitor on nuclear protein kinase activity indicated that phosphorylation of GAP and RAP is probably due to the presence of different
kinases in the tumor nuclei; the former is due to cAMP-independent protein
kinase and the latter is due to cAMP-dependent protein kinase. These results
led us to propose that an antagonistic action between cAMP and estrogen
in the growth control of a hormone-dependent mammary tumor is exerted
through a specific action on nuclear protein phosphorylation.

If one accepts the concept of gene transcription via a protein kinase-
dependent nuclear protein phosphorylation, then the interaction between
protein kinase and its substrate must have a high degree of specificity for

precise regulation to be achieved. Indeed, this has been found to be the case in (1): the recognition by protein kinase of a specific primary sequence of amino acids around the phosphorylation sites, e.g., presence of an arginine residue end terminal to the serine residue that undergoes phosphorylation (Langan, 1973); (2) specific substrate conformation (Bylund and Krebs, 1975); and (3) by the selective synthesis and activation of two general types of cAMP-dependent protein kinase, types I and II, in response to specific stimuli (Costa *et al.*, 1976).

3.3. Mechanism of cAMP and Estrogen Interaction

Two types of hormone–cell interaction involving steroid and nonsteroid hormones have been described. Steroid hormones enter the cell and bind to a specific extranuclear receptor protein to form a steroid–protein complex which then migrates to the nucleus where specific RNA synthesis is initiated (Jensen and DeSombre, 1972; O'Malley and Means, 1974). Certain nonsteroid hormones, such as catecholamines, trophic hormones, and polypeptides, act primarily at the cell surface to activate adenylate cyclase and thereby generate cAMP (Perkins, 1973). How does cAMP then mediate the diverse regulatory signals of hormones at the cellular level? The isolation of cAMP-dependent protein kinase by Walsh *et al.* (1968) and discoveries (Walsh *et al.*, 1968; Langan, 1968) of a wide substrate specificity of protein kinases led to the proposal by Kuo and Greengard (1969) that all cAMP effects in eukaryotic cells are mediated through protein kinase regulation in various tissues. Subsequently, the cAMP control of transcription via nuclear protein phosphorylation was suggested by the finding that nuclear proteins serve as substrate for cAMP-dependent protein kinase (Langan, 1968). However, it is difficult to explain the phosphorylation of nuclear proteins *in vivo* by a direct action of cAMP on nuclear protein kinase, since the kinase in isolated, intact nuclei has been found to be insensitive to stimulation by cAMP, in contrast to cytoplasmic kinase, which is sensitive to cAMP stimulation. A solution to this dilemma emerged from the discovery of the nuclear translocation of cytoplasmic cAMP-dependent protein kinase following membrane stimulation by trophic hormones (Jungmann *et al.*, 1975). The specific binding of cytoplasmic cAMP-binding protein and catalytic protein kinase subunit to chromatin acceptor sites has been shown to occur through cAMP stimulation both *in vivo* and *in vitro* (Jungmann and Kranias, 1977). Thus, it appears that the molecular mechanism underlying cAMP action is similar to that of steroid hormones whereby cAMP initially binds to a specific extranuclear receptor protein to form a cAMP–protein complex that then migrates to the nucleus, leading to gene transcription. How might cAMP and a steroid hormonee be interrelated in the regulation of gene expression and/or growth control? Data described in the preceding section lend support to the hypothesis that in hormone-dependent mammary tumors, the interaction of cAMP and estrogen may be antagonistically related. The inverse relationship between cAMP- and estrogen-binding activities found during growth and regression of DMBA tumors suggested that these binding proteins may interact in the growth control of this tumor. Moreover, an apparent antagonism between estrogen receptor and cAMP receptor protein was observed in their translocation from the cytosol to the nucleus (Bodwin et al., 1981a). In a hormone-dependent MTW9 mammary tumor cell-free system, cytosol activated with either [³H]17β-estradiol or [³H]cAMP was incubated with purified nuclei to determine the specific nuclear uptake of these receptor proteins. No competition was noted between estrogen and cAMP for each other's cytoplasmic binding proteins or the nuclear acceptor sites. However, the presence of 100 nM cAMP in the activated cytosol inhibited the nuclear uptake of [³H]17β-estradiol (5 nM) by 50% and the presence of 5 nM 17β-estradiol in the cytosol inhibited the nuclear uptake of [³H]cAMP (100 nM) by 50%

These results suggested that cAMP and estrogen interaction through their respective receptor proteins at the nuclear level may be involved in the control of hormone-dependent mammary tumor growth.

3.4. Estrogen Receptor/cAMP Receptor Ratio as a Probe of Hormone-Dependence

The inverse relationship between cAMP- and estrogen-binding activities is closely related to the hormone-dependency of mammary tumors in rats (Figure 1A) (Cho-Chung, 1978). Similar inverse relationships between estrogen receptor and cAMP receptor protein were also found in primary human breast tumor cytosols (Handschin et al., 1983). This suggests that the relative concentrations of estrogen receptor (ER) and cAMP receptor protein (CR) in

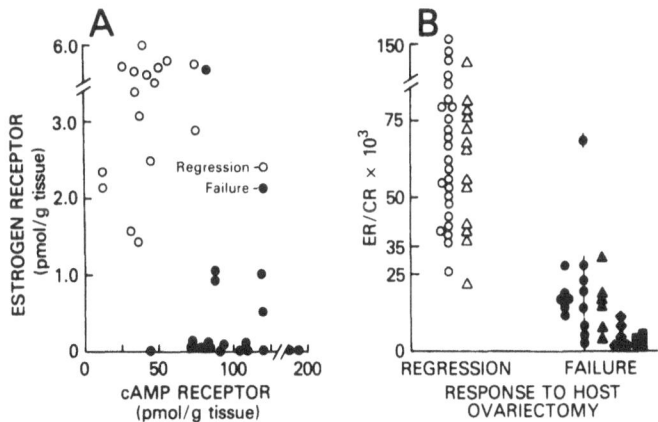

FIGURE 1. Relationship of estrogen- and cAMP-binding capacities to the response of tumors to host ovariectomy. Estrogen- and cAMP-binding activities in tumor cytosols were measured on biopsy specimens before ovariectomy. Tumor responses to ovariectomy are: regression, >50% decrease in tumor volume by day 6; failure, >60% increase in tumor volume by day 6. Tumors used are primary DMBA- and MNU-induced mammary carcinomas and transplantable DMBA #1 and MT13762 tumors (from Cho-Chung, 1978, and Bodwin et al., 1980).

tumor cytosol may be a more sensitive indicator of hormone-dependency than ER level alone. Indeed, this was proven to be true in rat tumor models. In a study of 70 rat mammary tumors, 95% of hormone-dependent tumors had an ER/CR ratio of 35×10^{-3} or more whereas 97% of hormone-independent tumors had an ER/CR ratio of less than 35×10^{-3} (Figure 1B) (Bodwin *et al.*, 1980). When ER alone was measured, hormone-dependency could only be predicted in 60% of the tumors. The ER/CR ratios were also elevated in normal estrogen target tissues as compared to nontarget tissues. Thus, the relative concentrations of ER/CR reflect the hormone-dependency of mammary tumors and normal tissues more accurately than does the concentration of ER alone.

These results were confirmed in a limited number of primary human breast cancers examined (Kvinnsland *et al.*, 1983). Patients with advanced, evaluable breast cancer were biopsied before the start of endocrine treatment, and ER and CR levels were measured. Sixteen of thirty patients (53%) had an objective response to endocrine treatment. When ER and CR were expressed as a ratio and this ratio was related to treatment response, it was found that all objective responders had ratio values above 2.5×10^{-3}. Nine of fourteen nonresponders had ER/CR ratios below this value. Thus, a threshold limit of 2.5×10^{-3} ER/CR ratio value correctly predicted the response to endocrine treatment in 25 of 30 patients (83%). These results suggest that CR measurements may be a tool to achieve a better selection of patients for endocrine therapy, and provide new data on important aspects of breast cancer.

4. cAMP RECEPTOR PROTEINS (CR)

In mammalian cells, cAMP interacts with its receptor protein (a high-affinity binding protein), the regulatory subunit of cAMP-dependent protein kinase (Kuo and Greengard, 1969; Krebs, 1972). The protein kinase has been purified from various tissues of several animal species and consists of two catalytic (C) and two regulatory (R) subunits. When cAMP binds to R, the holoenzyme (RC) dissociates, freeing C from R, thus activating the enzyme. The catalytically active C then phosphorylates specific proteins, thereby modifying their biological activity. Thus, the action of cAMP involves protein phosphorylation as proposed by Kuo and Greengard (1969).

Daniel *et al.* (1973) were the first to observe the relationship between the resistance to the cytotoxic effect of DBcAMP and aberrant CR in cultured mouse lymphoma cells. Subsequently, Simantov and Sachs (1975) found a similar relationship in a clone of neuroblastoma cells. A W256 rat mammary carcinoma line (*in vivo*) (Cho-Chung and Gullino, 1974b), unresponsive to DBcAMP, showed several qualitative and quantitative CR differences from a responsive line (Cho-Chung *et al.*, 1977c). A striking correlation between the heat stability of CR and DBcAMP-induced regression has also been found in other types of mammary tumors and hepatomas (Cho-Chung and Clair, 1977).

Furthermore, during DBcAMP-induced regression, the CR in W256 mammary tumors accumulated in the nuclei (Cho-Chung et al., 1977b). The accumulation of CR was not found in DBcAMP-unresponsive tumors that contained defective CR (Cho-Chung et al., 1977a). Thus, a correlation was found between a defective CR, incapable of accumulating in the nucleus, and cAMP-unresponsiveness in vivo. These data indicate that growth regulation by cAMP involves the CR and thus there may be no simple relationship between intracellular concentration of cAMP and the rate of cell replication (Cho-Chung, 1979a; Christoffersen and Brønstad, 1980).

4.1. cAMP Receptor Proteins (CR) and cAMP Responsiveness in Vivo

The molecular species of CR involved in tumor regression was examined in hormone-dependent DMBA-induced mammary carcinomas. The growing tumors contained two major CR with molecular weights of 39K and 56K in the cytoplasm but not in the nucleus (Cho-Chung, 1980a). The 56K protein is the regulatory subunit of cAMP-dependent protein kinase type II and the 39K protein is the proteolytic fragment of the 56K protein (Corbin et al., 1978; Weber and Hilz, 1979). Following DBcAMP treatment, the 56K protein increased in the cytoplasm of regressing tumors, whereas the 39K protein showed no change; and only the 56K protein appeared in the nuclei of regressing tumors (Cho-Chung, 1980a). The increase of 56K CR also occurred in tumors regressing after ovariectomy (Cho-Chung, 1980a), injections of tamoxifen or pharmacologic doses of estrogen (Bodwin et al., 1981b), and in tumor slices incubated with cAMP in the presence of benzamidine and arginine in vitro (Cho-Chung et al., 1979). In contrast, autonomously growing mammary tumors that fail to regress after ovariectomy or DBcAMP treatment contained the 56K protein in the cytoplasm but showed no increase of this receptor in either the cytosol or the nucleus (Cho-Chung, 1980b).

We speculated that the inability of the 56K CR of hormone-independent tumors to penetrate the nucleus may be due to a structural alteration of the protein. In fact, the 56K receptor of hormone-independent tumors was found to have a charge alteration as compared to the receptor of hormone-dependent tumors (Cho-Chung et al., 1981b). This charge alteration did not affect the cAMP-binding, but decreased the self-phosphorylation of the receptor. Self-phosphorylation [phosphorylation of the regulatory subunit of protein kinase by its own catalytic subunit (Erlichman et al., 1974)] has been shown to be characteristic of cAMP-dependent protein kinase type II from various tissues (Rubin and Rosen, 1975), and decreased self-phosphorylation correlates with a decreased ability of the CR to interact with the catalytic subunit of protein kinase (Corbin et al., 1978; Cho-Chung et al., 1981b).

Based on these data, we postulated (Cho-Chung, 1980b) that the CR that does penetrate into the nucleus must have two functional domains, one for cAMP-binding and the other for an interaction with the catalytic subunit of protein kinase. The CR of the hormone-independent tumors is deficient in its ability to be phosphorylated and to interact with the catalytic subunit of protein kinase and is incapable of migrating into the nucleus. The 39K CR, the proteolytic fragment of the 56K receptor, is also incapable of penetrating into the nucleus (Cho-Chung, 1980b). This protein retains the intact cAMP-binding, but has reduced ability to be phosphorylated and to be bound with the catalytic subunit of protein kinase. Another class of abnormal CR, AUT-PK85, has been isolated from adrenocortical carcinomas (Shanker et al., 1979); this receptor can bind cAMP and be autophosphorylated, but cannot interact with the catalytic subunit of protein kinase.

The above data are consistent with the hypothesis (Cho-Chung, 1982) that neoplastic growth, i.e., unrestrained growth, may be the consequence of an aberrant cAMP-dependent protein kinase system that is associated with the decreased amount of holoprotein kinase in the cell. As most of the cAMP-dependent protein kinase in normal cells is present in the form of holoenzyme (RC) (Krebs, 1972), the enzyme activity is stimulated by cAMP in vitro at least fivefold (Kuo and Greengard, 1969), and the amounts of subunits R and C and the proteolytic fragments of R are present in small fractions. In contrast to normal cells, the holoprotein kinase (RC) is greatly decreased in cancer cells. In most experimental tumors examined, cAMP-binding and cAMP-dependent protein kinase activities have been found to be lower than in normal tissues, and, in particular, the stimulatory effect of cAMP on the enzyme activity is decreased (see review by Cho-Chung, 1979a). A decrease of cAMP-dependent protein kinase, especially the type II enzyme, has also been reported in primary human mammary carcinoma (Handschin and Eppenberger, 1979). Compared with normal tissues, neoplastic tissues showed an impressively wide range of cAMP levels from very low to very very high (see review by Cho-Chung, 1979a). At low levels of cAMP, the amount of total cAMP-dependent protein kinase would be expected to be low, whereas at high levels of cAMP, the amount of holoenzyme (RC) should decrease due to its separation to the subunits, R and C (Krebs, 1972). Proteolysis potentiates the decrease of RC by an irreversible breakdown of the R subunit to its fragments, which cannot recombine with the C subunit (Corbin et al., 1978; Weber and Hilz, 1979). Indeed, the 39K CR is largely increased in tumors, as compared with normal tissues (Cho-Chung et al., 1981b; Handschin et al., 1983). The structural abnormality of R and C should also influence the interaction between the two subunits. Abnormal R has been shown to be correlated with resistance to cAMP in S49 lymphosarcoma mutant cells (Steinberg et al., 1977), a clone of neuroblastoma cells (Simantov and Sachs, 1975), and in hormone-independent mammary carcinomas (Cho-Chung et al., 1981b).

Hormone-dependent mammary carcinomas, which possess intact but decreased amounts of cAMP-dependent protein kinase, can undergo regression with the proper cAMP stimulation and the holoprotein kinase in these regressing tumors increases, thereby mimicking normal cells (Cho-Chung et al., 1978b; Cho-Chung, 1980b). Thus, the biochemical reversion of neoplastic to normal-like cells appears to depend on the relative cellular concentration of cAMP to cAMP-dependent protein kinase holoenzyme.

4.2. Nucleolar Localization of cAMP Receptor R^{II}

The molecular species and intracellular localization of CR in human breast cancer cells in culture were examined using affinity-purified antibodies (Kapoor and Cho-Chung, 1983a) directed against the purified CR (R^I and R^{II}) of bovine cAMP-dependent protein kinases type I and type II. The anti-R^I and -R^{II} antibodies specifically cross-reacted with the R^I and R^{II} CR of MCF-7 breast cancer cells (Kapoor and Cho-Chung, 1983b). Indirect immunofluorescence revealed that the R^{II} CR is specifically localized in the nucleoli of MCF-7 cells, whereas the R^I is diffusely localized in the nuclei (Figure 2) (Kapoor and Cho-Chung, 1983b). The localization of R^{II} CR on the mitotic spindles was also found for MDA-MB-231 human breast cancer cells (Kapoor and Cho-Chung, 1983c). Immunoprecipitation identified the molecular species of 50K R^{II} and 47K R^I in both cytosols and nuclear extracts

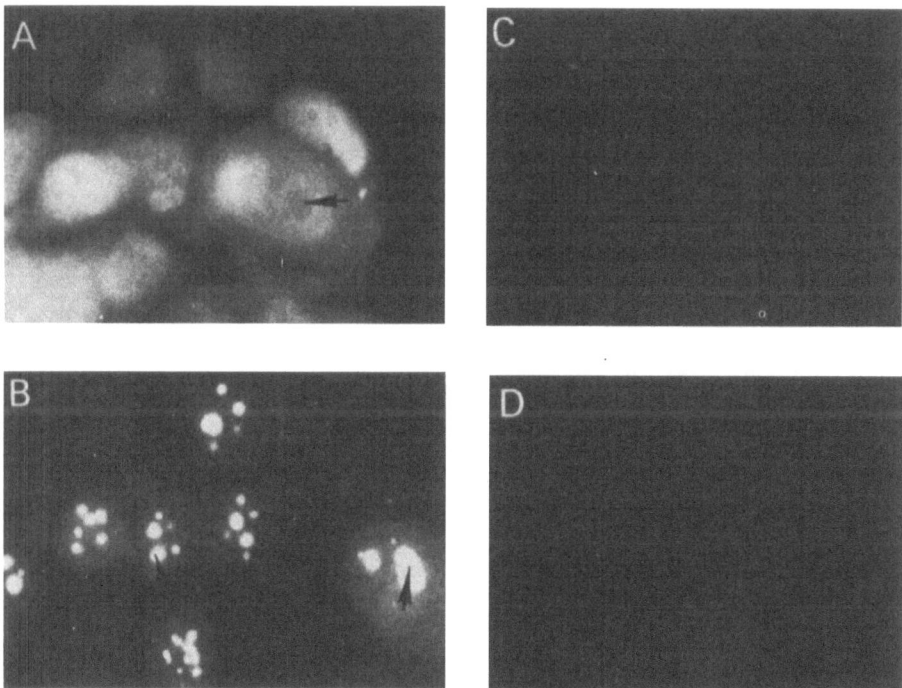

FIGURE 2. Immunocytochemical localization of R^I (A) and R^{II} (B) cAMP receptor proteins in MCF-7 cells. C, R^I antibody preabsorbed with R^I antigen; D, R^{II} antibody preabsorbed with R^{II} antigen. Arrowheads, nucleoli in nucleus, ×800 (from Kapoor and Cho-Chung, 1983b).

of MCF-7 and MDA-MB-231 cells (Kapoor and Cho-Chung, 1983b,c). The 50K and 52K R^{II} CR have also been detected in the cytosols of primary human breast tumors (Weber et al., 1981; Handschin et al., 1983).

During regression of MCF-7 tumors in nude mice following hormone withdrawal (Shafie and Grantham, 1981), the intensity of immunofluorescence of R^{II} increased dramatically in the nucleoli whereas that of R^{I} remained the same (Figure 3) (Kapoor et al., 1983). In the growing tumors, the 50K and 52K R^{II} CR were found in the cytosol but not in the nuclei: the growing tumor nuclei contained the low-molecular-weight 34K and 44K receptors, probably the proteolytic fragments of R^{II} (Kapoor et al., 1983). Following estrogen withdrawal, the 50K and 52K R^{II} proteins increased in the cytosol and newly appeared in the nuclei of the regressing tumors (Kapoor et al., 1983). Thus, the increase in the intensity of immunofluorescence in the regressing tumor nuclei was due to selective accumulation of the 50K and 52K R^{II} receptors. Hormone withdrawal, therefore, resulted in the specific transfer of the intact R^{II} CR from the cytoplasm to the nucleus. The results parallel the finding (Cho-Chung, 1980a), obtained with rat mammary tumors in vivo, that the nuclear translocation of the intact R^{II} CR correlates with the growth arrest induced by hormonal deprivation.

5. MECHANISM OF HORMONE-DEPENDENT MAMMARY TUMOR REGRESSION

The results of studies described to this point suggest that cAMP and its receptor protein play a key role in hormone-dependent mammary tumor regression. In regressing mammary tumors produced by hormone withdrawal (ovariectomy) or DBcAMP treatment, both cAMP-binding and cAMP-dependent protein kinase activities increased in the nucleus with new phosphorylation of 76K nuclear protein, RAP (Cho-Chung and Redler, 1977). Phosphorylation of RAP ceases when tumor growth is resumed following either the injection of estrogen or the cessation of DBcAMP treatment. Phosphorylation of RAP was also induced in regressing DMBA tumors following tamoxifen or high-dose estrogen injections (Bodwin et al., 1981b).

We have investigated the relationship between the transfer of cAMP-dependent protein kinase from the cytoplasm to the nucleus and the phosphorylation of nuclear proteins using the hormone-dependent mammary tumor model.

FIGURE 3. Immunocytochemical localization of R^{I} and R^{II} cAMP receptor proteins in growing and regressing MCF-7 tumors in nude mice. A and C, R^{II} localization in growing and regressing tumors, respectively; E and G, R^{I} localization in growing and regressing tumors, respectively. B, D, F, and H represent the phase-contrast pictures of A, C, E, and G, respectively. Arrowheads, nucleoli in nucleus (from Kapoor et al., 1983).

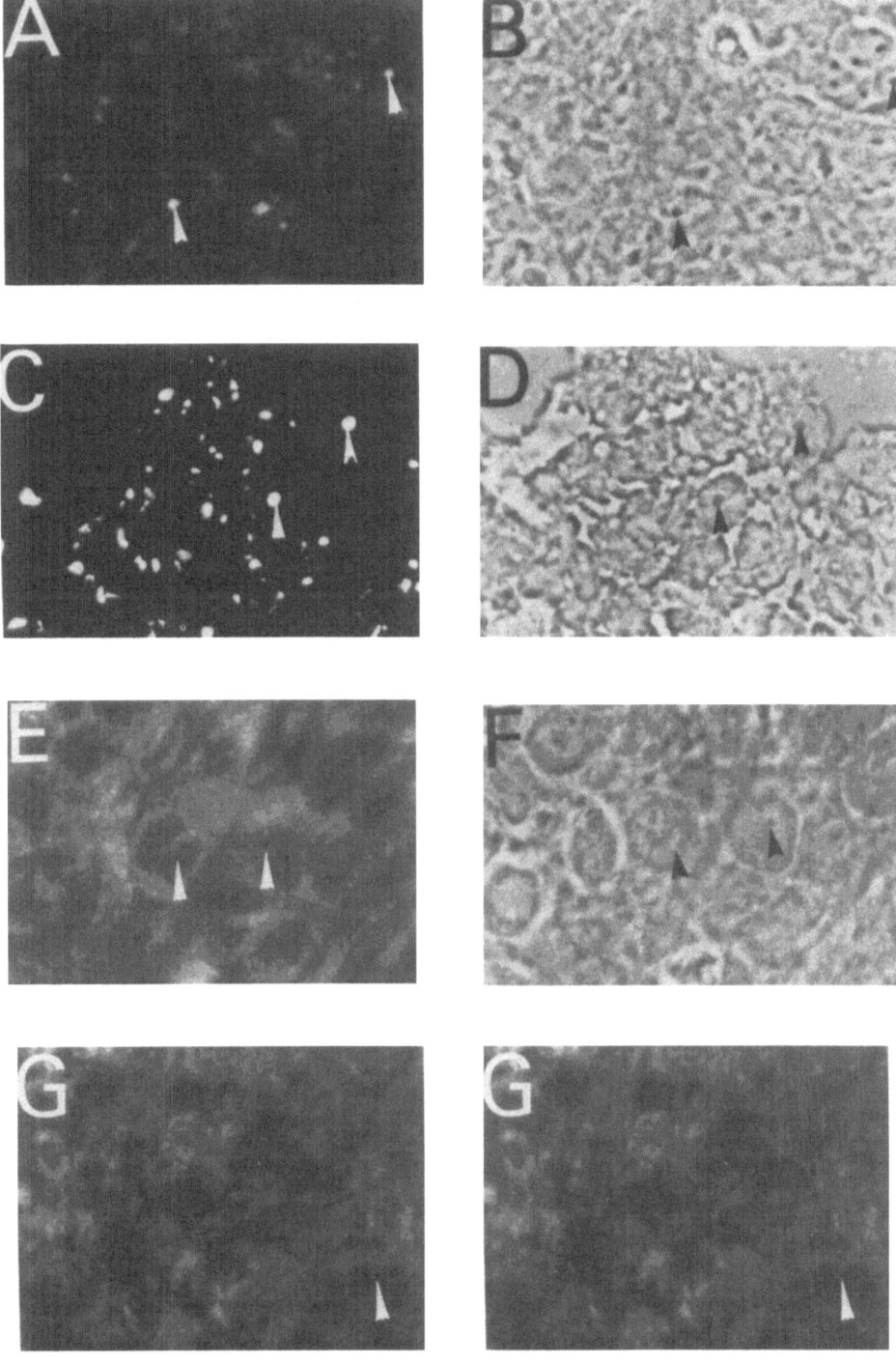

5.1. Nuclear Translocation of cAMP + Receptor Complex

Direct evidence that the cytoplasmic cAMP receptor–ligand complex enters the nucleus and binds with nuclear macromolecules has been obtained by the photoaffinity cross-linking technique using 8-azido [^{32}P]cAMP in the DMBA ttumor cell-free system. The nuclear binding of the 56K CR was accompanied by new phosphorylation of the 76K nuclear protein (Cho-Chung, 1980b). Moreover, the 56K CR that penetrated into the nucleus showed self-phosphorylation, indicating the coexistence of the cAMP-dependent protein kinase catalytic subunit in the stimulated nucleus. Since cAMP-dependent protein kinase activity is undetectable in growing DMBA tumor nuclei, but present in the tumor cytosol (Cho-Chung et al., 1978b), the enzyme is probably transferred from the cytosol to the nucleus. In fact, protein kinase extracted from the stimulated nuclei is cAMP-dependent as is that found in the cytosol; furthermore, it preferentially utilizes histone as exogenous substrate (Cho-Chung et al., 1978b). In contrast, the kinase extracted from growing tumor nuclei exhibits no cAMP stimulation and preferentially utilizes casein.

Binding of the 56K CR and phosphorylation of the 76K protein also occur (Cho-Chung et al., 1979) in DMBA tumor nuclei when the tumor cytosol is replaced by protein kinase type II holoenzyme of bovine heart. However, phosphorylation of the nuclear protein was not observed using only the catalytic subunit of the kinase. These results suggest that the protein kinase catalytic subunit cannot penetrate into the nucleus by itself; it must be combined with the CR, probably in an "activated" holoenzyme form (Cho-Chung et al., 1979). This apparent "activation" of the kinase is dependent on temperature and cAMP concentration: the binding of 56K CR and phosphorylation of 76K protein in the tumor nuclei require incubation at 23°C and occur maximally at a physiological level of cAMP (10^{-8} M) and minimally at both sub- and supraphysiological levels of cAMP (Cho-Chung, 1980b).

In hormone-independent mammary tumors that fail to regress following ovariectomy or DBcAMP treatment, neither nuclear translocation of CR nor phosphorylation of the 76K nucler protein occurs (Cho-Chung and Redler, 1977; Cho-Chung et al., 1978a). In an attempt to find an explanation for these results, a recombinant experiment was carried out using activated cytosol and isolated nuclei from hormone-dependent and -independent DMBA tumors (Cho-Chung, 1980b). It was found that the activated cytosol derived from the hormone-dependent tumor was able to induce phosphorylation of the 76K in the nuclei derived from both hormone-dependent and -independent tumors, whereas the activated cytosol derived from the hormone-independent tumor failed to induce phosphorylation of this protein in either hormone-dependent or -independent tumor nuclei. Moreover, the absence of phosphorylation of the 76K protein is correlated with diminished nuclear binding of the 56K CR. We interpreted these data to indicate that both nuclear binding of CR and subsequent phosphorylation of the 76K protein depend on the cAMP receptor complex of the cytosol, but not of the nucleus. The hormone-dependent tumor contains aberrant cytoplasmic CR (i.e., a charge alteration, decreased self-phosphorylation, and a decreased ability to interact with the catalytic subunit of protein kinase), which fails to penetrate into the nucleus and thus does not exhibit phosphorylation of the 76K protein.

Evidence from the experiments described above supports the hypothesis (Cho-Chung, 1980b) that translocation of cAMP receptor complex from the cytoplasm to the nucleus may be the triggering event leading to tumor regression *in vivo*.

5.2. Alteration in Gene Expression

The mechanism of cAMP action at the nuclear level, as demonstrated by the nuclear translocation of the cAMP receptor complex, is remarkably similar to that of steroid hormone action (Jensen and DeSombre, 1972; O'Malley and Means, 1974) at the nuclear level. Thus, an interrelationship between the action of cAMP and a steroid hormone in the expression of genetic information seems possible. We examined (F. L. Huang and Cho-Chung, 1982) whether the growth of hormone-dependent mammary tumors is under transcriptional control and whether regressions produced by ovariectomy and DBcAMP treatment are evoked by a similar mechanism. Poly(A)-containing RNAs isolated from growing and regressing DMBA tumors were translated in cell-free protein-synthesizing systems and their translation products were analyzed by SDS–polyacrylamide gel electrophoresis. Within 6 hr following DBcAMP treatment, the concentration of one protein band (20.5K) increased and those of two protein bands (22K and 35K) decreased in the regressing tumors as compared to the growing tumors (Figure 4). Strikingly, the translated protein patterns of the regressing tumors were identical whether regression was induced by ovariectomy or DBcAMP treatment (Figure 4). Thus, both DBcAMP treatment and ovariectomy may have resulted in the accumulation of at least one and the reduction of two mRNA species

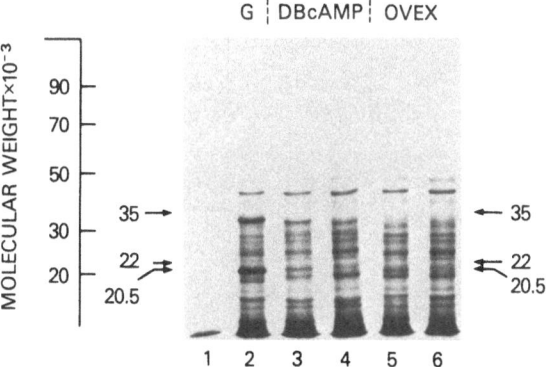

FIGURE 4. Autoradiograms of the *in vitro* translation products of mRNAs from growing and regressing DMBA mammary tumors. Track 1, the control (no mRNA added); track 2, with poly(A) RNA of growing tumors; tracks 3 and 4, with poly(A) RNAs of regressing tumors at 6 and 16 hr after DBcAMP treatment, respectively; tracks 5 and 6, with poly(A) RNAs of regressing tumors at 6 and 16 hr after ovariectomy, respectively. Translation is carried out in wheat germ extract (from F. L. Huang and Cho-Chung, 1982).

in the tumors. In contrast, autonomously growing tumors exhibited protein patterns appreciably different from that of hormone-dependent tumors, and the patterns did not change after ovariectomy or DBcAMP treatment. Moreover, the changing levels of transcription products in the regressing tumors are not associated with incipient cell death in general, since treatment with the cytotoxic chemotherapeutic agent, cyclophosphamide (10 mg/day per 200-g rat, s.c.), did arrest the growth of DMBA tumors, but had no effect on the translation products.

The results suggest that mammary tumor growth is subject to genomic regulation and that the same changes in gene expression occur in both DBcAMP- and ovariectomy-induced regression. It is probable that the antagonistic action between cAMP and estrogen is responsible for the differential genetic expression demonstrable during growth and regression of hormone-dependent mammary carcinoma.

5.3. Suppression of a Cellular Oncogene Expression

Differential gene expression observed between growing and regressing hormone-dependent mammary tumors described above suggested that an enhanced expression and suppression of genes associated with cellular proliferation or oncogenic expression may be involved in the growth/regression of mammary tumors.

The 22K protein is one of the two prominent in vitro translated proteins of the growing DMBA tumors as compared to the regressing tumors. We examined whether the 22K protein represents the 21K transforming gene product (p21) of a cellular ras proto-oncogene (c-ras) (Shih et al., 1979). The [^{35}S]methionine-labeled in vitro translation products from growing DMBA tumors were analyzed for p21 protein by immunoprecipitation with a rat monoclonal antibody directed against Harvey sarcoma virus-encoded p21 (Furth et al., 1982). A substantial amount of the 22K translated protein was specifically immunoprecipitated by the antibody and the immunoprecipitated band comigrated with the 22K translated protein on SDS–acrylamide

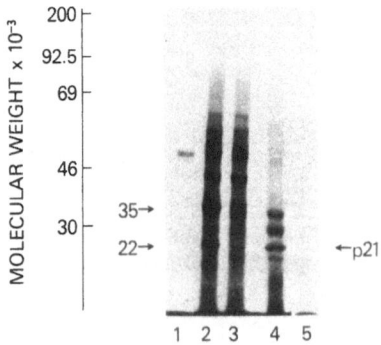

FIGURE 5. Immunoprecipitation of p21 from the in vitro translation products of DMBA-induced mammary tumors. Immunoprecipitation of p21 was carried out by the method of Furth et al. (1982). 1, No messenger; 2 and 3, in vitro translation products from growing and regressing (3 days after ovariectomy) tumors, respectively; 4 and 5, p21 immunoprecipitates of 2 and 3, respectively (from Cho-Chung and Huang, 1984).

gels (Figure 5) (Cho-Chung and Huang, 1984). The antibody detected no significant amount of p21 from the translation products of the regressing tumors (Figure 5). Quantitation by densitometry showed that the levels of p21 in the translation products of the regressing tumors at day 3 after ovariectomy or DBcAMP treatment were only 20% of those found in the growing tumors and that the levels of p21 in the growing tumors were sixfold greater than those found in the virgin rat mammary glands.

Injections of estradiol valerate into the ovariectomized hosts or cessation of DBcAMP treatment produced resumption of tumor growth and the tumors resumed p21 production. Moreover, approximately 12% of DMBA-induced tumors that have failed to regress and continued to grow after ovariectomy or DBcAMP treatment contained levels of translated p21 as low as those in virgin mammary glands and the p21 levels did not change after either ovariectomy or DBcAMP treatment. Thus, in the hormone-independent tumors, expression of the p21 is not elevated. These results suggest that enhanced expression of the cellular ras^H oncogene is associated with hormone-dependent growth of mammary carcinomas in vivo and that cAMP may act to suppress this oncogene. Because ras genes are members of a family of related human genes (Ellis et al., 1981), the involvement of this gene observed in the hormone-dependent growth of rat mammary carcinomas suggests the possibility that this oncogene might have a role in the growth of hormone-dependent human breast cancer.

The changes in ras gene expression observed during growth and regression of the mammary carcinomas appear to be due to modulation of the gene at a regulatory locus. It is conceivable that cAMP and a steroid hormone may counteract each other at a "regulatory locus" of the ras gene. We tested (Clair and Cho-Chung, 1984) this hypothesis in the clone 433 of NIH 3T3 cells.

The 433 cell line is a stable carrier of the molecular chimera with the ras gene of Harvey sarcoma virus (v-ras^H) linked to DNA containing the long terminal repeat (LTR) of mouse mammary tumor virus (MMTV); expression of the transforming ras gene in the 433 cells is strictly under the control of glucocorticoid hormone (A. L. Huang et al., 1981). Flat, contact-inhibited monolayers are observed in the absence of hormone; in the presence of dexamethasone, a synthetic glucocorticoid hormone (10^{-10}–10^{-6} M), the cells become round and refractile and float away from the substratum. This effect of dexamethasone was markedly inhibited when cAMP (10^{-4} M), DBcAMP (10^{-4} M), 8-azido cAMP (10^{-5} M), 8-Br cAMP (10^{-5} M), or cholera toxin (20 ng/ml) was added simultaneously with dexamethasone (10^{-8} M). When DBcAMP was added 2 days prior to the addition of dexamethasone, the dexamethasone effect was completely abolished; the cells exhibited flat, contact-inhibited monolayers just as the cells in the absence of dexamethasone. The phenotypic "switch" of 433 cells in response to glucocorticoid has been correlated with the induction of the 21K transforming protein (p21) of the v-ras^H gene. The level of p21 in 433 cells was determined using a monoclonal antibody against Harvey sarcoma virus-encoded p21. The results showed that p21 was induced by dexamethasone and DBcAMP blocked the p21 production.

Thus, cAMP can block the expression of a viral oncogene as well as its transforming activity. The inhibitory effect of cAMP on glucocorticoid-dependent expression of the viral ras gene in 433 cells seems to parallel the in vivo results (Cho-Chung and Huang, 1984) with hormone-dependent mammary carcinomas in rats, where an increased production of the c-ras^H mRNA appears to be dependent on the continuous presence of hormone. Hormone withdrawal following ovariectomy results in decrease of the ras mRNA concentration and tumor regression. Treatment of tumor-bearing animals with DBcAMP also results in inhibition of c-ras^H expression followed by tumor regression (Cho-Chung and Huang, 1984).

These results of in vivo and in vitro studies demonstrated the relationship between quantitative alteration of a cellular proto-oncogene expression and hormone-dependent cellular proliferation.

6. CONCLUSIONS

The studies described above show that cAMP plays the pivotal role in controlling the growth of mammary tumors. Animal experiments have shown that various cAMP derivatives inhibit tumor growtth in vivo. Differences in sensitivity of various tumors to cAMP have also been shown. Moreover, information exists about the molecular basis for resistance in certain neoplastic cells. The most common type of molecular lesion associated with the resistance to cAMP in neoplastic cells was found to be aberrant CR, the regulatory subunit of cAMP-dependent protein kinase. this means that as long as the integrity of the CR is preserved, tumors should undergo regression with the proper cAMP stimulation.

In rat mammary tumor models, DBcAMP produces growth arrest in hormone-dependent tumors and some hormone-independent tumors. Moreover, this growth inhibition is synergistically enhanced by L-arginine. Growth of human breast cancer cells (MCF-7) in culture is also synergistically inhibited by DBcAMP and L-arginine.

In hormone-dependent mammary carcinomas, the action of cAMP is antagonistic to the estrogen action. This antagonism is expressed in the amount of the respective receptor proteins in the cytoplasm, their nuclear translocation, phosphorylation of specific nuclear proteins, and regulation of gene expression, especially the cellular ras^H oncogene expression. That cAMP suppresses the hormone-stimulated enhancement of the c-ras^H gene expression in mammary carcinoma suggests an essential role of cAMP in the regulation of cellular proliferation. Elucidation of the precise role of cAMP in the regulation of the cellular proto-oncogene expression in vivo may contribute to understanding the etiology of hormone-dependent mammary cancer.

These results suggest a therapeutic potential for cAMP in the treatment of breast cancer in humans. DBcAMP and L-arginine may be substituted for the antiestrogens and other cytotoxic drugs.

REFERENCES

Bodwin, J. S., Clair, T., and Cho-Chung, Y. S., 1978, Inverse relation between estrogen receptors and cyclic adenosine 3',5'-monophosphate-binding proteins in hormone-dependent mammary tumor regression due to dibutyryl cyclic adenosine 3',5'-monophosphate treatment or ovariecttomy, Cancer Res. 38:3410–3413.

Bodwin, J. S., Clair, T., and Cho-Chung, Y. S., 1980, Relationship of hormone-dependency to estrogen receptor and adenosine 3',5'-cyclic monophosphate-binding proteins in rat mammary tumors, J. Natl. Cancer Inst. 64:395–398.

Bodwin, J. S., Hirayama, P. H., and Cho-Chung, Y. S., 1981a, Cyclic AMP-binding protein and estrogen receptor: Antagonism during nuclear translocation in a hormone-dependent mammary tumor, Biochem. Biophys. Res. Commun. 103:1349–1355.

Bodwin, J. S., Hirayama, P. H., Rego, J. A., and Cho-Chung, Y. S., 1981b, Regression of hormone-dependent mammary tumors in Sprague–Dawley rats as a result of tamoxifen or pharmacologic doses of 17β-estradiol: Cyclic adenosine 3',5'-monophosphate-mediated events, J. Natl. Cancer Inst. 66:321–326.

Bylund, D. B., and Krebs, E. G., 1975, Effect of denaturation on the susceptibility of proteins to enzymic phosphorylation, J. Biol. Chem. 250:6355–6361.

Cho-Chung, Y. S., 1974, In vivo inhibition of tumor growth by cyclic adenosine 3',5'-monophosphate derivatives, Cander Res. 34:3492–3496.

Cho-Chung, Y. S., 1978, Antagonistic action between cyclic adenosine 3',5'-monophosphate and estrogen in rat mammary tumor growth control, Cancer Res. 38:4071–4075.

Cho-Chung, Y. S., 1979a, Cyclic AMP and tumor growth in vivo, in: Influence of Hormones on Tumor Development (J. A. Kellen and R. Hilf, eds.), Volume 1, CRC Press, Boca Raton, Fla., pp. 55–93.

Cho-Chung, Y. S., 1979b, Minireview: On the interaction of cyclic AMP-binding protein and estrogen receptor in growth control, Life Sci. 24:1231–1240.

Cho-Chung, Y. S., 1980a, Cyclic AMP and mammary tumor regression, Cell. Mol. Biol. 26:395–403.

Cho-Chung, Y. S., 1980b, Cyclic AMP and its receptor protein in tumor growth regulation in vivo, J. Cyclic Nucleotide Res. 6:163–177.

Cho-Chung, Y. S., 1982, Mode of cyclic AMP action in growth control, in: Hormonal Regulation of Mammary Tumors (B. S. Leung, ed.), Volume II, Eden Press, Montreal, pp. 155–177.

Cho-Chung, Y. S., and Clair, T., 1977, Altered cyclic AMP-binding and db cyclic AMP-unresponsiveness in vivo, Nature 265:452–454.

Cho-Chung, Y. S., and Doud, F. J., 1978, Antagonistic action between cyclic AMP and estrogen in phosphorylation of mammary tumor nuclear proteins, Cancer Lett. 5:219–224.

Cho-Chung, Y. S., and Gullino, P. M., 1973, Mammary tumor regression. VI. Synthesis and degradation of acid ribonuclease, J. Biol. Chem. 248:4750–4755.

Cho-Chung, Y. S., and Gullino, P. M., 1974a, In vivo inhibition of growth of two hormone-dependent mammary tumors by dibutyryl cyclic AMP, Science 183:87–88.

Cho-Chung, Y. S., and Gullino, P. M., 1974b, Brief communication: Effect of dibutyryl cyclic adenosine 3',5'-monophosphate on in vivo growth of Walker 256 carcinoma: Isolation of responsive and unresponsive cell populations, J. Natl. Cancer Inst. 52:995–996.

Cho-Chung, Y. S., and Huang, F. L., 1984, Enhanced expression and suppression of c-ras[H] oncogene during growth and regression of hormone-dependent mammary tumors, in: Advances in Gene Technology: Human Genetic Disorders (F. Ahmad, S. Black, J. Schultz, W. A. Scott, and W. J. Welam, eds.), ICSU Press, Miami, pp. 142–143.

Cho-Chung, Y. S., and Redler, B. H., 1977, Dibutyryl cyclic AMP mimics ovariectomy: Nuclear protein phosphorylation in mammary tumor regression, Science 197:272–275.

Cho-Chung, Y. S., Clair, T., and Huffman, P., 1977a, Loss of nuclear cyclic AMP-binding in cyclic AMP-unresponsive Walker 256 mammary carcinoma, J. Biol. Chem. 252:6349–6355.

Cho-Chung, Y. S., Clair, T., and Porper, R., 1977b, Cyclic AMP-binding proteins and protein kinase during regression of Walker 256 mammary carcinoma, *J. Biol. Chem.* **252:**6342–6348.

Cho-Chung, Y. S., Clair, T., Yi, P. N., and Parkison, C., 1977c, Comparative studies on Cyclic AMP binding and protein kinase in cyclic AMP-responsive and unresponsive Walker 256 mammary carcinomas, *J. Biol. Chem.* **252:**6335–6341.

Cho-Chung, Y. S., Bodwin, J. S., and Clair, T., 1978a, Cyclic AMP-binding protein: Inverse relationship with estrogen-receptors in hormone-dependent mammary tumor regression, *Eur. J. Biochem.* **86:**51–60.

Cho-Chung, Y. S., Clair, T., and Zubialde, J. P., 1978b, Increase of cyclic AMP-dependent protein kinase type II as an early event in hormone-dependent mammary tumor regression, *Biochem. Biophys. Res. Commun.* **85:**1150–1155.

Cho-Chung, Y. S., Archibald, D., and Clair, T., 1979, Cyclic AMP receptor triggers nuclear protein phosphorylation in a hormone-dependent mammary tumor cell-free system, *Science* **205:**1390–1392.

Cho-Chung, Y. S., Clair, T., Bodwin, J. S., and Hill, D. M., 1980, Arrest of mammary tumor growth in vivo by L-arginine: Stimulation of NAD-dependent activation of adenylate cyclase, *Biochem. Biophys. Res. Commun.* **95:**1306–1313.

Cho-Chung, Y. S., Clair, T., Bodwin, J. S., and Berghoffer, B., 1981a, Growth arrest and morphological change of human breast cancer cells by dibutyryl cyclic AMP and L-arginine, *Science* **214:**77–79.

Cho-Chung, Y. S., Clair, T., Schwimmer, M., and Steinberg, L., 1981b, Cyclic adenosine 3′,5′-monophosphate receptor proteins in hormone-dependent and -independent rat mammary tumors, *Cancer Res.* **41:**1840–1846.

Cho-Chung, Y. S., Clair, T., Shepheard, C., and Berghoffer, B., 1983, Arrest of hormone-dependent mammary cancer growth in vivo and in vitro by cholera toxin, *Cancer Res.* **43:**1473–1476.

Christoffersen, T., and Brønstad, G. O., 1980, A commentary on the role of cyclic nucleotides in cell growth and malignancy, *Prog. Pharmacol.* **4:**117–135.

Clair, T., and Cho-Chung, Y. S., 1984, Suppression of v-ras^H oncogene linked to the mouse mammary tumor virus promoter by cyclic AMP, *Proc. Am. Assoc. Cancer Res.* **25:**67.

Corbin, J. D., Sugden, P. H., West, L., Flockhart, D. A., Lincoln, T. M., and McCarthy, D., 1978, Studies on the properties and mode of action of the purified regulatory subunit of bovine heart adenosine 3′,5′-monophosphate-dependent protein kinase, *J. Biol. Chem.* **253:**3997–4003.

Costa, E., Kurosawa, A., and Guidotti, A., 1976, Activation and nuclear translocation of protein kinase during transsynaptic induction of tyrosine 3-monooxygenase, *Proc. Natl. Acad. Sci. USA* **73:**1058–1062.

Daniel, V., Litwack, G., and Tomkins, G. M., 1973, Induction of cytolysis of cultured lymphoma cells by adenosine 3′,5′-cyclic monophosphate and the isolation of resistant variants, *Proc. Natl. Acad. Sci. USA* **70:**76–79.

Dubpernell, S. A., and Gavurin, L., 1978, The effect of cyclic AMP on the growth and morphology of a normal human fibroblast parent strain and its transformed progeny line, *Cell Differ.* **7:**375–386.

Ellis, R. W., DeFeo, D., Shih, T. Y., Gonda, M. A., Young, H. A., Tsuchida, N., Lowy, D. R., and Scolnick, E. M., 1981, The p21 src genes of Harvey and Kirsten sarcoma viruses originate from divergent members of a family of normal vertebrate genes, *Nature* **292:**506–511.

Erlichman, J., Rosenfeld, R., and Rosen, O. M., 1974, Phosphorylation of a cyclic adenosine 3′,5′-monophosphate-dependent protein kinase from bovine cardiac muscle, *J. Biol. Chem.* **249:**5000–5003.

Furth, M. E., Davis, L. J., Fleurdelys, B., and Scolnick, E. M., 1982, Monoclonal antibodies to the p21 products of the transforming gene of Harvey murine sarcoma virus and of the cellular ras gene family, *J. Virol.* **43:**294–304.

Handschin, J. C., and Eppenberger, U., 1979, Altered cellular ratio of type I and type II cyclic AMP-dependent protein kinase in human mammary tumors, *FEBS Lett.* **106:**301–304.

Handschin, J. C., Handlaser, K., Takahashi, A., and Eppenberger, U., 1983, Cyclic adenosine 3′,5′-monoposphate receptor proteins in displastic and neoplastic human breast tissue cytosol and their inverse relationship with estrogen receptors, *Cancer Res.* **43:**2947–2954.

Holmgren, J., 1981, Actions of cholera toxin and the prevention and treatment of cholera, *Nature* **292**:413–417.

Huang, A. L., Ostrowski, M. C., Berard, D., and Hager, G. L., 1981, Glucocorticoid regulation of the Ha-MuSV p21 gene conferred by sequences from mouse mammary tumor virus, *Cell* **27**:245–255.

Huang, F. L., and Cho-Chung, Y. S., 1982, Dibutyryl cyclic AMP treatment mimics ovariectomy: New genomic regulation in mammary tumor regression, *Biochem. Biophys. Res. Commun.* **107**:411–415.

Huggins, C., Grand, L. C., Brilliantes, F. P. 1961, Mammary cancer induced by a single feeding of polynuclear hydrocarbons, and its suppression, *Nature* **189**:204–207.

Jensen, E. V., and DeSombre, E. R., 1972, Mechanism of action of the female sex hormones, *Annu. Rev. Biochem.* **41**:203–230.

Jungmann, R. A., and Kranias, E. G., 1977, Minireview: Nuclear phosphoprotein kinases and the regulation of gene transcription, *Int. J. Biochem.* **8**:819–830.

Jungmann, R. A., Lee, S. G., and DeAngelo, A. B., 1975, Translocation of Cytoplasmic protein kinase and Cyclic adenosine monophosphate-binding protein to intracellular receptor sites, *Adv. Cyclic Nucleotide Res.* **5**:781–306.

Kapoor, C. L., and Cho-Chung, Y. S., 1983a, Affinity purification of antibodies of regulatory subunits of cAMP-dependent protein kinase using cross-linked immunoabsorbent, *J. Immunol. Methods* **57**:215–220.

Kapoor, C. L., and Cho-Chung, Y. S., 1983b, Compartmentalization of regulatory subunits of cyclic adenosine 3′,5′-monophosphate-dependent protein kinases in MCF-7 human breast cancer cells, *Cancer Res.* **43**:295–302.

Kapoor, C. L., and Cho-Chung, Y. S., 1983c, Mitotic apparatus and nucleoli compartmentalization of 50,000-dalton type II regulatory subunit of cAMP-dependent protein kinase in estrogen receptor negative MDA-MB-231 human breast cancer cells, *Cell Biol. Int. Rep.* **7**:49–60.

Kapoor, C. L., Grantham, F., and Cho-Chung, Y. S., 1983, Appearance of 50,000- and 52,000-dalton cAMP receptor proteins in the nucleoli of regressing MCF-7 human breast cancer upon estrogen withdrawal, *Cell Biol. Int. Rep.* **7**:937–946.

Kim, U., and Furth, J., 1960, Relation of mammotropes to mammary tumors. IV. Development of highly hormone dependent mammary tumors, *Proc. Soc. Exp. Biol. Med.* **105**:490–492.

Kojima, R., Shimada, L., and Asano, H., 1973, Effects of oral administration of arginine on tumor bearing mice, *Exp. Anim.* **22**:237–242.

Krebs, E. G., 1972, Proteind kinase, *Curr. Top. Cell. Regul.* **5**:99–133.

Kuehl, F. A., Jr., Ham, E. A., Zanetti, M. E., Sanford, C. H., Nicol, S. E., and Goldberg, N. D., 1974, Estrogen-related increases in uterine guanosine 3′,5′-cyclic monophosphate levels, *Proc. Natl. Acad. Sci. USA* **71**:1866–1870.

Kuo, J. F., and Greengard, P., 1969, Cyclic nucleotide-dependent protein kinase. IV. Widespread occurrence of adenosine 3′,5′-monophosphate-dependent protein kinase in various tissues and phyla of the animal kingdom, *Proc. Natl. Acad. Sci. USA* **64**:1349–1355.

Kvinnsland, S., Ekanger, R., Døskeland, S. O., and Thorsen, T., 1983, Relationship of cyclic AMP binding capacity and estrogen receptor to hormone sensitivity in human breast cancer, *Breast Cancer Res. Treat.* **3**:67–72.

Langan, T. A., 1968, Histone phosphorylation: Stimulation by adenosine 3′,5′-monophosphate, *Science* **162**:579–581.

Langan, T. A., 1973, Protein kinases and protein kinase substrates, *Adv. Cyclic Nucleotide Res.* **3**:99–153.

Levy, H. M., Montanez, G., Feaver, E. R., Murphy, E. A., and Dunn, M. S., 1954, Effect of arginine on tumor growth in rats, *Cancer Res.* **14**:198–200.

Matusik, R. J., and Hilf, R., 1976, Relationship of adenosine 3′,5′-cyclic monophosphate and guanosine 3′,5′-cyclic monophosphate to growth of dimethylbenz(α)anthracene-induced mammary tumors in rats, *J. Natl. Cancer Inst.* **56**:659–661.

Milner, J. A., and Stepanovich, L. V., 1979, Inhibitory effect of dietary arginine on growth of Ehrlich ascites tumor cells in mice, *J. Nutr.* **109**:489–494.

Nakanishi, K., 1969, Studies on tumor growth inhibition of arginine imbalanced diet, *Osaka Univ. Med. J.* **21**:193–204.

O'Malley, B. W., and Means, A. R., 1974, Female steroid hormones and target cell nuclei: The effects of steroid hormones on target cell nuclei are of major importance in the interaction of new cell functions, *Science* **183**:610–620.

Pastan, I., and Perlman, R. L., 1972, Regulation of gene transcription in *E. coli* by cyclic AMP, *Adv. Cyclic Nucleotide Res.* **1**:11–16.

Pastan, I., Johnson, G. S., and Anderson, W. B., 1975, Role of cyclic nucleotides in growth control, *Annu. Rev. Biochem.* **44**:491–522.

Perkins, J. P., 1973, Adenyl cyclase, *Adv. Cyclic Nucleotide Res.* **3**:1–64.

Prasad, K. N., 1975, Differentiation of neuroblastoma cells in culture, *Biol. Rev.* **50**:129–165.

Puck, T. T., 1979, Studies on cell transformation, *Somatic Cell Genet.* **5**:973–990.

Robinson, G. A., Butcher, R. W., and Sutherland, E. W., 1971, *Cyclic AMP*, Academic Press, New York.

Rubin, C. S., and Rosen, O. M., 1975, Protein phosphorylation, *Annu. Rev. Biochem.* **44**:831–887.

Shafie, S., and Brooks, S. C., 1977, Effect of prolactin on growth and the estrogen receptor level of human breast cancer cells (MCF-7), *Cancer Res.* **37**:792–799.

Shafie, S. M., and Grantham, F. H., 1981, Role of hormones in the growth and regression of human breast cancer cells (MCF-7) transplanted to nude mice, *J. Natl. Cancer Inst.* **67**:51–56.

Shafie, S. M., Cho-Chung, Y. S., and Gullino, P. M., 1979, Cyclic adenosine 3′,5′-monophosphate and protein kinase activity in insulin-dependent and -independent mammary tumors, *Cancer Res.* **39**:2501–2504.

Shanker, G., Ahrens, H., and Sharma, R. K., 1979, Novel protein kinase, AUT-PK85, isolated from adrenocortical carcinoma: Purifiction and characterization, *Proc. Natl. Acad. Sci. USA* **76**:66–70.

Shih, T. Y., Weeks, M. O., Young, H. A., and Scolnick, E. M., 1979, Identification of a sarcoma virus coded phosphorprotein in nonproducer cells transformed by Kirsten or Harvey murine sarcoma virus, *Virology* **96**:64–69.

Simantov, R., and Sachs, L., 1975, Temperature sensivitity of cyclic adenosine 3′,5′-monophosphate-binding proteins and the regulation of growth and differentiation in neuroblastoma cells, *J. Biol. Chem.* **250**:3236–3242.

Steinberg, R. A., O'Farrell, P. H., Friedrich, U., and Coffino, P., 1977, Mutations causing charge alterations in regulatory subunits of the cyclic AMP-dependent protein kinase of cultured S49 lymphoma cells, *Cell* **10**:381–391.

Takeda, Y., Tominago, T., Tei, N., Kitamura, M., Taga, S., Murase, J., Taguchi, T., and Miwatani, T., 1975, Inhibitory effect of L-arginine on growth of rat mammary tumors induced by 7,12-dimethylbenz(α)anthracene, *Cancer Res.* **35**:2390–2393.

Walsh, D. A., Perkins, J. P., and Krebs, E. G., 1968, An adenosine 3′,5′-monophosphate-dependent protein kinase from rabbit skeletal muscle, *J. Biol. Chem.* **243**:3763–3765.

Weber, W., and Hilz, H., 1979, Stoichiometry of cAMP binding and limited proteolysis of protein kinase regulatory subunits RI and RII, *Biochem. Biophys. Res. Commun.* **90**:1073–1081.

Weber, W., Schwoch, G., Schroder, H., and Hilz, H., 1981, Analysis of cAMP-dependent protein kinases by immunotitration: Multiple forms—multiple functions, in: *Cold Spring Harbor Conference on Cell Proliferation*, Volume 8, Cold Spring Harbor Laboratory, Cold Spring Harbor, N.Y., pp. 125–140.

CHAPTER 8

CELLULAR HETEROGENEITY OF HUMAN TUMORS
Implications for Understanding and Treating Cancer

HARRY K. SLOCUM, GLORIA H. HEPPNER, and
YOUCEF M. RUSTUM

1. INTRODUCTION

Among the "seven warning signals" of cancer, the American Cancer Society lists "a lump or thickening in the breast or elsewhere." In the case of a malignant neoplasm, we know that the "lump" represents uncontrolled cellular growth that is not working in the best interests of the host or, ultimately, of itself. As indicated by long-standing observations on the behavior of human tumors (Foulds, 1969, 1975; Bodenham, 1968), a change in a single cell may suffice to begin the neoplastic process (Fialkow, 1979; cf. Woodruff, 1983), but the result is far from a mass of homogeneous progeny. The heterogeneous nature of human tumors was deemphasized early in modern treatment, as investigators worked to find therapeutically exploitable differences between "the normal cell" and "the cancer cell." This approach was less successful than hoped, because differences between malignant and normal cells have turned out to be more quantitative than qualitative (Markert, 1982; Nicolson, 1984a). Even more damaging to a simple "exploitable difference" approach is evidence, now accumulating, that significant differ-

HARRY K. SLOCUM and YOUCEF M. RUSTUM • Department of Experimental Therapeutics and Grace Cancer Drug Center, Roswell Park Memorial Institute, Buffalo, New York 14263. GLORIA H. HEPPNER • Michigan Cancer Foundation, Detroit, Michigan 48201.

ences may exist between malignant cells even within the same tumor. These differences may be greater than the differences between a given malignant and a corresponding normal cell. Although the problem of tumor cell heterogeneity has been a focus of intense research interest for a relatively short time (Heppner, 1984), it is now getting such attention as to generate numerous reviews from various points of view (Heppner, 1984; Heppner and Miller, 1983; Nicolson, 1984a; Spremulli and Dexter, 1983; Woodruff, 1983; Brattain et al., 1984; Fidler and Hart, 1982; Weiss, 1980; Henson, 1982; Fidler and Berendt, 1982), has been a central issue in recent symposia (Fidler and White, 1980; Owens et al., 1982; Nicolson and Milas, 1984), and is the subject of over 300 papers published since 1978 (Poste, 1984).

A population is considered heterogeneous if it is "composed of unlike or unrelated parts" (Friend and Guralnik, 1960). The cells comprising human tumors are unlike, but certainly not unrelated. Simply stating that "one cell is different from another" has no meaning until the cellular features being compared, and the precision with which they can be measured, are defined. When viewed in sufficient detail, each tumor cell may be unique (Heppner, 1984). The type of heterogeneity we are most interested in, however, and the kind with the greatest consequences for cancer therapy, is that manifested by heritable differences in cell behavior that become apparent during attempts by the host (or clinician) to limit the disease. Nonheritable differences, such as those imposed by immunologically privileged sites, sanctuaries isolated from chemotherapy, and cell cycle, are consequences of the time and space circumstances in which the cell finds itself. These may have important clinical implications, but are unlikely to result in relapse into resistant disease and tumor progression (Foulds, 1969, 1975; Nowell, 1976, 1982, 1983; Sinkovics, 1979). If the mechanism of resistance is not heritable, one would expect to be able at least to reduce tumor burdens consistently with repeated courses of therapy. Instead, the common observation is, even in a disease initially responsive to therapy (Abeloff et al., 1979b; Livingston, 1979; Minna et al., 1980, 1982), that relapse occurs into resistant, fatal disease (Greco and Oldham, 1981; Baylin et al., 1984). Effects of sanctuary or cell cycle may be overcome by changes in drug delivery or timing, but no change in delivery or timing of a drug at concentrations to which the cell is inherently resistant will improve therapy. In fact, in the face of heritable drug resistance, the more effectively a drug is used, the more effectively it will select for drug-resistant variants (Nowell, 1976, 1982; Kerbel and Davies, 1982).

Although the majority of observations forming the basis for our understanding of tumor cell heterogeneity have been obtained through the use of animal model tumors (Poste, 1984), considerable data also exist of heterogeneity in human tumors, whether in culture, growing as xenografts, or direct from biopsy. These studies are the emphasis of this review.

Observations of far-reaching significance need not be made with sophisticated technology. As Woodruff (1983) points out, "an ordinary camera and a few rolls of black and white film" were all that Bodenham (1968) required to document behavior of cutaneous metastases of malignant melanoma "strongly suggestive of phenotypic diversity . . . . Some nodules may regress while new ones are appearing in their vicinity and the total number of nodules is increasing." Such clinical observations, carefully noted, keep laboratory research in relevant context and provide productive leads. In turn, "clinical benefit [will be] the fringe benefit derived from biological hypothesis testing" (Fisher, 1984).

2. HETEROGENEITY OBSERVED IN HUMAN TUMORS

2.1. Histopathology

The earliest observations of human tumor heterogeneity were made by histopathologists (Henson, 1982). As Henson states: "An old observation by pathologists has become a new paradigm for cell biology. This paradigm–the heterogeneity of tumors—borrows from patholgists what they have long observed: that tumors are histologically and functionally heterogeneous."

Considerable evidence of histological and morphological heterogeneity in human tumors continues to be reported. Recently, Day (1981) reviewed observations of histological heterogeneity of gastric tumors. J. R. Shapiro et al. (1984) noted extensive regional heterogeneity of high-grade gliomas and considered that no one region was representative of the whole tumor. Bigner et al. (1981) also reported morphological heterogeneity in surgical biopsies of human glioma. Importantly, this histological heterogeneity was not maintained during growth of the biopsies as xenografts in nude mice. Bernal et al. (1983) identified and separated two morphologically distinct cell populations apparently cocultivated through many passages in a human neuroblastoma cell line. Morphological and ultrastructural heterogeneity was noted by McDowell et al. (1981) in a bronchial carcinoid tumor. Scheen et al. (1984) observed morphological heterogeneity of malignant lymphomas developing extracutaneously in patients with mycosis fungoides. Molenaar et al. (1983) described cytohistological heterogeneity of follicular center cell lymphomas and indicated that the cellular composition affected immunological and histochemical features. In a companion paper, van den Berg et al. (1983) related heterogeneity observed to clinical behavior.

Heterogeneity in histological pattern of multiple samples of breast cancer has been reviewed by Parbhoo (1981). In an attempt to limit this as a problem in histological grading, Geier et al. (1979) developed an objective technique to demonstrate cytological uniforrmity between cells from areas with markedly different histology. Sharkey (1983) assessed differentiation in a series of breast cancers in order to investigate whether the traditional practice of grading a tumor based on its least differentiated areas was appropriate, and concluded that the heterogeneity found indicated that all areas of the tumor should be considered in the final grading.

Gleason has developed a grading system for adenocarcinoma of the prostate that, by taking heterogeneity into account, divides patients into prognostically relevant groups (Gleason, 1977; Gleason et al., 1974). The behavior of prostate tumors seems to be predicted more accurately by averaging of "best" and "worst" parts, rather than by ignoring heterogeneity and considering only the least differentiated area. Interestingly, the histology of primary prostatic tumors as rated by the Gleason score seems to be reproduced by metastatic tumors in the same patient (Kramer et al., 1981). As has been shown in animal systems (Fidler and Hart, 1982), metastases need not be less heterogeneous than the primaries from which they derive.

Small-cell lung carcinoma has proven to be a fruitful ground for investigation of heterogeneity related to treatment response and progression (Minna et al., 1980, 1982; Baylin, 1980; Baylin et al., 1975, 1978, 1980, 1984; Hirsch et al., 1983). Small-cell lung carcinoma is generally very sensitive to initial therapy (Livingston, 1978; Abeloff et al., 1979a,b; Minna et al., 1980, 1982; Baylin, 1980; reviewed by Greco and Oldham, 1981), but almost inevitably recurs (Greco and Oldham, 1981). Non-small-cell lung carcinoma, although generally a less virulent disease, is much less responsive to chemotherapy or radiation therapy. Whereas tumors from a small minority (less than 1%) of small-cell lung cancer patients reveal a mixture of small-cell and non-small-cell (squamous or adenocarcinoma) histology at initial diagnosis, fully one-third of treated cancers examined at autopsy show either a combination histology (Matthews, 1979; Minna et al., 1982) or a totally non-small-cell histology (Abeloff et al., 1979a; Brereton et al., 1978). It appears possible that therapy selects a resistant subpopulation of cells that ultimately kill the patient. Minna et al. (1982) reported mixed large-cell and small-cell type histology in about 12% of patients diagnosed with small-cell lung carcinomas. Such patients showed poorer response to combination chemotherapy and had shorter median survival times than did patients with uniform histology. The presence of the large-cell histology does not preclude potential cure, however, as 10% of long-term survivors in the NCI registry are of this mixed histology (Matthews, 1979; Minna et al., 1982).

Shifts between small- and large-cell variants have been reported in lung cancer cell cultures and nude mouse xenografts (Gazdar et al., 1981a; Goodwin et al., 1983). The large-cell variants are composed of a cell type found in patients (Goodwin et al., 1983), display cell surface proteins characteristic of both small-cell and non-small-cell lung carcinoma (Goodwin et al., 1983; Baylin et al., 1984), and bear chromosomal and biochemical markers relating them to small-cell carcinoma (Gazdar et al., 1981a; Minna et al., 1982).

Okabe et al. (1983) reported isolation of 25 clones from a xenografted human sarcoma of the stomach. These clones were divisible into two morphological types: criss-crossed arrays and multilayers with high terminal density (type 1) and well-organized monolayers ("fingerprint whorls") with lower saturation density (type 2). Most type 1 clones formed tumors in nude mice, and did so with uniform histology, namely poorly differentiated sarcoma with some features of smooth muscle cells. Type 2 clones were not tumorigenic in nude mice.

One-hundred and ten patients with high-grade soft-tissue sarcomas were studied by Wilson *et al.* (1984), and of 14 patients with recurrent or persistent tumor, 7 had low-grade recurrences. All of the patients with low-grade recurrences had been treated with chemotherapy, with or without radiotherapy. One patient had evidence of mixed high- and low-grade tumor before initial surgery, but this was not noted in the others. Perhaps the recurrences were due to the emergence of an occult, low-grade population less sensitive to therapy.

Adenocarcinoma of the colon is another common human tumor in which extensive evidence of heterogeneity in histology (and many other characteristics) is available (see reviews by Brattain *et al.*, 1984; Dexter, 1984). Dexter *et al.* (1981) reported heterogeneity in the histological features of an adenocarcinoma of the sigmoid colon, xenografts of the tumor grown in nude mice, and morphological distinction between two clones from the DLD-1 cell line established from the original tumor. Tumors produced in nude mice by these clones exhibited distinct histological patterns reminiscent of two patterns seen in the original neoplasm. Brattain *et al.* (1981) also reported establishment of variant cell lines from a primary cell culture of a single human colonic carcinoma. Three morphological variants, isolated by density gradient centrifugation, retained their morphology during subsequent passage. The variants produced distinct histological patterns in nude mice. These lines were morphologically similar to cells seen in primary cultures of the original tumor. The authors warned, however, that the cultures had been carried for an extended period since isolation, and the characteristics of the variant cells might be different from properties of cells in the parental cancer. Indeed, tracing heterogeneity observed in materials derived from human tumors back to the original tissues is a major consideration in the demonstration of tumor heterogeneity. Histology and morphology are among the characteristics that are most easily related to original tissues.

2.2. Biochemistry

Although a great deal of effort has been expended on the search for biochemical differences between malignant and normal tissues that might allow selective action of appropriately designed drugs (Mihich, 1973; Bodansky, 1975; Chabner, 1983), traditional biochemical approaches ignore tissue heterogeneity since they average the activities of all cell populations within the tissue. Other techniques, such as subpopulation isolation, flow cytometry, immunohistochemistry, or cloning, are necessary to reveal biochemical differences among cancer cells.

Siegal *et al.* (1981) used immunohistochemistry to monitor stages of neoplastic transformation of human breast tissue. Heterogeneous distributions of tumor cells capable of making type IV collagen and laminin were noted, and some tumor cells apparently made, but failed to deposit, extracellular matrix components, which then accumulated in the cytoplasm.

Biochemical heterogeneity has been demonstrated for other human cancers also. Baylin and Mendelsohn (1982) have described heterogeneity in medullary thyroid carcinoma, pointing out the unusual suitability of this type of cancer for such studies: the normal parent cell and its biochemical markers are known and biochemical changes can be associated with aggressiveness and progression. In Baylin's study, the parental cell was found to produce calcitonin and L-dopa decarboxylase, but diamine oxidase activity was present in appreciable amounts only in the tumor (Baylin, 1980), and could be used to clearly distinguish microscopic carcinoma from areas of C-cell hyperplasia (Mendelsohn et al., 1978; Baylin et al., 1979). Heterogeneity among tumor cells was noted by immunohistochemical staining for calcitonin production (Lippman et al., 1982). Patients whose tumor cells showed the greatest heterogeneity had virulent disease, and 5/16 of them died within 1–5 years of removal of primary tumor. All of the 11 patients whose tumors showed homogeneous staining patterns for calcitonin, however, were still alive over a similar time period. The authors concluded that biochemical progression away from the parental cell phenotype is related to degree of virulence of the disease, and that changes in individual biochemical markers signal changes in tumor development.

A common embryonal origin for medullary thyroid carcinoma, small-cell lung carcinoma, and certain normal cells of neural crest origin in various organs, has been proposed because they share "APUD" characteristics, i.e. amine precursor uptake and decarboxylase activities, and secretion of polypeptide hormones (Pearse, 1969; Baylin and Mendelsohn, 1982; Minna et al., 1982; Baylin et al., 1975, 1984). Baylin and co-workers reported a variable content of histaminase, L-dopa decarboxylase, and calcitonin within small-cell carcinoma of the lung (Baylin, 1980; Baylin et al., 1978; Abeloff et al., 1979a), having previously found differences between primary and metastatic small-cell lung tumors (Baylin et al., 1975, 1978). L-Dopa decarboxylase was present in all forms of lung cancer (Baylin et al., 1980), as was diamine oxidase, indicating small-cell lung carcinoma is not necesarily of unique histogenic origin among bronchogenic carcinomas. Human small-cell lung cancers established in culture had higher L-dopa decarboxylase levels than did solid tumors in vivo, but most of the cultured lines were derived from pleural fluids, not solid tissues.

Cultured small-cell lung carcinoma lines were examined by Minna et al. (1982) for expression of L-dopa decarboxylase. Up to eightfold variations in enzyme content were seen among clones from these lines, but compared to large-cell variants, all 48 subclones had high L-dopa decarboxylase activity. Large-cell variants occasionally arose from small-cell cultures; when this occurred, L-dopa decarboxylase was lost. The large-cell variants still had some small-cell markers, however, including intermediate levels of neuron-specific enolase (Marangos et al., 1982) and high levels of the BB isoenzyme of creatine kinase (Gazdar et al., 1981b).

Minna et al. (1980, 1982) have also examined hormone secretion by small-cell lung carcinoma. Clones of cells isolated from established lines showed heterogeneity in production of ACTH, arginine vasopressin, and calcitonin. Some clones produced only one or two of the hormones, others produced all three. The authors proposed that *in vivo* this heterogeneity may make clones interdependent by a "cross-feeding" effect. Thus, a given subpopulation not making a required peptide hormone such as arginine vasopressin (Minna *et al.*, 1982) may be getting it from a second subpopulation, while the first may make another hormone required for tumor cell growth (Moody *et al.*, 1981). Such tumor subpopulation interactions are discussed more fully below.

The lactate dehydrogenase (LDH) isoenzyme patterns of tissue taken from three regions of the same uterine sarcoma have been reported to be substantially different (Nelson *et al.*, 1984). Cell lines derived from tumors directly (but not from the three pieces just mentioned) also were heterogeneous.

Although systems to study human prostatic cancer *in vitro* have been developed (Stone *et al.*, 1978; Kaighn *et al.*, 1979; Hoehn *et al.*, 1980; Horoszewicz *et al.*, 1980) including squamous cell carcinoma of the prostate (Grossman *et al.*, 1984), thus far these have not been used to characterize biochemical heterogeneity. The Dunning R-3327 rat prostatic adenocarcinoma line (Dunning, 1963), considered in many respects to be a good model of human disease, has been the subject of a series of investigations into heterogeneity and progression (Isaacs, 1982) and recently into the biochemistry of progression as related to metastatic potential (Lowe and Isaacs, 1984). Spontaneous conversion of a slow-growing tumor to a faster-growing and eventually highly metastatic tumor, was accompanied by a shift in the biochemical profile toward an increase in proteolytic enzyme activities (elastase, chymotrypsin). This occurred simultaneously with appearance of anaplasia, karyotypic changes (Wake *et al.*, 1982; Isaacs *et al.*, 1982), and loss of hormone dependency.

Intratumoral heterogeneity in alkaline phosphatase activity in ovarian cancer was reported by Haskill *et al.* (1983) using flow cytometry for enzyme and DNA content quantitation. The tumor cells in ascites fluid from a patient with ovarian carcinoma consisted of two populations with respect to levels of alkaline phosphatase, and the solid tumor was more heterogeneous, containing three such populations.

Spears *et al.* (1984) reported a lack of heterogeneity in thymidylate synthase activity among repeat biopsies of human colon and breast carcinoma, and normal human liver, during therapy with 5-fluorouracil. Larner and Rutherford (1982) have employed micromethods to assess heterogeneity of 3':5'-nucleotide phosphodiesterase in human breast tumors, using neighboring frozen histological sections to document histology. It would be of interest to apply similar methods to the study of thymidylate synthase, to see if enzymatic homogeneity would still be demonstrated in areas of histological heterogeneity.

Flow cytometry is a potent technique for demonstrating cellular heterogeneity in regard to determinants of response to chemotherapy. Monoclonal antibodies have already been developed for dihydrofolate reductase (Grill *et al.*, 1984) and used for immunostaining in a semiquantitative way to demonstrate heterogeneity associated with methotrexate resistance in human

leukemia. Alabaster et al. (1984) have described a method of probing metabolism of individual cells by measuring intracellular pH by flow cytometry.
Although it may ultimately prove to be critical to assess cells individually
for such biochemical/metabolic characteristics, an analysis of individual cell
metabolism cannot reveal cell–cell metabolic interactions such as may occur
within tissues. For example, cells lacking an enzyme needed for purine
salvage (hypoxanthine-guanine phosphoribosyltransferase) can use another
cell's metabolism to provide needed precursors for DNA synthesis (Cox et
al., 1976; Loewenstein, 1979; van Zeeland et al., 1972; Subak-Sharpe et al.,
1969), overcoming the effect of an antimetabolite that would have been lethal
to the mutant cell in isolation. Thus, we must understand not only the types
of cells comprising heterogeneous tissues, and how they function as individuals, but also their behavior in combination (Fisher, 1984; Heppner, 1984;
Heppner and Miller, 1983).

2.3. Antigenic Heterogeneity

The antigenicity of human tumor cells has been assessed in two ways.
The first is immunogenicity in the patient and may be directly relevant to
the host's ability to restrict (or possibly enhance) tumor growth immunologically. The second is antigenicity in a foreign host (another species or
"hybridoma" culture), used to create antibodies for use as tools to describe
moieties that are not necessarily relevant to host immunological responses.
Although antigenic expression can be dependent on cell cycle (Everson et
al., 1974), cell size, and other nonheritable factors (Bahler et al., 1984), cell
surface characterization can be a versatile and sensitive method of identifying
subpopulations of cells. These subpopulations, whether relevant to host
immunological response or not, may display other heritable characteristics
necessary to the host's attempt to limit the disease.

Byers and Johnston (1977) reported an interesting example of antigenic
heterogeneity in osteogenic sarcoma. This tumor grows radially outward,
and the cells are held in a bony matrix; thus, the youngest cells in the tumor
are located at the periphery. By sampling cells from the center, middle area,
and edges of the tumor, and testing them for binding of autologous or marker
antibody, the authors demonstrated higher antigenic density on cells more
recently derived in the tumor. While the access of the immune system to
the tumor may be limited by the bony matrix, it appears that the most exterior
cells become more immunogenic as the tumor grows. Selection, however,
need not favor either the most or the least immunogenic cells. Prehn (1982),
reviewing work with sarcomas induced in animals by 3-methylcholanthrene,
pointed out that cells of intermediate immunogenicity seemed to have an
overall growth advantage. He predicted that tumors of high and low immunogenicity might progress toward some intermediate level, and that each
tumor–host system may have its own optimum.

A number of normal as well as tumor-associated antigens have been found to be heterogeneous in distribution in human tumors. Daar and Fabre (1983) reported intralesional and interlesional heterogeneity of HLA-DR antigen expression in human colorectal cancer cells. Brattain et al. (1983) found a large difference in carcinoembryonic antigen (CEA) expression by two clones derived from a primary culture of human colon carcinoma. Rognum et al. (1983) also found heterogeneous expression of HLA-DR and CEA in human large-bowel carcinoma, and related this and DNA content to disease progression. These authors noted that Duke's stage A and B cancers showed more heterogeneity in expression of both HLA-DR and CEA than did Duke's C and D disease. Well-differentiated tumors were heterogeneous in CEA and HLA-DR expression ("patchy") and were usually near diploid, whereas poorly differentiated tumors were quite uniform in staining, and all were aneuploid. Ejeckam et al. (1979) reported heterogeneity of CEA expression in gastric cancer, and Hockey et al. (1984) found differences in binding of a monoclonal antibody against CEA by cells in primary versus metastatic lesions from individual gastric cancer patients. Differential localization of CEA and a pancreas-associated antigen was noted in pancreatic tumor xenografts by Tan et al. (1981).

Weiss et al. (1981) reported heterogeneous distribution of β_2-microglobulin in human breast cancer. Hand et al. (1983), using a series of monoclonal antibodies to tumor-associated antigens, demonstrated heterogeneity among subpopulations of cells from the human mammary tumor cell line, MCF-7. Clones of MCF-7 were distinguished by at least four distinct antigenic phenotypes; some clones were unstable in this regard after repeated passage. Cell lines and fresh tissue sections from human breast tumors were studied by Natali et al. (1983a), using fluorescent-labeled monoclonal antibodies. They found highly variable fluorescence intensity among cells within the same tumor, and also found marked heterogeneity in antibody binding in sections of normal tissue. Peterson et al. (1983) similarly described phenotypic variability in surface antigen expression of both normal and malignant breast epithelial cells in culture. The rate of generation of new antigenic variants was higher in cultures of malignant cells than in normal cells, consistent with Nowell's hypothesis of the role of genetic instability in the evolution of tumor heterogeneity (Nowell, 1976, 1982, 1983). As the authors noted, however, all of the cultures of malignant cells studied were long term, and all of the normal breast epithelia were short-term cultures. Furthermore, the rate of variant generation was surprisingly high in the normal cell cultures. Smith et al. (1984) have reviewed in detail the use of monoclonal antibodies to characterize malignant and nonmalignant human mammary epithelia.

Hirohashi et al. (1984) recently reported that distribution of precursor antigen I (MA), a blood group antigen, was markedly heterogeneous in individual cases of adenocarcinoma of the lung. A panel of monoclonal antibodies was employed by Rosen et al. (1984) to characterize human small-cell lung carcinoma in culture. Large-cell variants in culture, which appeared less differentiated and exhibited amplified c-myc oncogenes, failed to express several of the antigens tested, or expressed them at lower levels than the majority small-cell population.

Heterogeneity in expression of membrane-associated antigens of human malignant melanoma cell lines (Sorg et al., 1978; Burchiel et al., 1982) and tumor cells directly from melanoma patients (Albino et al., 1981) has been reported. Also, Natali et al. (1983b) reported antigenic heterogeneity of skin tumors of nonmelanocyte origin.

2.4. Estrogen Receptors

Estrogen receptors can be distributed heterogeneously among cells within individual human breast tumors (Hawkins et al., 1977; Pertschuk et al., 1978; King and Greene, 1984; Adams and Emerman 1984) and human endometrial tumors (Castagnetta et al., 1983). Brennan et al. (1979) reported variability among multiple metastases from individual breast cancer patients, although others have found a general concordance among multiple metastatic sites (Allegra et al., 1980). Harland et al. (1983) reported that the receptor status of breast cancers could change through time, and concluded that biopsy is most appropriately done at the time endocrine therapy is proposed.

Allegra et al. (1980) also reported a marked decrease in estrogen receptor concentration after hormonal therapy, and Yang and Samaan (1983) found a reduction in estrogen receptor concentration in established human breast cancer cell lines after exposure to anticancer drugs. Although the results of Allegra et al. (1980) could be due to selection for receptor-negative cells during therapy, the effect of the cytotoxic drugs was reversible and attributed to inhibition of protein synthesis. Evidence of heterogeneity of receptor regeneration capacity and chemotherapeutic sensitivity among the cells tested, however, was presented by the authors.

Molecular heterogeneity of estrogen receptors per se was discussed by Clark et al. (1983), who presented evidence of two types of receptors, differing in ligand affinity, from breast tumors. Whether these receptors are distributed heterogeneously on different populations of cells in the same tumor is unknown.

2.5. Tumorigenicity in Nude Mice

The ability of cells to form tumors in animals has long been used as evidence of malignant transformation, and the immunodeficiency of the athymic nude mouse has to some extent made this definition applicable to human tumors. Some complications in the system exist, however, as some nonmalignant lesions will form tumors in nude mice (Smith et al., 1984), human material injected into nude mice may result in murine tumors (Kuo et al., 1984; Bowen et al., 1983; Beattie et al., 1982; Goldenberg and Pavia, 1981), and some, indeed most, human malignant tumors grow only rarely as xenografts and these metastasize at very low frequency. Cells taken directly from metastases are reported to metastasize more readily in nude mice than do cells from primary cancers (Kozlowski *et al.*, 1984). Furthermore, clones of human tumor cells display heterogeneity in tumorigenicity, indicating possible variation in the way tumor cells interact with host factors such as natural killer cells, active in nude mice (Hanna, 1980).

Okabe *et al.* (1983) reported that clones isolated from a human sarcoma cell line varied in their ability to form tumors in nude mice, and increased tumorigenicity was generally associated with a less-structured morphology in culture. Interestingly, the parent cell line was originally derived from a nude mouse xenograft.

The human bladder cell line EJ was cloned by Hastings and Franks (1983), and one clone of seven was unable to produce tumors in nude mice, although it grew with high cloning efficiency in soft agar.

Aubert *et al.* (1980) observed that human malignant melanocytes of primary and metastatic melanoma from the same patient were heterogeneous in their ability to produce tumors in nude mice.

2.6. Karyotype

The concept of karyotypic progression (reviewed by Wolman, 1983) involves the selection within malignant tumors of cells of variant karyotypes (Wolman, 1983; Smith *et al.*, 1984; Hart, 1983). Selection of cells exhibiting variant karyotypes has been reported in the Dunning rat prostatic carcinoma model (Isaacs, 1982; Isaacs *et al.*, 1982; Wake *et al.*, 1982), where conversion to a fast-growing, androgen-independent, metastasizing tumor is accompanied by a change from diploid to aneuploid karyotype, and appearance of specific chromosomal changes. A change in karyotype in ovarian cancer was observed by Siracky (1979) during successive biopsies in the course of therapy. Siracky also observed changes in nuclear morphology of endometrial cancer cells during progesterone therapy.

Clones of cells from individual human tumors have been observed to be heterogeneous in karyotype. Brattain *et al.* (1983) described karyotypic differences, albeit slight, in two clones from a human colorectal cell line, and J. R. Shapiro *et al.* (1981) demonstrated marked heterogeneity in karyotype among clones derived from single human malignant gliomas. The latter authors also demonstrated that both explant growth and growth of cells dispersed from the tissues resulted in karyotypically heterogeneous cultures. They took a unique approach, however, and related the karyotypes found in culture to a "reference set" obtained with cells freshly disaggregated from the surgical specimens. They reported that heterogeneous stem lines derived from dispersed cells (but not explants) were present in the original tumor, dispelling claims that the karyotypic abnormalities seen were artifacts of the passage of cells *in vitro*. In a follow-up study J. R. Shapiro *et al.* (1984) described anatomical segregation of karyotypically distinct subpopulations in high-grade gliomas.

Ochi *et al.* (1984) sampled metastatic melanoma lesions from one patient on three separate occasions, while the patient was undergoing chemotherapy. They reported two clones identified karyotypically, with some chromosomal markers in common. Predominance of one clone over the other in any given lesion appeared to be associated with specific histological and morphological characteristics, and different chemotherapeutic sensitivity.

Ohno (1971), in an early review of karyotyping of human malignant cells, commented that well-advanced solid tumors showed such diverse heterogeneity that it was often impossible to define a stem like karyotype. Chen (1978) commented similarly about heteroploid cell lines established from solid tumors, but also reported on the remarkable stability of karyotype in a human melanoma cell line, having observed that abundant cells with identical karyotype could be found in cultures derived from the same line but maintained separately in vitro for over 2 years. Chen et al. (1982) reported that established human colorectal carcinoma lines with heterogeneous karyotypes could be divided into those that were karyotypically stable, unstable, or of intermediate stability.

Sandberg (1982) noted a narrow distribution of modal chromosome number in cells of normal tissue, and a relatively wide variation in modal number in cells from malignant tissues. He proposed that this heterogeneity in karyotype was responsible for the wide variety of phenotypes in advanced tumors. It is possible, however, that much of the karyotypic heterogeneity observed contributes little to the biological behavior of a tumor. Stitch and Steele (1962) observed that cells in telophase, which have just finished division, were much more uniform in DNA content than were cells in mitosis. Thus, many cells that contribute to karyotypic analysis may actually be incapable of completing the division process, and remain in mitotic arrest. Although these cells may be produced often, due to genetic instability (Nowell, 1976, 1982, 1983), lethal gene configurations (Smith et al., 1984) may remove them from the genetically influential proliferative population. This view is consistent with observations utilizing flow cytometry, since the peaks of DNA histograms generally display much sharper distribution of DNA content than would be expected from typical karyotypic analyses (Barlogie et al., 1983; Frankfurt et al., 1984a).

2.7. DNA Content

Measurement of DNA content alone does not have the sensitivity of karyotypic analysis for demonstrating subtle genomic changes. Small deletions, or chromosomal rearrangements, with no change in DNA content at all, may be the most significant events in cancer development (Cairns, 1981; Wolman, 1983). However, karyotyping can yield information only about cells in metaphase, a select population of cells with unknown proliferative potential, and is limited to observing a relatively small sample of the population. Furthermore, present cytogenetic techniques are not successful with all tumors. By contrast, DNA content can be assessed by slide microspectrophotometry (Pollister and Ris, 1947), and by flow cytometry with a high probability of success.

Microspectrophotometric analysis may be applied to smears or histological sections (Atkin and Richards, 1956; Atkin et al., 1966), and DNA content determined semiquantitatively by Feulgen stain, on cells that are identified by standard histological criteria as tumor or stromal cells. Although studies examining a large number of cases have been conducted (Atkin and Kay, 1979), until automated image analysis is combined with this technique, the number of cells that can be examined for each tumor will be limited.

Flow cytometry has the capability of measuring DNA content very precisely and quickly in large numbers of cells, and thus can generate a DNA histogram to which a more significant proportion of the cells in a tumor contributes. Multiple-parameter flow cytometry can give additional information about the individual cells examined (Dethlefsen et al., 1980; Barlogie et al., 1983; Benson et al., 1984; Tanke et al., 1983), and so distinguish between tumor and normal cells with diploid DNA content. As mentioned earlier, considerable variation in DNA content among tumor cells in histological sections of human tumors is observed using slide cytometry (Stitch and Steele, 1962), the greatest heterogeneity being reported in metaphase and interphase cells. Using flow cytometry, Teodori et al. (1983) found wide-ranging heterogeneity in DNA content in cells of non-small-cell lung carcinoma. Vindelov et al. (1980) reported that 74% of small-cell lung carcinoma samples contained DNA-aneuploid cells, and 21% had two different aneuploid clones. They also reported dissimilarity in DNA content among metastatic foci within the same patient. Petersen et al. (1981) reported that 19 of 62 samples of human colorectal carcinomas contained two or three subpopulations with different DNA content. However, the more common finding is that suspensions of cells from human solid malignancies contain only cells with normal diploid and one aneuploid DNA content (Frentz and Moller, 1983; Nervi et al., 1982; Perez et al., 1981; Friedlander et al., 1984; Frankfurt et al., 1984a). When an aneuploid peak is evident in the histogram, a diploid peak is almost always present, and usually represents normal cells in the tumor (Perez et al., 1981; Barlogie et al., 1980; Frankfurt et al., 1984a,b). It may contain tumor cells as well, however (Frankfurt et al., 1984b). Frankfurt et al. (1984a) observed a case of sarcoma in which the primary tumor contained cells with aneuploid and diploid DNA content. A metastatic lesion from the same patient was diploid only, implying that tumor cells with diploid DNA content, and metastatic potential, were present in the primary along with the aneuploid population.

Frankfurt et al. (1984a) observed multiple aneuploid clones in individual tumors, but this was relatively rare (30/656 tumors). Multiple aneuploidy occurred most often in colorectal carcinoma and sarcoma. Minna et al. (1982) described two aneuploid stem lines in a pleural effusion from a patient with small-cell lung carcinoma. A culture from the effusion contained both lines, but 12 clones from this culture each contained one line only; none were bimodal.

Primary and metastatic specimens were obtained from 15 patients in the study of Frankfurt et al. (1984a). In 12 of these the same aneuploid stem line predominated in both the primary and metastatic tumors. In one case, a renal carcinoma, the primary appeared to be diploid, but the metastasis contained two aneuploid lines. Either these were present in the primary at a proportion too small to detect by the method employed (<5%), or arose later during the development of the metastasis. One sarcoma, mentioned previously, contained aneuploid cells in the primary while the cells in the metastasis had a diploid DNA contant. An interesting case of colon carcinoma contained two aneuploid lines in the primary, only one of which was represented in the liver metastasis obtained at the time of primary surgery.

Flow cytometry can also be used to identify cells with S-phase DNA content. Variation in the fraction of tumor cells with S-phase DNA content may be considerable, even when the ploidy index is stable (Friedlander et al., 1984), but the S-phase fraction has been reported to be relatively homogeneous in one normal tissue (bladder epithelium) by Farsund and Hostmark (1983). A cell with S-phase DNA content may not necessarily be synthesizing DNA, however, and a fluorescent probe of bromodeoxyuridine incorporation has been developed (Raza et al., 1984; Raza and Preisler, 1984) that should allow flow cytometry to be used to measure S-phase indices more accurately.

DNA content appears to be relatively homogeneous within subpopulations of a given ploidy by flow cytometry. Multiple-parameter flow cytometry, or secondary characterization of cells sorted by flow systems, may reveal additional variations within populations of similar DNA content.

Subpopulations of cells may be isolated by cell sorting for further analysis, as described by Tanke et al. (1983), who combined cell sorting with image cytometry. This may help overcome the problem of insensitivity of flow cytometry for displaying small differences in DNA content.

2.8. Chemotherapeutic Sensitivity

Relapse from initial responsiveness to chemotherapy into resistant disease is commonly thought to be due to the presence of resistant cells capable of repopulating the tumor after treatment. Talmadge et al. (1984) have demonstrated that murine melanoma cells recently established in culture can rapidly develop heterogeneity in chemotherapeutic sensitivity after cloning. Trope (1980) reviewed evidence for heterogeneity in sensitivity to chemotherapy among cells from individual tumors. A number of groups have employed incorporation of radiolabeled thymidine in vitro as a measure of drug effect. Trope et al. (1975) used this method to demonstrate anatomical segregation of cell populations of human adenocarcinoma of the colon and stomach, heterogeneous in their response to a variety of anticancer drugs.

Trope et al. (1979) also reported similar findings for ovarian cancer, and Biorklund et al. (1980) found that three of seven non-Hodgkin's lymphomas displayed such heterogeneity. Siracky (1979) employed the same approach and demonstrated heterogeneity among different regions, and within ascites cells, of an ovarian carcinoma.

Inhibition of colony formation on plastic was employed by Barranco et al. (1972, 1973) to demonstrate heterogeneity in sensitivity to arabinosyl-cytosine, 1,3-bis-(2-chloroethyl)-1-nitrosourea, and bleomycin in four established lines from a single nodule of human melanoma. Sensitivity of cultured cells to drugs must be interpreted carefully, however, as the work of Talmadge et al. (1984) indicates. Berry et al. (1975) also showed instability in drug sensitivity, studying freshly explanted cultures from an ovarian carcinoma after only two serial subpassages. This was not a cloned culture, however, and selection for subpopulations during passage may partly explain the results.

Colony formation in semisolid media is another system for measuring sensitivity to chemotherapeutic agents (see Section 7.2). Using this approach, Schlag and Schreml (1982) reported that cells from primary and metastatic human tumors differed in their drug sensitivity profile. Bertelsen et al. (1983) published similar findings comparing drug sensitivity of cells from primary and metastatic lesions from a variety of cancers. Overall, in 49 patients from whom primary and metastatic tumor material could be successfully assayed and compared, 35% showed a difference in chemotherapeutic sensitivity between cells from primary and metastatic locations.

Selby et al. (1979) also noted differences in chemosensitivity of primaries and metastases in a human tumor that metastasized when xenografted in nude mice. After chemotherapy of the xenograft in vivo, drug effect was measured in a colony formation assay in diffusion chambers containing soft agar, implanted intraperitoneally into preirradiated strain C57 mice. Metastatic cells were generally more sensitive, showing a steeper dose–response curve than were the cells from primary implants. In this case an element of drug delivery was involved, as treatment was done in vivo, and all of the metastases were smaller, better-perfused lesions than the primaries. Both drug delivery and intrinsic cellular resistance may also have played a role in the observations of Slack and Bross (1975) in their survey of clinical drug responsiveness of 1687 tumors entered in phase II trials. Again, metastases were generally more sensitive, but the study was a statistical one and was not designed to define mechanisms.

Shapiro and co-workers (J. R. Shapiro et al., 1981, 1984; W. R. Shapiro et al., 1981; Yung et al., 1982) have reported on chemosensitivity of cultured clones of human glioma. They employed two in vitro methods, cell count (attachment) 24 hr after drug exposure, and colony formation on plastic. Heterogeneity of drug responsiveness in both assays was seen among clones from single human glioma lesions. Since, as was mentioned earlier, the clones all bore marker karyotypes present in cells of the orginal tumor, it is unlikely that the variants were generated due to the in vitro environment.

2.9. Oncogene Expression

Detection of the expression of oncogenes in tumor cells depends upon knowledge of the nature of the products encoded by the genes. There may be variations in quality or quantity of proteins normally produced by cells of various types (Weinberg, 1980; Rigby, 1982; Nicolson, 1984a). To date the question of heterogeneity in oncogene expression has received little specific attention. However, Albino *et al.* (1984) recently reported that of five cell lines originating from separate metastases of a melanoma patient, only one contained activated *c-ras*. The lines did share an antigen not present on the patient's fibroblasts, B cells, or 45 allogeneic melanoma cell lines. The authors concluded that *c-ras* expression was not required for initiation or maintenance of tumor in this patient, and might simply have been the consequence of genetic instability in the malignancy. Of course, one cannot rule out the possibility that the gene could have been expressed during initiation, and was later shut off.

3. METHODS TO DEFINE HETEROGENEITY IN HUMAN TUMORS

The most precise methods of defining cellular heterogeneity are those that evaluate individual cells. These generally must either have the capability of rapid evaluation, or settle for examining small numbers of cells. Subpopulation isolation or enrichment may be less precise, but may make traditional biochemical approaches workable in spite of heterogeneity, and may provide starting material to make true cell-by-cell methods more practical.

3.1. Isolation of Tumor Subpopulations

A simple Ficoll–Hypaque step gradient is sufficient to isolate populations of malignant cells from peripheral blood and bone marrow of leukemic patients for use in predicting duration of remission induced by arabinosyl-cytosine/anthracycline chemotherapy (Rustum and Preisler, 1979; Preisler *et al.*, 1985). Leukemic cells, however, are much easier to isolate than are the malignant cells of solid tumors. The obvious first problem with solid tissues is the necessity to disaggregate the cells (Waymouth, 1974; Pretlow *et al.*, 1975).

Studying cells in suspension has a number of advantages. Cells can be characterized on an individual basis by, for example, cytochemistry, flow cytometry, or cloning, and their heterogeneity defined. Cell suspensions can be characterized in a variety of assays, and the results compared directly, without the sampling errors inherent in assays conducted on separate tissue pieces. Cell suspensions can be subjected to density gradient and sedimentation velocity centrifugation, cell sorting, and other separation methods to prepare subpopulations for further study.

Tumor disaggregation, however, has attendant disadvantages. The cells of tumors are not independent entities and intercellular relationships are disrupted during successful disaggregation. Furthermore, certain cell interactions can make successful disaggregation and cell subpopulation separation enormously difficult (Pretlow et al., 1975; Shortman, 1972). Philosophically, a purely reductionist approach to understanding tumors by studying their isolated cells may be doomed to failure since a cancer is a tissue and its biology must be defined in terms of tissue biology (Heppner, 1984). Some understanding of the cells as individuals is, however, clearly a prerequisite for understanding their interactions.

Slocum et al. (1981a) reported a method of removing cells from tumor tissues that has proven useful for a wide variety of tumor types (Table I). Cells are obtained in two steps: the first is mechanical release during slicing, similar to the technique of Lasfargues (1973) for "spilling" cells from breast tumors (see also Leibovitz, 1975). After mechanically derived cells have been removed, remaining tissue, not amenable to further cell release by simple cutting, is exposed to a crude enzyme mixture. Although the mixture contains collagenase, it is likely not the collagenolytic activity that is responsible for the disaggregating activity, since other collagenolytic enzymes differ widely in their ability to disaggregate human tumor tissues (Slocum, unpublished observation).

Further mincing before the enzymatic step does not yield significant numbers of cells. The fact that some cells are available from the tumor by cutting and others require enzymatic intervention is apparently a reflection of heterogeneity in firmness of cell binding in tumor tissue.

The number of cells obtained by any disaggregation procedure ought to be documented on a "per gram of tissue basis" so some estimate of the

TABLE I
Cell Yields from Tumor Specimens

Tumor	n	Cell yield (millions/g)[a]	
		Median	Range
Prostate	49	42.0	11.0–100
Breast	111	42.3	2.9–800
Sarcoma	144	56.0	4.1–420
Colorectal	133	60.1	2.8–610
Ovarian	82	66.4	7.9–2100
Bladder	69	67.0	6.3–600
Renal	62	69.1	3.7–320
Melanoma	103	84.5	6.6–1300
Lung	70	95.0	13.0–620
Total	823	66.4	2.9–2100

[a]Total from mechanical and enzymatic steps, expressed per gram of tissue slices disaggregated.

fraction of cells recovered from the tissue can be made (Helms et al., 1975; Brattain et al., 1977a; Hemstreet et al., 1980; Slocum et al., 1981a; Besch et al., 1983). Unfortunately, little information is available on the number of cells comprising human tumors. A 1-g tumor is estimated to contain about 10^9 cells (DeVita et al., 1975), but there is obvious variation in cellularity among tumors of different histological types. Stephens et al. (1977) used DNA content analysis to estimate the cellularity of line B16 murine melanoma tumors, and found 4×10^8 cells/g wet wt tissue. Similarly, Reinhold (1965) reported approximately 5×10^8 cells/g for a rat rhabdomyocarcoma (B1112) by dry weight and DNA content analyses. If these figures are of general validity, the yields of cells from human tumors by current techniques may be 5–10%. Thus, the selective pressures exerted by disaggregation may result in a very distorted view of the cells comprising a tumor, even if the cells obtained are unaffected by the procedure. Appreciable numbers of subpopulations may be entirely missed if they are unusually susceptible to damage, or resistant to release, by a given disaggregation procedure. Careful characterization of the types of cells in the resultant suspension is obviously critical to further attempts to isolate and characterize subpopulations (Pretlow et al., 1975, 1976).

The cells obtained in the two steps of this disaggregation procedure are qualitatively alike, but quantitatively dissimilar. The mechanical step yields larger numbers of DNA-aneuploid cells, when an aneuploid population is present in the tumor (Frankfurt et al., 1984a), but most cells released in this step fail to exclude trypan blue (Slocum et al., 1980, 1981a,b; Table II). Thus, cells obtained in the first step are useful for DNA flow cytometry, but for assays requiring viable cells, the cells derived in the enzymatic step give a higher probability of success (Wake et al., 1981; Kusyk et al., 1979).

Surprisingly, a low percentage of cells viable by dye exclusion do not depress colony-forming capacity in soft agar (Slocum et al., 1980, 1981a,b; Cowan et al., 1984). This is probably due to the relative insensitivity of the trypan blue test (lower limit 1% if 100 cells counted) compared to the colony formation assay (10–30 colony-forming units/500,000 cells plated = 0.006%). Nonetheless, this implies that the subpopulation of cells responsible for colony formation is not well represented by the viability of the general population of cells in the suspension.

Our experience (Slocum et al., 1983) has been that cells obtained in the enzymatic step are more suitable for cell separation methods such as equilibrium density gradient centrifugation in Ficoll (Pretlow et al., 1975) or Percoll (Pertoff et al., 1977), sedimentation velocity in linear Ficoll gradients (Pretlow et al., 1975), or centrifugal elutriation (Keng et al., 1981a,b) than are the mechanically released cells. During elutriation, buffer flows through the centrifuge head in a direction opposing the centrifugal force on the cells (Keng et al., 1981a). In this way, cells are separated primarily based on their size, although density also contributes. In our hands, elutriation of cell suspensions composed of mostly dye-admitting cells (more than 60%) is unsuccessful due to irreversible aggregation of cells in the centrifuge (Slocum

TABLE II
Dye Exclusion of Cell Suspensions Obtained in
Each Step of the Disaggregation Procedure

Tumor	Disaggregation step[a]	Dye exclusion (%)	
		Median	Range
Colorectal	M	14	0–84
	E	79	10–97
Breast	M	12	1–68
	E	77	1–97
Bladder	M	24	3–73
	E	75	2–100
Lung	M	23	1–97
	E	85	3–99
Melanoma	M	13	1–74
	E	74	5–98
Prostate	M	11	2–59
	E	75	7–96
Ovarian	M	15	2–96
	E	79	32–100
Sarcoma	M	14	11–54
	E	81	1–99
Renal	M	19	0–85
	E	85	5–99
Total	M	14	0–97
	E	79	0–100

[a]M, mechanical step (first step of disaggregation procedure);
E, enzymatic step (second step of disaggregation procedure).

et al., 1983). Although high trypan blue exclusion ratios may permit success, they unfortunately do not guarantee it.

Heterogeneity in size of cells from human tumor lines has been reported (Burchiel et al., 1982; Okamura et al., 1981), but little data are available concerning the sizes of malignant cells obtained directly from human tumors (Ashton et al., 1975). We have been unable to perform cell sizing by Coulter analysis on suspensions directly after disaggregation, due to large amounts of subcellular-sized particles generated during the disaggregation procedure in both the mechanical and enzymatic steps. This complication cannot be overcome by "dialing out" the lower channels in the analysis to ignore small particles, because they are so numerous compared to the cells that the probability of coincidental passage is high, and they appear as a population whose larger members approach cell size (Figure 1, solid line). When small particles are eliminated by elutriation, however, the distribution of cell sizes becomes evident (Figure 1, dashed line), and appears quite heterogeneous, even when cytological evaluation indicates the fraction is free of aggregates and nearly 100% tumor cells (H. K. Slocum, M. Gamarra, and E. Nava, unpublished observation).

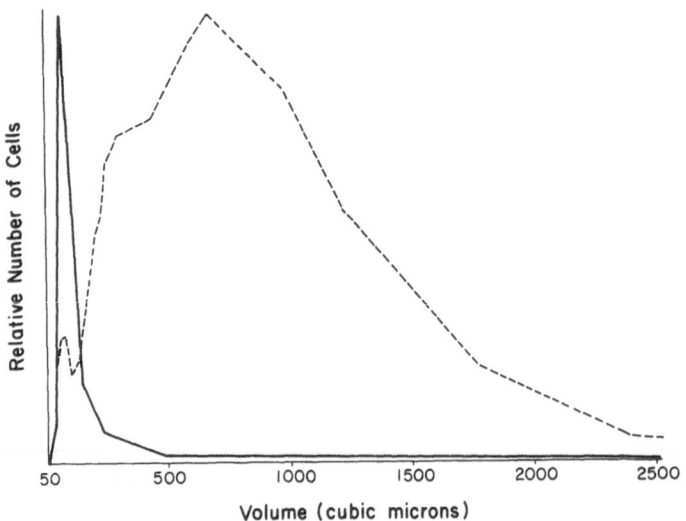

FIGURE 1. Sizing histogram of cell suspensions before (——) and after (-----) elutriation, generated by a C-1000 channelyzer and ZBI Coulter counter with 140-μm aperture, aperture current and amplification both = 1, base channel threshold = 2, window width = 100.

We have found centrifugal elutriation quite useful for enriching cell suspensions for DN/.-aneuploid populations. In some cases this has reduced heterogeneity by virtually eliminating cells of diploid DNA content. In 30 cases in which (1) DNA-aneuploidy was present in the unseparated starting suspension, (2) elutriation yielded at least 2 million cells in the fraction of interest, and (3) the DNA content of the fraction was measurable by flow cytometry, enrichment for DNA-aneuploid cells was obtained in every case. The median percentage of DNA-aneuploid cells was 45% in starting material, and 81% in fractions. In the best case, a cell suspension from a gastric adenocarcinoma in which 17% of the cells were DNA-aneuploid in the starting material, elutriation resulted in virtually complete isolation of the DNA-aneuploid population. In an instance of an ovarian adenocarcinoma in which 38% of the cells contained only 11% more DNA than the diploid population, again a near purification of the aneuploid population was achieved. Although these occasions of apparent purification of subpopulations by DNA content do not mean that this technique can be applied in general to provide homogeneous populations, enrichment of aneuploid cells may be useful for providing starting material for more specific cell separation techniques. Cell sorting, for example, may be impractical if applied to starting material of unrestricted heterogeneity, but may become possible if preceded by elutriation or some other enrichment technique.

Walle and Niedermayer (1984) reported the use of density gradients of Percoll for separation of DNA-aneuploid and diploid cells of human acute lymphoblastic leukemia. Pretlow and co-workers have used "isokinetic" linear gradients of Ficoll to partially purify subpopulations of cells from human tumors (Pretlow et al., 1976), including colon carcinoma (Brattain et al., 1977a,b), renal cell carcinoma (Hemstreet et al., 1980), and benign prostatic hyperplasia (Helms et al., 1975).

Some of the technical problems encountered in cell subpopulation isolation have been reviewed (Pretlow et al., 1975; Shortman, 1972) and recent advances in technology are the subject of a series of volumes (Pretlow and Pretlow, 1984; see also Bloemendal, 1977; Catsimpoolas, 1977).

3.2. Flow Cytometry and Other "Cell-by-Cell" Methods

The importance of employing methods capable of examining cells individually in research aimed at clinical benefit in cancer has been stressed (Tanneberger, 1979; Fisher, 1984). Advances in flow cytometric techniques promise to be most useful in this regard. Barlogie et al. (1983) have reviewed the recent use of flow cytometry in clinical cancer research. The heterogeneity in DNA content of cells from human tumors has been mentioned earlier (see Section 2.7), and most of those data were generated by flow methods.

Other cellular features are now becoming the subject of flow cytometry of human tumor cells. Melamed et al. (1977) described the use of acridine orange to stain DNA and RNA simultaneously as an approach to using flow cytometry to automate cytology. Simultaneous measurement of DNA, RNA, and cell size has been used to identify quiescent and proliferative cell populations in clones from a single mouse mammary tumor (Dethlefsen et al., 1980), and may provide an added dimension to the approach described by Melamed et al. (1977). In addition, Frankfurt (1980) has shown that double-stranded RNA content is increased in proliferating murine tumor cells, and Barlogie et al. (1983) have extended this observation to human tumors. Monoclonal antibody technology has been combined with flow cytometry to characterize antigenic heterogeneity in human tumor cell lines and clones (Burchiel et al., 1982; Cillo et al., 1984). Metabolic heterogeneity has been demonstrated by Alabaster et al. (1984) by measuring intracellular pH by flow cytometry. Simultaneous measurements of DNA content and enzyme markers by flow cytometry has demonstrated intratumoral heterogeneity in ovarian carcinoma (Haskill et al., 1983).

Using simultaneous multiple-parameter analysis and Hoechst dye 33342, Benson et al. (1984) measured DNA, RNA, and protein content to define subpopulations and characterize progression in the Dunning rat prostatic carcinoma model. Frankfurt (1983) used the Hoechst 33342 dye to characterize permeability of HeLa cells, and related this to sensitivity of the cells to the cytotoxic effects of adriamycin. Also, adriamycin itself is fluorescent, and can be used to look for transport-resistant variants. The Hoechst dye method may prove to be of great utility in identifying drug-resistant variants in human tumors, as it has been related to multiple drug resistance in an animal model tumor (Lalande et al., 1981).

4. ORIGIN OF TUMOR HETEROGENEITY

4.1. Derivation of Tumors

The extensive cellular heterogeneity of cancers raises questions about the mechanism of neoplastic variations. Although multiple-cell (polyclonal) origin of tumors is the earliest possible source of heterogeneity among malignant cells, three lines of evidence have been cited in favor of a unicellular origin for malignant tumors (Nowell, 1976): karyotype, immunoglobulin production, and isoenzyme analysis.

Chromosomal aberrations common to otherwise heterogeneous tumor cells were noted by Makino (1957) who identified a stem line origin in ascitic rat tumors. The Philadelphia chromosome in chronic myelogenous leukemia is an example of karyotypic identification of a stem line in human disease (Nowell and Hungerford, 1960; Rowley, 1973), and other examples have been reviewed recently (Wolman, 1983). Ohno (1971), however, as mentioned earlier, observed extreme heterogeneity of karyotype in advanced solid tumors and found it impossible to identify a stem line karyotype.

Homogeneous immunoglobulin production in plasma cell malignancies has been noted (Linder and Gartler, 1965; Fialkow, 1974; Milstein et al., 1967) and is consistent with clonal origin.

The most systemic study of the clonal origin of tumor cells is the work of Fialkow (1970, 1979). This work has used isoenzyme analysis to trace cellular origin. Fialkow (1970, 1979) demonstrated homogeneous expression of glucose-6-phosphate dehydrogenase isoenzyme in cancer cells from women whose normal tissues were chimeric for two forms of the enzyme (A and B) due to random inactivation of one of the X chromosomes in their cells (the glucose-6-phosphate dehydrogenase locus is on the X chromosome). This provides evidence for the unicellular origin of the tumors, since mixed expression of isoenzymes in tumor tissue would be expected in heterozygous individuals if the tumor were polyclonal. The technique of isoenzyme analysis, however, is much more easily applied to leukemias than solid tissues, due to the problems of tissue preparation mentioned earlier and the presence of large numbers of normal cells. Further, as discussed by Woodruff (1983), none of the evidence for unicellular origin is absolute, as multiple cells with the same marker could have been transformed simultaneously, or one transformed cell among many may have outgrown the others early in the tumor's history. Nor do the studies indicate a unicellular origin of all types of cancer. Mixed A/B tumors have been reported in human colon, cervical, and breast carcinoma (Kerbel et al., 1983). Evidence supporting polyclonal origin for other tumors also exists. Murine fibrosarcomas induced by methylcholanthrene have been reported to be multicellular in origin (Reddy and Fialkow, 1979). Certain human tumors such as prostatic (Byar and Mostofi, 1972; Isaacs, 1982) and breast (Fisher et al., 1975; Parbhoo, 1981; Fisher, 1984) carcinomas, show apparent multifocal areas of tumor involvement. Thus, polyclonal origin may be a contributor to tumor heterogeneity in some tumor types.

The question of the clonality of primary tumors is recapitulated in the case of metastasis. Evidence for clonal origin of metastases has been presented in several experimental systems including B-16 (Poste et al., 1982; Talmadge et al., 1984) and K-1735 (Talmadge et al., 1984) murine melanomas, and human tumors xenografted in nude mice (Spremulli and Dexter, 1983). Direct evidence in human disease was reported by Frankfurt et al. (1984a), who observed a single aneuploid population in a metastatic lesion, while the primary tumor sampled simultaneously displayed two aneuploid populations. Fialkow (1979) also observed one isoenzyme type per metastasis in the majority of colon cancer patients in the study.

4.2. Heterogeneity of Cells of Normal Tissues

It should be kept in mind while considering clonal versus polyclonal origins for tumors, that the entire human organism is clonal in origin, and yet indisputably heterogeneous (Heppner, 1984). Even within a tissue, cellular heterogeneity is apparent. Natali et al. (1983a) and Peterson et al. (1983) reported antigenic heterogeneity in both normal and cancerous human breast epithelial cells in culture. Griffen et al. (1981) described variation in steroid 5α-reductase activity in cloned human skin fibroblasts. Heterogeneity in lineages derived from a common stem cell has been most well documented in the hemopoietic system (Till and McCulloch, 1980). Okamura et al. (1981) reported heterogeneity in cell size, proliferative activity, deoxynucleotidyl transferase, and isoenzymes of adenosine deaminase in human thymocytes and a T-lymphoblast cell line, MOLT-3. Barrett and Metcalfe (1984) and Shanahan et al. (1984) have recently reviewed heterogeneity in mast cells. Heterogeneity of natural killer cells in culture (Hercend et al., 1983) and in blood and tissues (Pizzolo et al., 1984) has been reported. Although heterogeneity may be more extensive in malignant tissues (Nicolson, 1984a), clearly it is not unique to tumors (Heppner, 1984).

4.3. Genetic Instability

Although cellular heterogeneity is a feature of normal tissues, the extent of diversity in neoplasia suggests that special mechanisms may be operating in cancer cells. Nowell (1976, 1982, 1983) has cited evidence for increased genetic instability in malignant cells and incorporated this concept into a hypothesis to explain tumor heterogeneity and progression. An increased frequency of mitotic errors in many neoplastic cell populations was cited by Nowell (1982), and a greater susceptibility of aneuploid cells to further chromosomal rearrangements has been reported (Hogstedt and Mitelman, 1981; Seabright, 1976). Sandberg (1982) called attention to abnormalities of the mitotic process in cancer cells (Oksala and Therman, 1974) as a possible source of karyotypic heterogeneity, and noted that no form of therapy appears "capable of modifying the tumor karyotype in the direction of normality." W. R. Shapiro et al. (1981) reported constant chromosomal rearrangement in most clones of human glioma cells in vitro. Siracky (1979) observed changes in karyotypes in ovarian cancer successively during therapy. Isaacs (1982) has discussed spontaneous karyotypic changes associated with androgen-independent growth and progression in Dunning prostatic carcinoma (Wake et al., 1982; Isaacs et al., 1982). Although Chen et al. (1982) reported stable modal chromosome numbers for four of nine established human colorectal cell lines, two others were of intermediate stability and three were unstable. Ohno (1971), noting extreme diversity of karyotype in advanced solid tumors, discussed the effect of hyperploidy on expression of mutations. The point was made that hyperploidy might provide protection from some recessive lethal mutations, and yet not forfeit all recessive mutations. Since a lost chromosome is not regained by duplication, what is left may contain a mutation otherwise masked by the dominant allele. Smith et al. (1984) recently discussed genetic instability in human breast cancer cells, noting that many of the aneuploid cells generated may have lethal gene configurations. Sager (1982) made a similar point in considering that heterogeneity must have natural limits, since only cells well adapted to their environment will succeed. Thus, mechanisms of variant generation in maligant cells may be even more prolific than we commonly observe, since selective pressures would tend to limit some variations.

Elucidating the underlying genetic and epigenetic changes that mediate the evolution of tumor cell heterogeneity is one of the biggest challenges in molecular biology (Baylin and Mendelsohn, 1982). Many tumor cell factors could contribute to these mechanisms, including mutation or other alterations in DNA or its repair, chromosomal rearrangements, oncogene expression, and any defect in control of gene transcription or translation (Nicolson, 1984a; Nowell, 1976, 1982, 1983). Diversification of normal cells, such as B cells for immunoglobulin secretion, involves genetic rearrangements that may also play a role in the generation of tumor cell variants (Nicolson, 1984a). The insertion of oncogenes or other promoters at specific locations could result in the rapid diversification of phenotypes observed in tumors (Nicolson, 1984a,b). It is not known whether oncogene expression is a cause (Nicolson, 1984b) or a consequence (Albino et al., 1984) of tumor cell genetic instability. Frost and Kerbel (1983) have suggested that DNA hypomethylation and consequent gene derepression may play a major role in variant generation in tumors (see also Feinberg and Vogelstein, 1983; Heppner, 1984). Feinberg and Coffey (1982) have pointed out the importance of DNA rearrangements, particularly as they affect the nuclear matrix and control of DNA structure and function. Transposable elements can also induce mutation at a high frequency (Green, 1980).

A basic question concerning genetic instability of tumor cells has been the contribution of point mutations relative to other genetic or epigenetic mechanisms. The low frequency of point mutations compared to the apparent rate of variant generation in neoplastic populations would seem to argue against this mechanism as the major contributor (Dulbecco et al., 1981; Chow and Greenberg, 1980). It is possible, however, that transformed cells may be hypermutable (Frank and Williams, 1982). In addition, tumor-associated host cells may contribute to mutation rates and the generation of tumor cell variants (Heppner and Miller, 1983). Heppner and co-workers (Loveless and Heppner, 1983; Heppner et al., 1984) observed mutagenic activity of macrophages isolated from murine tumors with metastatic capability.

Elmore et al. (1983) pointed out the factors affecting apparent mutation frequencies, including karyotype (ploidy), efficiency of the assay employed for recognition of mutants, saturation density (i.e., the total number of cell generations possible in a given vessel), cloning efficiency, growth rate, and cell–cell interactions. Considering these factors, these authors observed little difference in the mutation frequency of normal versus SV40-transformed human fibroblasts. Cifone and Fidler (1981) have reported that highly metastatic murine melanoma and fibrosarcoma cells have a higher spontaneous mutation rate than do their nonmetastatic, but tumorigenic counterparts. Although this observation was not repeated in metastatic versus nonmetastatic mouse mammary tumor lines, it was found that the metastatic lines were more sensitive to induced mutation than were the less malignant lines (Yamashima and Heppner, unpublished observations), suggesting that endogenous mutagens could play a role in tumor progression. It seems likely that in this, as in all other aspects of tumor biology, different mechanisms of variant formation will be operative, to different extents, in different tumors, but the net effect will be the same: an increasing number of cellular subpopulations.

Goldie and Coldman (1979, 1983, 1984) have presented an integration of somatic mutation theory with the time-dependent processes of variant generation and progression of neoplastic populations. They have pointed out that the number of divisions of a stem cell required to generate a given number of stem cell progeny depends on the probability of self-renewal (PSR), i.e., the likelihood of another stem cell being produced, instead of a daughter committed to differentiation and limited proliferation. For example, 30 replications of a stem cell with a PSR of 1.0 would produce 10^9 stem cell progeny, but 1200 replications would be required if the PSR were 0.51. This has the effect of magnifying the apparent mutation rate in the stem cell compartment, since the probability of the formation of a varient depends on the number of cell divisions at risk. The lower the PSR, the more slowly growing the tumor, and the greater the heterogeneity. Thus, a tumor whose stem cell PSR is low should grow slowly, and should contain a large number of variant stem cells. Applying this model to clinical drug resistance, however, does raise some questions. Partially responsive tumors regrowing after therapy, or tumors undergoing sudden bursts of growth such as chronic myelogenous leukemia in blast crisis, represent tumors with relatively short doubling times, and yet as Goldie and Coldman (1983) noted, are not generally characterized by chemotherapeutic responsiveness. Also, one would expect a normal stem cell compartment, such as bone marrow, to have a PSR closer to 0.5 (Till and McCulloch, 1980; Mackillop et al., 1983; Buick and Pollak, 1984), but variant generation resulting in acquired drug resistance after therapy is not reported for normal tissues. Thus, it seems necessary to invoke a mechanism of accelerated variant generation in tumor cells, or a mechanism preventing variant generation in normal stem cells. Indeed, Cairns (1975) has discussed ways in which normal stem cell populations might be protected from genetic variation. In Cairns's model, normal tissue structure is postulated to provide an environment to allow segregation of old and new DNA strands, so that the immortal stem cells do not encounter the risk of errors in DNA replication. Further, normal tissue structure may provide an environment in which competition between stem cells, and therefore operation of selective pressures, is reduced by territorial restriction. In a tissue with no organized geometry, such as bone marrow, Cairns suggested that a restriction of the number of immortal stem cells may be the mechanism of risk reduction.

With rare exceptions, such as osteogenic sarcoma, wherein the cells are embedded in a bony matrix, one may not assume that any region of a given tumor is populated only by the progeny of stem cells in that region. During embryonic development, mammalian cells are able to migrate extensively (Markert, 1984). Tumor cells, which seem to display many embryonic features, may also be motile. Hastings and Franks (1983) isolated a highly motile clone, three clones of intermediate motility, and three static clones from a human bladder cancer cell line (EJ). Vlodavsky *et al.* (1980) observed human tumor cells migrating out of clusters within minutes of plating on extracellular matrix-coated vessels. Strauli and Haemmerli (1984) have recently reviewed the role of cancer cell motility in invasion. Motility of cells of human tumors could bring cells together from previously more homogeneous areas, and foster cell–cell interactions that otherwise could not occur.

An additional factor in the consideration of the role of mutation in the generation of tumor heterogeneity is the differential effect of similar mutations in different cells. A nonmalignant human disease, osteogenesis imperfecta, provides evidence that mutations that result in a structural change in a single protein may cause very different effects in different cells. Thus, mutation altering the structure of type I procollagen produces a disease that affects primarily skin, tendons, and ligaments, while a similar change to another part of the same molecule produces a disease of the bone (Prockop, 1984). Mutations in heterogeneous malignant cells, even if affecting similar molecules, may also manifest themselves in a heterogeneous manner.

4.4. Epigenetic Mechanisms

Buick and Pollak (1984) have recently discussed the relationship of clonogenic cells, stem cells, and oncogenes, and suggested that neoplasia represents a derangement of the processes that control the entry of the cell into the division cycle, and the production of progeny committed to differentiation (control of PSR). Endogenous and exogenous growth factors and the process of differentiation may play major roles in the generation of heterogeneity.

The production of growth factors by a cell may influence its own or another cell's behavior. The influence of growth factors may be controlled by the production or down-regulation of growth factor receptors (Buick and Pollak, 1984; Haigler, 1983; Erickson et al., 1982). Brattain et al. (1983) described extra No. 7 chromosomes in two lines derived from the same human primary colon tumor, and noted that epidermal growth factor receptor (EGFR) is a product of this chromosome. Chen et al. (1982) noted the extra chromosome No. 7 in eight of nine human colorectal carcinoma lines, and observed that No. 7 was the most commonly modified chromosome of these lines. The presence of a growth factor receptor may be a useful marker of proliferative propensity of stem cells, but may play a completely different role in certain differentiated cells (Buick and Pollak, 1984; Johnson et al., 1980). Thus, the same growth factor may contribute to phenotypic heterogeneity by influencing cell behaviors other than proliferative activity.

Growth factors produced by cells may affect the behavior of other cell populations, making subpopulations within a tumor interdependent for expression of specific phenotypes. Salomon et al. (1984) reported several transforming growth factors in the human breast cancer cell line MCF-7, noting that this suggests heterogeneity within the line. Minna et al. (1982) reviewed the production of hormones by clones of human small-cell lung cancer cells, and postulated cross-feeding effects, with some clones capable of producing calcitonin, bombesin (Moody et al., 1981), ACTH, or arginine vasopressin essential for the proliferation of other clones not capable of producing them. Levine et al. (1984) reported the presence of both stimulatory and inhibitory activities in individual extracts of rat ascites fluids, implying complex interactions of cells and cell products in control of cell growth. Todaro and co-workers (Todaro et al., 1982; Sherwin et al., 1983) demonstrated transforming growth factor-like activities in the urine of pregnant, as well as tumor-bearing, humans. Thus, factors controlling growth and differentiation in tumors may be those involved in normal development and growth control.

Tumor cells may display differentiation capabilities similar to nonmalignant stem cells. In the proper environment, a tumor cell may even produce progeny capable of differentiating into normal cells, as evidenced by blastocyst control of a transplanted embryonal carcinoma cell to form a chimeric but otherwise normal mouse (Pierce and Wells, 1982; Brinster, 1974; Mintz and Illmensee, 1975). Pierce and Wallace (1971) reported the regeneration of "pearls" of normal squamous epithelium through differentiation of squamous cell carcinoma (see also Pierce, 1974), and Pierce and Dixon (1959) reported the maturation of embryonal carcinoma to teratocarcinoma (reviewed by Pierce and Wells, 1982). Differentiation of malignant to benign cells has been reported for teratocarcinoma and squamous cell carcinoma (Pierce and Wallace, 1971; reviewed by Heppner and Miller, 1983), and differentiation of tumor cells to other malignant variants (Heppner and Miller, 1983) has been reported in murine myeloma (Daley, 1981), rat and mouse mammary adenocarcinomas (Dulbecco et al., 1981; Hager et al., 1981), and a rat neurotumor (Imada and Sueoka, 1978). Clearly, the differentiation process can potentially produce a wide range of phenotypic diversity, although not all routes of development are available to cells in all differentiation states (Markert, 1982).

The microenvironment of the cell may have a profound influence on phenotype also (Schirrmacher, 1980; Nicolson, 1984a), although the mechanisms of this interaction are largely undefined (Milas, 1984; Nicolson, 1984a). The extracellular matrix (ECM) and stromal elements play a major role in differentiation of normal cells (Saxen et al., 1976; Bissell et al., 1982). The ECM is gaining increasing usage as a substrate for primary cell culture (Vlodavsky et al., 1980; Crickard et al., 1983). Semisolid media for cell culture have also been reported to influence the growth potential of human tumor cells in vitro (Pavlik et al., 1983), and have been reported to cause terminal differentiation in malignant human keratinocytes (Rheinwald and Beckett, 1980). In this latter case the cultured cells were heterogeneous in their response to semisolid media, some exhibiting terminal differentiation after only a few hours' exposure to that environment.

Local conditions of oxygen tension and nutrient supply can modulate cell phenotype, and change response to anticancer drugs or irradiation. Human colon carcinoma xenografts respond differently to photon irradiation under various circumstances of O_2 delivery, nutrient supply, and waste product or dead cell accumulation (Leith et al., 1984). Deficiencies in oxygen tension, or single amino acids, have been shown to increase genetic instability in vitro (Nowell, 1982). Heterogeneous blood flow (Blasberg et al., 1980) and nutritional and gas gradients are known to exist in solid tumors (Vaupel et al., 1981; Tannock, 1968; Heppner and Miller, 1983). Remarkable oscillations in oxygen microenvironment have been observed in mammalian cell cultures (Werrlein and Glinos, 1974). Potentiation of therapy by selective attack on hypoxic cells has been proposed (Teicher and Sartorelli, 1982; Wheeler et al., 1984; Kennedy et al., 1981).

Rubin and Chu (1984) have recently demonstrated that slight modification of the culture environment, such as 33% hypertonicity, can result in heritable changes in cells in vitro, reinforcing the conclusion that microenvironmental differences can result in persistent tumor cell heterogeneity. The change in local environment encountered by metastasizing tumor cells may contribute to heterogeneity. It may also be a critical determinant of a cell's ability to metastasize in a given locale (Markert, 1982; Weiss, 1980; cf. Nicolson and Custead, 1982).

Cell–cell interactions, such as mast cell production of leukotrienes (Lewis and Austen, 1981; Shanahan et al., 1984) and macrophage production of mutagens (Loveless and Heppner, 1983; Heppner et al., 1984), also contribute to the microenvironment, and may have a marked influence on cells locally.

4.5. Cell Fusion

The extreme of cell–cell interaction, and a potentially powerful means of variant generation, is cell fusion. Somatic cell hybridization with subsequent loss of some chromosomes could combine genetic information between tumor cells, or between tumor and normal cells, resulting in enormously variable genotypes, even though some marker chromosomes might be conserved. Ber et al. (1978) demonstrated fusion of murine tumor cells with host cells. Lala et al. (1980) used histocompatibility profiles to monitor fusion of Ehrlich ascites tumor cells and host cells in vivo. Similarly, Weiner et al. (1972) demonstrated tumor–host cell fusion using a T6 translocation as a marker. Marshall et al. (1982) used phosphoglucose isomerase isoenzymes and the T6 translocation as markers, to demonstrate spontaneous fusion of murine tumor and host cells in vitro. Hu and Pasztor (1975) reported in vivo hybridization of cultured murine melanoma cells and isogeneic normal cells, and Goldenberg et al. (1974) reported in vivo hybridization of human tumor and normal hamster cells. The acquisition of metastatic capability has been attributed to hybridization of nonmetastatic tumor cells with normal host spleen B lymphocytes (De Baetselier et al., 1981), possibly T lymphocytes (De Baetselier et al., 1984), and unspecified host cells (Lagarde et al., 1983) in model systems (reviewed by Larizza and Schirrmacher, 1984).

In an X-linked chimeric situation, analogous to the glucose-6-phosphate dehydrogenase situation in humans (Fialkow, 1979), Woodruff (1983) observed individual clones of mixed isoenzyme type in a murine fibrosarcoma, and concluded that this was due either to fusion of type A and B cells, or chromosome replication without cell division, and reactivation of an inactive X chromosome. Kerbel et al. (1983) proposed a similar explanation for the observed mixed A/B tumors in human colon, cervical, and breast carcinomas. Atkin (1979) has reported premature chromosome condensation in carcinoma of the bladder as presumptive evidence of the fusion of malignant and normal human cells.

5. CELL–CELL INTERACTION IN HETEROGENEOUS TUMORS

As mentioned earlier, cancers are tissues, not accumulations of independent cells. Cellular interactions introduce an unwelcome complication into the problem of malignancy, magnifying by orders of magnitude the difficulty in defining the factors controlling tumor behavior. Normal and tumor cells are known to influence each other's growth (Ranadive and Bhide, 1962), probably by interactions similar to those in normal development (Deuchar, 1975). Eosinophils (Pretlow et al., 1984), mast cells (Farram and Nelson, 1980), macrophages (Heppner et al., 1984; Loveless and Heppner, 1983; Fidler and Kleinerman, 1984), and various classes of lymphocytes (Heppner et al., 1984) infiltrate tumors (Nicolson, 1984a) and profoundly influence cells in their proximity. The interactions of tumor cells with normal cells of the tissue in which the tumor arose, or to which it metastasized, are largely undefined. Normal cells are certainly present in most biopsy specimens. It has been shown by cytological analysis that in the presence of aneuploid cells, a diploid peak in flow cytometric histograms generally represents normal cells (Frankfurt et al., 1984a,b; Perez et al., 1981). Frankfurt et al. (1984a) in a large series of fresh specimens of tumors of various types, observed a diploid component in 97% of the 430 suspensions that displayed aneuploid populations.

The mechanisms by which malignant cells may interact with each other or with normal cells are multiple. Cell–cell interactions may occur via soluble molecules secreted by one population and influencing another. The production of growth factors by clones of tumor cells with potential cross-feeding effect has already been mentioned (Minna *et al.*, 1982; Moody *et al.*, 1981). The biochemical signals involved in control of myeloproliferation (Bloch, 1984; Moore, 1984; Till and McCulloch, 1980) are a complex system of proliferation factors, growth factors, and differentiation factors. These are probably involved in cell–cell interaction in myeloid leukemia (Bloch, 1984; Moore, 1984) and possibly other tumors as well (Buick and Pollak, 1984; Mackillop *et al.*, 1983).

Plasminogen activator and the fibrinolysis system have for some time been postulated to be related to the metastatic process in cancer (reviewed by Cederholm-Williams, 1981; Markus, 1983, 1984). An enigma in this hypothesis is the notion that while a cell's fibrinolytic activity may be important to release it from the primary tumor, the same activity would make it difficult for the cell to arrest in the tissue of the metastatic site (Markus, 1984). Markus *et al.* (1983) examined plasminogin activator secretion in short-term organ cultures of primary and metastatic human cancer. Whereas the activity found in the tissue was similar in primaries and metastases, the *rate of secretion* of plasminogen activator by the metastatic tissue was 1/20th the rate exhibited by the primary tissues. The authors proposed that the cells originating the metastasis, which were able to escape the primary due to the high plasminogen activator environment, did not themselves secrete the enzyme and were thus able to lodge in the distant site. Thus, the heterogeneity in plasminogen activator secretion could be responsible for success in the overall metastatic process, through "cooperation" of unlike cells. This model would predict that metastases need not be an enriched source of cells for further metastases, and indeed this was the finding of Sugarbaker *et al.* (1971) in an experimental system. This also implies that transplantable animal metastases should not become increasingly efficient at producing metastases upon serial transplantation subcutaneously (Weiss, 1980), even though their ability to produce metastases after intravenous injection may be enhanced (Fidler and Kripke, 1977). However, if a metastasis developed cellular heterogeneity in plasminogen activator-secreting ability during its growth, it might then become a source of metastases comparable to the primary.

Additional evidence that tumor cells may cooperate in the production of metastases has been provided by F. R. Miller (1983) in a mouse mammary tumor system. Miller injected a nonmetastasizing line of tumor cells subcutaneously into mice, and when the tumor developed, injected another, metastasizing, line intravenously. As might be expected, metastases in the lung were produced, but unexpectedly, these metastases contained cells of both lines. Thus, cells that by themselves could not metastasize, did so in the presence of metastatic cells. The mechanism of this interaction is not known.

Important cell–cell interactions can occur through direct intercellular contact. Rubin and Chu (1982) reported that crowding of highly transformed 3T3 mouse fibroblasts can reverse the transformed phenotype in vitro. The authors demonstrated that this was not due to depletion of any essential nutrient from the medium, as cells in the uncrowded periphery incorporated tritiated thymidine, and medium that had been in contact with crowded cultures for 17 hr was still able to support greater than 30-fold growth of initially sparse populations.

The most intimate cell–cell contact short of cell fusion is probably the gap junction (Gilula, 1974), whereby the cytoplasm of two cells is connected. Gap junctions have been observed in cancer cells (Johnson and Sherridan, 1971; Azarnia and Larsen, 1977), and have been postulated to play a role in control of cell growth (Loewenstein, 1979). Metabolic cooperation (Subak-Sharpe et al., 1969; van Zeeland et al., 1972; Cox et al., 1976; Loewenstein, 1979) may occur between cells of different biochemical capabilities. Enucleated human fibroblasts, for example, have been shown to be capable of providing IMP from hypoxanthine to cells lacking hypoxanthine-guanine phosphoribosyltransferase, under conditions blocking the de novo synthesis of purines (Cox et al., 1976). Thus, the capabilities of one cell type theoretically can be provided to any cell type (capable of producing a gap junction) in a tumor, and antimetabolite therapy might be circumvented (or augmented) by this mechanism (Miller et al., 1981).

Normal growth, development, and tissue maintenance are phenomena requiring extensive cell–cell interaction, and malignant growth should be expected to be similarly interactive as well (Heppner and Miller, 1983; Miller et al., 1980), albeit with different results, Heppner and co-workers (Heppner et al., 1980, 1983; Heppner, 1982; Heppner and Miller, 1983) reported interactions in cell cultures wherein one population could stimulate or inhibit another's growth. Other cellular characteristics are also subject to cell–cell interactive modulation (Heppner et al., 1980, 1983; Heppner, 1984). Chemosensitivity may be changed in vivo or in vitro (Miller et al., 1981; Heppner et al., 1983) by interaction of heterogeneous populations. Poste et al. (1984) have recently reviewed extremely interesting work demonstrating that heterogeneity stabilizes metastatic potential of murine tumor cells in vitro and in vivo. Similar results were reported by Miner et al. (1982). Cillo et al. (1984) reported that although cloned human melanoma cell lines were of variable antigenic phenotype, two uncloned parental lines were stable over more than 100 passages in vitro. Whatever mechanisms are active in generating heterogeneity, at least some of them apparently are responsive to control by cell–cell interactions.

6. PROGRESSION AND TUMOR HETEROGENEITY

Foulds (1954, 1969, 1975) thoroughly documented the concept of "neoplastic progression," describing tumor development as a series of qualitative changes from type A lesions, wherein the most subtle of neoplastic changes begin, to type C lesions, which are clinically evident malignant neoplasms. The major issue in Foulds's work, particularly the second volume (1975), is the observed changes that occur in progression to type C lesions.

Although Foulds noted a degree of randomness in neoplastic development, overlaid on the A–B–C schema, progression is not totally random. Evidence from several experimental systems indicates that patterns of progression occur, including changes after Foulds's stage C is achieved. Vaage (1980) reported a consistent pattern of changes in individual C3H mammary tumors. Kiang et al. (1982) also reported systematic changes in characteristics of GR mouse mammary tumors during independent transplantations. Welch and co-workers (Neri et al., 1982; Welch and Nicolson, 1983; Welch et al., 1983) have reported that mouse mammary adenocarcinoma clones undergo changes at predictable passage numbers in vitro. Chen (1978) reported nonrandomness in karyotypic diversification of human melanoma stem lines in vitro.

Foulds's (1975) observations documented detailed changes in human and animal tumors from early neoplasia to the recognition of a malignancy. There is no reason to believe that the mechanism of tumor development changes qualitatively with the advent of clinically recognizable disease, and the recent emphasis in the application of Foulds's concepts has been to the processes occurring later in neoplasia, such as development of metastases and clinical resistance to therapy (Nowell, 1976, 1982; Nicolson, 1984a; Heppner and Miller, 1983; Weiss, 1980, 1983).

The possible mechanisms of tumor progression are basically two. Theoretically, one could imagine some sort of field change in which an entire neoplastic cell population would be altered in essential characteristics. Nowell (1976), however, succinctly described another mechanism, which depends on underlying heterogeneity in the tumor population. As described above, Nowell postulated that a fundamental "genetic instability" in tumor cells would lead to the production of new, multiple variants. The qualitative changes in tumor behavior seen in progression would therefore be a reflection of shifts in the distribution of variant populations within the neoplasm as a whole. Both innate tumor cell factors and microenvironmental factors would contribute to these shifts by influencing the degree of variant production and by selection of dominant populations. The random aspects of progression would seem to argue for the selection of randomly generated variants as the basic mechanism (Nowell, 1976, 1982; Goldie and Coldman, 1983, 1984; Talmadge et al., 1984). Talmadge et al. (1984) observed some degree of randomness in chemotherapeutic sensitivity of murine cancer metastatic cells with some clones becoming more sensitive to adriamycin while others became resistant. Clinical observation, however, and the reproducible predictable changes in phenotype during progression mentioned earlier (Vaage, 1980; Kiang et al., 1982; Chen, 1978) indicate stochastic processes cannot fully explain the data.

Consistent with the argument for selection of preexisting populations (Nowell, 1976; Fidler and Kripke, 1977) is the observation that the phenotypes observed to dominate late in development can be shown to be present early. J. R. Shapiro et al. (1981) carefully documented the presence of "reference" karyotypes in human malignant gliomas, to relate these to the karyotypes observed later in cultures from cell suspensions derived from individual tumors. However, these workers also observed development of karyotypes in explant cultures that were not demonstrable in the reference set.

Abeloff et al. (1979a) concluded that lesions of non-small-cell lung carcinoma found at autopsy in small-cell lung cancer patients after unsuccessful therapy were most likely due to emergence of a preexisting population, because foci of non-small-cell tissue were observed in untreated patients who died with small-cell histology. Biochemical tracking of small-cell lung progression in vivo and in vitro has been reported by Baylin and co-workers (Abeloff et al., 1979a; Baylin et al., 1975, 1980, 1984) and Minna et al. (1982).

Of course, demonstration of preexistence of eventually dominant phenotypes does not prove the selection hypothesis, nor does it define the role of fluctuating environmental conditions in changing tumor cell behavior (Weiss, 1980). Fidler and Kripke (1977) demonstrated that preexisting variants were the source of metastases in a murine melanoma, but whether this is the case in naturally occurring metastases has been questioned (Weiss, 1980, 1983; Weiss et al., 1983).

Although it would seem that selection of variants must certainly play a role in tumor progression, the existence of cellular interactions of the type described in the previous section implies that a great deal more than simple competition is involved in the selection process. Orderly and repeatable patterns described by Foulds (1975) and others (Vaage, 1980; Kiang et al., 1982; Chen, 1978), and work to further test and extend Foulds's hypotheses (Nowell, 1976, 1982, 1983; Nicolson, 1984a; Heppner and Miller, 1983; Weiss, 1980, 1983; Wolman, 1983) indicate that random variant generation and selection occur in the context of developmental-type processes, contributed to in a yet underfined way by the interactions of heterogeneous populations in complex microenvironments.

7. IMPLICATIONS FOR CANCER THERAPY

In his monumental work on neoplastic development, Foulds (1975) discusses the importance of critically evaluating hypotheses of neoplasia in the context of clinical observations, as well as in the context of established biological principles. Fisher (1984) has also emphasized the interdependence of clinical and laboratory research. The concepts of tumor heterogeneity have important implications for therapy of human disease (Calabresi et al., 1979; Calabresi and Dexter, 1982; Goldie, 1982, 1983; Fidler and Poste, 1982a,b; Trope, 1980, 1982; Dolnick and Bertino, 1982). The degree to which theories of tumor development and origins of heterogeneity fit clinical observation must be critically evaluated, and implications of such theories must be tested in appropriately designed clinical trials.

7.1. Clinical Resistance

Local tumors may be removed by surgery or irradiation, and the problems of heterogeneity overcome by elimination of all cells in the tumor. Unfortunately, in more than half of all cases, malignant diseases are disseminated at the time of diagnosis, and systemic therapy must be applied (Perloff et al ., 1982). Most commonly, chemotherapy, often with combinations of drugs, is the approach of choice. In the cancers that affect the largest number of people, however, such as lung, breast, colon, and prostate carcinomas (American Cancer Society, 1982), ways to improve the success of chemotherapy are still being sought (DeVita, 1983; Frei, 1980). Even with initially sensitive tumors, such as small-cell lung carcinoma (Greco and Oldham, 1981), relapse to resistant disease usually occurs. Many tumor types are poorly responsive at the outset, and become more resistant after or during therapy (Sinkovics, 1979; Goldie and Coldman, 1983; Curt et al., 1984; Poste and Fidler, 1980).

Failure of chemotherapy might in principle be due to a variety of mechanisms, only some of which are dependent upon cellular heterogeneity. Effective concentrations of drug may not be delivered to the target cells (Segre, 1979; Morasca, 1979; Alberts et al., 1980). Also, the same drugs may be metabolized differently by different patients. For example, duration of response has been shown to vary among patients with acute nonlymphocytic leukemia treated with arabinosylcytosine (ara-C)/anthracycline combination chemotherapy, depending on the retention of the active antimetabolite, arabinosylcytosine triphosphate (ara-CTP), in their leukemic cells (Rustum and Preisler, 1979; Preisler et al., 1984). Patients could be classified into three main groups based on the ability of their cells to transport and activate ara-C, and retain ara-CTP. Also, in recent results employing high doses of ara-C as a single agent, significant variation in the in vivo metabolism of ara-C and retention of ara-CTP among different patients was observed (Y. M. Rustum, unpublished observations).

Even if all cells of a tumor are sensitive in isolation, interaction of populations in the tumor as a tissue could in principle cause clinical resistance. For example, metabolic cooperation though gap junctions (Gilula, 1974; Subak-Sharpe et al., 1969; Cox et al., 1976) might allow a subpopulation to escape the effect of an antimetabolite. On the other hand, intercellular metabolism might make some cells subject to damage by a toxic metabolite created by another cell's metabolism. Also, it has been demonstrated that intercellular interactions affecting drug sensitivity do not necessarily require cell–cell contact (B. E. Miller et al., 1981).

Heterogeneous oxygenation of tumors may result in hypoxic subpopulations that are temporarily nonproliferating and thus less sensitive to chemotherapy (Kennedy et al., 1981; Teicher and Sartorelli, 1982; Wheeler et al., 1984). Noncycling G1-phase cells have been reported in exponentially growing 3T3 mouse fibroblasts (Sturani et al., 1984), and cell cycle heterogeneity may be therapeutically significant in breast (Meyer et al., 1984) and other human tumors (Torosian et al., 1984). Arguing against cell kinetics as a major source of drug resistance, however, Goldie and Coldman (1984) have pointed out that regrowing populations of relapsing tumors have a high percentage of proliferating cells, yet often show the greatest drug resistance.

Variant tumor cells with increased content of dihydrofolate reductase due to gene amplification provide the basis for resistance to methotrexate in some human tumor cell lines (Dolnick and Bertino, 1982), and in acute lymphocytic leukemia (Grill et al., 1984).

Variation in drug uptake or responsiveness probably need not be extreme to make a significant difference clinically. Resistance of three orders of magnitude can be observed in vitro (Dolnick and Bertino, 1982; Hakala, 1973), and in vitro even a fivefold resistance may seem insignificant. Clinically, however, where the problems of host toxicity are of overriding importance, a twofold difference in drug dose may make a significant difference in therapeutic index (Frei and Canellos, 1980; Cortes et al., 1979). Thus, levels of resistance that are undetectable in standard in vitro systems may be critical in vivo.

Development of resistance to combinations of anticancer agents has been studied in mice with L1210 leukemia by Schmid et al. (1976), and was shown to occur more quickly if the agents were given sequentially than if they were administered simultaneously. This effect has been explained by the opportunity for rapid generation of variants in regenerating populations of restricted heterogeneity (Fidler and Poste, 1982a; Poste et al., 1981, 1984; Wright, 1982) and the high probability that some of these will be resistant to any given drug (Goldie and Coldman, 1979, 1983, 1984).

The mechanisms of drug resistance in human tumors are multifaceted, and there is no reason to discount the possibility that multiple mechanisms occur within the same tumor. Goldie and Coldman (1984) have emphasized the role of individual cells' sensitivity and resistance in clinical responsiveness; Heppner and co-workers (Heppner, 1984; Heppner and Miller, 1983) have stressed the role of cellular interactions.

An interesting analogue to neoplasia as a model of the interaction of heterogeneous cells was recently reviewed by Dvorak (1984). Trypanosoma cruzi is a protozoan parasite responsible for Chagas' disease in humans, and can also infect other vertebrates, such as mice. It displays clonal heterogeneity as great as that of tumor cells with respect to variation in DNA content, cell cycle time, and antigenicity. Since the agents causing the disease can be studied in laboratory animals, and display considerable heterogeneity, this disease might provide a very interesting system to study the effect of heterogeneity on therapeutic attempts against disease-causing eukaryotic cells other than cancer cells.

7.2. Predictive Tests for Cancer Chemotherapy

Since the advent of chemotherapy, *in vitro* tests of drug efficacy have been sought. The approach has been reasonably successful for choosing antibiotics to treat microbial infections. The problem in cancer is much more difficult due to (1) difficulty in identifying and isolating cancer cells, (2) heterogeneity of cancer cells, (3) difficulty in growing or otherwise maintaining cancer cells during the test, and (4) lack of drugs able to kill or influence cancer cells specifically. Predictive tests are sought to screen new agents for anticancer activity (Fidler and White, 1980; Shoemaker *et al.*, 1984; Weisenthal, 1981) and to choose chemotherapy for individual patients (Salmon, 1980; Von Hoff *et al.*, 1981b; Von Hoff, 1983; Selby *et al.*, 1983). A number of authors have recently reviewed the general subject of *in vitro* tests for cancer chemotherapy (Von Hoff and Weisenthal, 1980; Hamburger, 1981; Mattern and Volm, 1982; Osieka *et al.*, 1984; Weisenthal and Lippman, 1985; Tanneberger and Nissen, 1983; Hoffman *et al.*, 1984; Kaufmann, 1980). Our concern in this review is with the implications of heterogeneity for the design, conduct, and interpretation of such tests.

Anatomical segregation of heterogeneous subpopulations creates the potential for sampling error with small biopsies, regardless of the predictive assay employed (Siracky, 1979; Trope, 1982). The potential for error becomes even greater when prediction of the sensitivity of a metastatic lesion is demanded of a test of a primary or other metastatic tumor (Bertelsen *et al.*, 1983; Fidler and Poste, 1982a; Schlag and Schreml, 1982). Fidler and Poste (1982a) have pointed out that most currently employed screens of potential anticancer drugs monitor the effect of the drug on primary tumors, but metastatic tumors may be quite different from their primaries. If metastatic lesions differ from primaries in some consistent way in their drug responsiveness, monitoring the response of *metastases* will be required. Otherwise, agents active against metastases specifically (a most valuable class of agents, should such agents exist) might be missed in initial screening.

Tests employing cell suspensions from solid tissues introduce a further source of sampling error, since only cells that can survive the disaggregation procedure will be available for assay (Slocum *et al.*, 1981a,b; Waymouth, 1974), and these cells may be a very small percentage of cells comprising the tumor.

The earliest predictive tests employed tumor tissues, homogenates, or short-term cultures in biochemical assays, and took little or no account of cellular heterogeneity. Several tests showed encouraging results in small numbers of patients (Dendy, 1976; Hall, 1971, 1974), but never proved useful (or possibly were never attempted) in large enough trials to gain wide acceptance. Biochemical testing of cell suspensions has succeeded in acute myelogenous leukemia for prediction of duration of remission induced by ara-C/anthracycline combination chemotherapy (Rustum and Preisler, 1979; Preisler *et al.*, 1984). Identification of biochemical determinants of drug action in solid tumors has not yet reached the same stage, however, partly due to the greater difficulty in isolating and characterizing tumor cells from solid tissues.

As discussed earlier, the approaches that allow cell-by-cell analysis are most likely to allow definition of the role of heterogeneity in determining responsiveness, and thus are likely to produce the most informative predictive tests. Colony-formation assays, also called "clonogenic" or "stem cell" assays, represent one such approach.

The relative merits of colony-formation versus other types of predictive assays have been reviewed (Weisenthal and Lippman, 1985). Two assays of drug sensitivity employing vital dye exclusion as end points have recently been described (Weisenthal et al., 1983; Durkin et al., 1979), although demonstration of lack of sensitivity of a dye exclusion test in comparison to growth assays (Roper and Drewinko, 1976) has rendered such approaches unpopular (Weisenthal and Lippman, 1985).

Major impetus to the clinical application of colony-formation assays in semisolid medium was given by Salmon and co-workers (Hamburger and Salmon, 1977; Hamburger et al., 1978; Salmon, 1980) who applied a two-layer soft agar assay to the prediction of chemotherapeutic responsiveness in human tumors, initially multiple myeloma and ovarian carcinoma.

Clinical application of this type of test has recently been reviewed (Salmon, 1980; Ajani et al., 1983; Johnson and Rossof, 1983; Von Hoff, 1983; Editorial, 1982; Kern et al., 1983; Niell et al., 1983; Salmon et al., 1983; Salmon and Trent, 1984; Lieber and Kovach, 1982). Clinical correlations of drug responsiveness with the results of this assay (Von Hoff et al., 1981b; Bertelsen et al., 1984; Moon et al., 1981; Welander et al., 1983) provide the biological foundation for utilizing the method to examine the cell biology and biochemistry responsible for drug action in human tumors. If the test provides useful information to clinicians, the basis for this fact may allow insight into determinants of drug action in the target cells of human tumors. Clinical correlations, however, must be interpreted cautiously. Most often, advanced solid tumors are unresponsive to chemotherapy, and in vitro prediction of resistance is of little value in demonstrating the validity of a test. Any test tht predicted resistance most of the time would likely correlate well with clinical observations. The convincing data must be in correctly predicting sensitivity, and this is a most challenging task, as failures of drug delivery or other extracellular factors may spoil the correlation of even a very accurate test of cellular sensitivity. Further, clinical trials have a certain degree of bias toward responsiveness, as therapeutic response is the desire of all involved (Warr et al., 1984). This bias is unlikely to be reduced if clinical personnel are aware of the results of an in vitro test they hope will work, and in prospective trials of an assay this situation must be considered.

Although growth in semisolid media has been associated with tumorigeneity (Freedman and Shin, 1974; Mattern and Volm, 1982; Macpherson, 1973; Hamburger, 1981; Pavlik et al., 1983), not all tumor cells will grow in soft agar (Pavlik et al., 1983; Neugut and Weinstein, 1979; Thomson and Meyskens, 1982; Rheinwald and Beckett, 1980), and some nonmalignant cells will form colonies (Asano and Mandel, 1981; Hamburger et al., 1978; Von Hoff et al., 1981a; Tisman et al., 1982). Establishment of colonies as the progeny of tumor cells is thus important (Salmon, 1980).

The "stem cell" basis for such assays is hypothetical, but not without evidence (Mackillop et al., 1983; Buick and Mackillop, 1981; Thomson and Meyskens, 1982). Colony formation has been variously defined to require two to eight divisions from a single cell (Weisenthal and Lippman, 1985; Preisler, 1980; Courtenay and Mills, 1978; Hamburger and Salmon, 1977; Rosenblum et al., 1981). Colony size is theoretically important in establishing the proliferative capacity of a colony-forming cell as consistent with that generally expected of a stem cell (Mackillop et al., 1983), and practically important because even cells lethally irradiated may divide a certain number of times before "dying" (Kallman, 1984; Hurwitz and Tolmach, 1969; Thompson and Suit, 1969). However, establishing the number of cells in a colony from its size can be a complex endeavor, varying from one tumor to another (Meyskens et al., 1984).

In practice, the definition of responsiveness in vitro is never complete inhibition of colony formation, but is empirically determined (Salmon, 1980) to maximize correlation with clinical response. As Brattain et al. (1981) have pointed out, minority populations that are drug resistant may go undetected in such tests. Indeed, growth of 30% of colony-forming units after drug exposure is generally allowed in a "positive" in vitro test (Salmon, 1980; Von Hoff et al., 1981b). In theory, a single clone of resistant cells could result in relapse after chemotherapy (Nowell, 1976). It must be kept in mind, however, that clinical correlations thus far made with any in vitro assay have been for objective responses, involving reduction in gross tumor mass, not for cures, which theoretically require obliteration of proliferative potential in all tumor stem cells.

Another consideration is change in cellular phenotype during the test, which can happen very rapidly in semisolid media (Nicolson, 1984a; Nicolson et al., 1983; Rheinwald and Beckett, 1980). Rheinwald and Beckett (1980) observed loss of proliferative potential in subpopulations of malignant human keratinocytes after only a few hours' suspension in semisolid medium. The authors attributed this effect to terminal differentiation. It appears that response of cells to the semisolid medium environment, or effects of anticancer drugs on differentiation state, could markedly influence the outcome of colony-formation assays in agar.

Changes in media (Pavlik et al., 1983; Pavelic et al., 1983; Hamburger et al., 1981; Buick and Fry, 1980), modification of disaggregation technique (Leibovitz et al., 1983; Slocum et al., 1980; Gioanni and Lalanne, 1982), or use of other versions of the basic semisolid medium assay (Courtenay and Mills, 1978; Courtenay et al., 1978) have all been shown to influence colony formation. Although low plating efficiencies may in part be due to inherently small numbers of "stem cells" (Salmon, 1980; Mackillop et al., 1983; Hamburger, 1981), there has been a widespread effort to improve the system and increase plating efficiency (Editorial, 1982; Mattern and Volm, 1982; Hamburger, 1981). Changes in the assay that allow greater numbers of cells to form colonies, however, will not necessarily "improve" the assay in the sense of correctly determining chemosensitivity of cancer cells in patients, and clinical correlates for any "improved" assays will have to be done independently.

In theory, if a small subpopulation of cells is responsible for the growth potential of tumors, and for growth in the in vitro assay, it should be possible to improve plating efficiencies by isolation of appropriate subpopulations. Mackillop et al. (1982) employed differential centrifugation to isolate colony-forming cells from human ovarian carcinoma cells obtained from ascites fluids. Karp et al. (1984) recently employed isokinetic Ficoll gradients (Pretlow et al., 1975) to separate clonogenic multiple myeloma cells from granulocyte–macrophage colony-forming units, and observed that the normal cells proliferated only when separated from the tumor cell population. In an attempt to isolate colony-forming subpopulations from human tumors, we are employing counterflow centrifugation (elutriation), but have not achieved increased colony-forming efficiencies in subpopulations, although enrichment for aneuploid cells has been observed (see Section 3.1). It is possible that the elutriation procedure adversely affects the colony-forming subpopulation. However, trypan blue exclusion of these cell suspensions, and nucleoside triphosphate pools, energy charge, and tumorigenicity of cells from several animal model tumors, were not adversely affected by the same procedure (Slocum and Rustum, unpublished observations).

Seeking an alternative explanation for lack of colony-forming capacity of elutriated fractions, we noted that the elutriator markedly depletes aggregates from cell suspensions, since it separates particles primarily based on size (Keng et al., 1981a; Slocum et al., 1984). Multicell aggregates, which are always present to some extent in cell suspensions derived from epithelial solid tumors (Rupniak and Hill, 1980; Agrez et al., 1982; Slocum et al., 1984), could be the source of most or all colonies in an agar assay (Agrez et al., 1982; Mattern and Volm, 1982; Slocum et al., 1984). When plating efficiencies are low, even a small percentage of aggregates in cell suspensions from human tumors could totally account for colony formation. By following colony formation by serial photomicrography, we have confirmed the report of Agrez et al. (1982) that colony formation from aggregates occurs. In examination of 159 pairs of photographs of 26 cell suspensions plated in soft agar, we have not yet observed colony formation by single cells (Slocum et al., 1984). Heterogeneity within colonies (Cillo et al., 1984; Durie et al., 1982) is also consistent with possible multicellular origin. Aggregates may be at a growth advantage since the cells within them may be protected from some of the trauma of the disaggregation procedure. Also, although not all cells within the aggregate may proliferate, cell–cell interactions may be important to colony formation and confer advantages to aggregates.

To assess the role of aggregates in colony formation, we have depleted suspensions of aggregates by filtration through meshes with openings of 30 μm and added the aggregate-loaded meshes to experimental plates as shown in Figure 2. Since aggregates do form colonies directly, one would not expect to totally restore colony counts. An effect of aggregates in support of colony formation, however, would result in partial restoration of colony-forming capacity. Indeed, this was the result obtained (Figure 3); aggregate depletion reduced colony formation significantly by threefold, and loaded meshes partially restored colony formation by twofold (Slocum et al., 1984).

Although aggregate growth may contribute to colony formation in all cases except those in which rigorous evaluation of plates at time zero indicates the monodisperse nature of the tumor cells, this does not preclude the use of agar assays containing aggregates for prediction of clinical responsiveness. However, detailed analysis of colony-forming units cannot be made in a nonclonal assay, as multiple colony-forming units may be present in one aggregate. Also, the number of cell divisions required for a colony of a given size is impossible to determine, unless a colony starts as an individual cell, or its formation can be traced to an aggregate of known size.

The presence of colony-forming units in aggregates implies that the optimal method of reducing the content of aggregates in cell suspensions is by disaggregation, not by elimination of aggregates by filtration or other means. Indeed, Leibovitz et al. (1983) have reported that more complete disaggregation of cells by a medium designed to disaggregate intestinal epithelia (Carter et al., 1982) can improve the colony-forming capacity of cells freshly disaggregated from human tumors.

Plated aggregates of sufficient size to be considered colonies can create an artifact in colony-formation assays, creating an apparent drug (or radiation)-resistant population (Editorial, 1982). Use of vital dyes to establish the

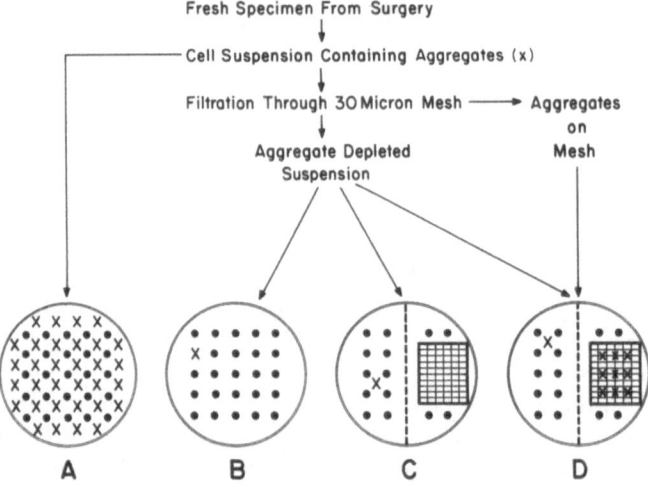

FIGURE 2. Experimental design to define the role of aggregates in a colony formation assay. Cell suspensions were depleted of aggregates by filtration through 30-μm nylon mesh, and colony formation compared when aggregate-loaded or empty meshes were embedded on one side of the agar plate.

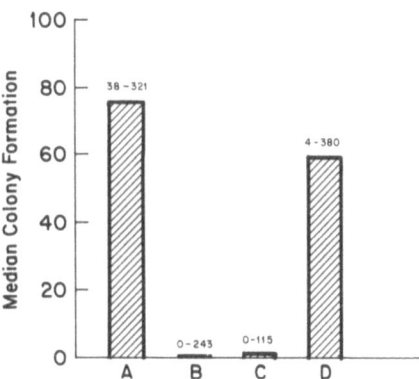

FIGURE 3. Effect of aggregates on colony formation in soft agar. A-D refer to plate types indicated in Figure 2: A, control suspension; B, aggregate depleted suspension; C, aggregate depleted suspension with empty mesh embedded; D, aggregate depleted suspension with loaded mesh embedded. Aggregate depletion (B and C) markedly reduced colony formation compared to controls (A), and presence of aggregates on meshes embedded in the agar partially restored colony-forming capacity (D). Ranges of colony counts for each category are indicated above each column.

metabolic capability of colonies (Klebe, 1984; Alley et al., 1982), time-zero counting, and positive controls (Shoemaker et al., 1984) are currently under investigation as ways to eliminate this artifact.

Plating cells from human tumors onto feeder layers (Smith et al., 1981, 1984; Brattain et al., 1983) or onto ECM (Crickard et al., 1983) may represent the basis of assays similar in principle to semisolid medium assays, if the complication of growth of nonmalignant cells can be adequately dealt with.

Approaches to predictive assays, which seek to take advantage of, rather than eliminate, intercellular interactions, are: the growth of tumors as xenografts in immune-deficient mice (Mattern and Volm, 1982; Steel et al., 1983; Houghton and Houghton, 1983), xenografts under the renal capsule of normal mice (Bogden et al., 1979; Bogden and Von Hoff, 1984), and the explanting of tumor tissue in gels containing ECM components (J. Yang et al., 1980; B. E. Miller et al., 1983). It is hoped that drug effects closer to those occurring in vivo may be achieved if cellular interactions are not disrupted. This advantage, and the reduced trauma and selection that cells face, may make these assays better predictors of chemotherapeutic responsiveness. They will require further probing, however, to yield information about intracellular or intercellular mechanisms responsible for drug sensitivity.

8. FUTURE DIRECTIONS

The concepts of cellular heterogeneity of cancer impact on future use of currently available therapy, the search for new therapeutic agents, and the design of future treatment strategies.

The rapid generation of variants in tumors implies that even tumors that are not very large are likely to contain therapeutically resistant cells capable of causing a relapse to clinically resistant disease (Goldie, 1982, 1983; Poste and Fidler, 1980; Poste and Greig, 1982; DeVita, 1983; DeVita et al., 1975). Therefore, optimal use of currently available agents would likely be by their application in combination (DeVita et al., 1975; DeVita, 1983; Poste and

Greig, 1982; Teicher and Sartorelli, 1982; Calabresi *et al.*, 1979; Calabresi and Dexter, 1982; Goldie, 1982, 1983) as soon as possible, prior to, or immediately after reduction in tumor burden by surgery or radiation therapy. Non-cross-resistant therapies thus applied may eliminate subpopulations of tumor cells that otherwise will be the source of resistant clones producing a resistant tumor.

Identification of mechanisms of resistance may provide a biochemical basis for overcoming heterogeneity, provided that the number of basic mechanisms of resistance is limited (Goldie and Coldman, 1984; Curt *et al.*, 1984; Teicher and Sartorelli, 1982; Ling *et al.*, 1984). Design of "second-generation" drugs, analogous to the synthetic modification of antibacterial antibiotics (Goldie and Coldman, 1984), may then be a fruitful approach. Combinations of anticancer drugs and other pharmacological agents, such as the use of calcium channel blockers to overcome pleiotropic drug resistance (Rogan *et al.*, 1984), or the combination of 5-fluorouracil with leucovorin (Madajewicz *et al.*, 1984; Evans *et al.*, 1981), represent another approach made possible by identification of drug resistance mechanisms. This approach also may make possible the design of protocols to overcome what Martin *et al.* (1985) have termed "quantitative heterogeneity" at the cellular level. Combination chemotherapy has been for many years based on qualitative heterogeneity (Martin, 1958), combining agents individually effective against subpopulations of tumor cells. Quantitative differences in cells whose resistance is qualitatively similar, however, may necessitate increasing the effectiveness of specific agents in combinations, rather than simply adding more different agents with individual activity. In fact, the quantitative aspects of drug resistance may be exacerbated if adding new agents necessitates reducing the dose of others in the combination. Rather than increasing dosages, however, which may cause unacceptable toxicity, Martin *et al.* (1983a,b, 1985) suggest biochemically "modulating" the effects of agents based on known mechanisms of action, even if this means including agents that by themselves do not have antitumor activity.

Malignant cells may be making abnormal use of the normal genome (Markert, 1982), and failure to commit to differentiation may be the basic defect in neoplasia (Petricciani, 1980; Buick and Pollak, 1984; Nicolson, 1984a,b; Sachs, 1980; Bloch, 1984). Bloch (1984) has suggested that this defect may not be irreversible, although it is possible that at some point during tumor progression the defect does become irreversible (Nicolson, 1984a; Sachs, 1980). Therapy based on correcting the abnormality, i.e., inducing normal differentiation (Bloch, 1984; McCulloch *et al.*, 1978; Moore, 1984), is in principle very attractive, since it is not aimed at killing large numbers of cells, and may thus largely avoid host toxicity. Malignant cells have been reported to differentiate under various conditions, some to malignant variants (Heppner and Miller, 1983; Bennett *et al.*, 1978; Dulbecco *et al.*, 1981; Hager *et al.*, 1981; Imada and Sueoka, 1978; Daley, 1981), and some to benign cells (Pierce and Wallace, 1971; Pierce, 1974). Whether malignant cells of human tumors can give rise to normal tissues is a long-standing question (Woodruff, 1983).

The microenvironment may markedly influence the differentiation state of cells in vitro or in vivo (Nicolson, 1984a; Saxen et al., 1976; Bissell et al., 1982). As mentioned earlier, murine embryonal carcinoma cells can be controlled by a blastocyst environment to produce normal mouse tissues (Brinster, 1974; Mintz and Illmensee, 1975; Pierce et al., 1979; Pierce and Wells, 1982), but groups of tumor cells may be too large to control (Brinster, 1974; Papaioannou et al., 1975; Pierce and Wells, 1982) and even individual cells may vary in their ability to respond to the blastocyst environment (Illmensee, 1978; Papaioannou et al., 1979; Pierce and Wells, 1982).

As mentioned earlier, transformed murine 3T3 fibroblasts may be induced to reverse the transformed phenotype when crowded in vitro (Rubin and Chu, 1982), and malignant human keratinocytes displayed heterogeneity in reaction to suspension in a semisolid medium, some undergoing terminal differentation within 3 hr of exposure to the anchorage-preventing environment (Rheinwald and Beckett, 1980). Dexter et al. (1979) reported that the human colorectal cell lines they studied lost the ability to grow in soft agar and lost tumorigenicity in nude mice, in response to exposure to the organic solvent N,N-dimethylformamide. Similarly, Leith et al. (1981) used N,N-dimethylformamide to induce differentiation in mouse mammary adeno-carcinoma cell lines. The resulting cell populations were more uniform in their response to X-irradiation. Although the concentration of this organic solvent used in vitro is unlikely to be useful clinically, these studies suggest that the use of differentiation-inducing agents to reduce heterogeneity, and thus create more uniform responsiveness to therapy, may be a productive approach (Heppner and Miller, 1983; Calabresi et al., 1979).

The factors that control differentiation and proliferation in human myeloid cells are coming to be understood (McCulloch et al., 1978; Bloch, 1984; Moore, 1984), and may form the basis for new approaches to therapy of myeloid leukemia. Induction of differentiation may become an adjuvant therapy to current chemotherapy (Moore, 1984). Bloch (1984), however, has pointed out that cytotoxic therapy may antagonize attempts to restore normal differentiation, by adversely affecting cells producing important differentiation or proliferation factors. An important advantage in differentiation-inducing therapy may be the production of normal regulatory factors by leukemic cells induced to differentiate (Bloch, 1984; Maeda and Ichikawa, 1980).

Another relatively new approach to therapy is the activation of tumoricidal macrophages, which apparently can be therapeutically successful even when the tumor cells display considerable phenotypic diversity (Fidler and Raz, 1981; Poste and Fidler, 1980; Fidler and Poste, 1982b; Miner et al., 1983; Miner and Nicolson, 1983; Fidler and Kleinerman, 1984). The therapeutic specificity and effectiveness thus far demonstrated against heterogeneous experimental tumors make this approach extremely interesting.

Other approaches, based on heterogeneity already defined in human tumors, involve the targeting of cells in oxygenated and hypoxic compartments in the tumor (Kennedy et al., 1981; Teicher and Sartorelli, 1982; Wheeler et al., 1984), or targeting aneuploid cells (Spremulli and Dexter, 1983). The importance of aneuploid cells as therapeutic targets, however, is not established (Wolman, 1983; Smith et al., 1984).

Better definition of heterogeneity in human tumors and its significance will no doubt suggest other approaches to therapy. In vitro drug tests and screens that examine cells on an individual basis will accrue benefits similar to those described in earlier sections for defining heterogeneity in general. Multiple-parameter flow cytometry (Melamed et al., 1977; Dethlefsen et al., 1980; Barlogie et al., 1983; Benson et al., 1984; Tanke et al., 1983; Frankfurt, 1983; Haskill et al., 1983) offers the possibility of studies in cellular pharmacology, which could help define subpopulations, and cell sorting may make controlled mixing of subpopulations a workable technique to define subpopulation interactions. Automated image analysis combined with the techniques of autoradiography (Stephen and Ambrose, 1983), monoclonal antibody staining, and fluorescence microscopy may prove useful in defining therapeutically important subpopulations, and assessing drug effects (Wolf and Aronson, 1961) in the often very small numbers of cells available from human tissues. Improvements in techniques to obtain greater numbers of cells from tissues, with minimum damage, and improved culture methods for human tumor cells should also improve our ability to obtain the most information from small biopsy samples.

The general principles being defined for tumor cell heterogeneity suggest that interference with the process of variant generation and outgrowth would be advantageous (Calabresi et al., 1979; Leith et al., 1981; Poste and Greig, 1982; Curt et al., 1984; Nowell, 1976, 1982, 1983). Control of variant generation apparently involves subpopulation interactions (Poste and Greig, 1982) that, if better understood, might be exploitable therapeutically.

Future strategies in design of cancer treatment must include consideration of heterogeneous response to therapy at the cellular level. Currently available agents should be utilized according to our understanding of variant generation and response. New agents with activity against heterogeneous systems should be sought. New approaches should target variant generation as a component of clinical resistance. Also, it should be kept in mind that the ultimate objective clinically is to interrupt, or redirect, the biological processes that are responsible for morbidity and mortality. It is possible that annihilation of all tumor cells is unnecessary if invasion and metastases can be prevented or arrested, or differentiation of malignant cells to more benign behavior can be achieved.

9. CONCLUDING REMARKS

Heterogeneity of the cells comprising human tumors has been noted in studies of histopathology, biochemistry, antigenicity, receptor status, tumorigenicity (as xenografts), DNA content, karyotype, chemotherapeutic sensitivity, and oncogene expression. This heterogeneity generally exceeds that exhibited by the cells of normal tissues, and appears to be due to a genetic instability associated with malignancy. Progression of tumors beyond the lower limits of clinical detection to advanced, therapeutically recalcitrant lesions, appears to involve selection of increasingly autonomous, therapeutically resistant cells arising out of a sea of variants. Understanding the sources of and control of variant generation and outgrowth, and definition of mechanisms of drug resistance commonly exhibited by variants, will greatly assist in design of better systemic therapy.

In addition to understanding the parts, however, we must understand the whole. Interactions between tumor cells, and between tumor and normal cells, are presently poorly defined, but probably represent a very significant determinant of tumor behavior. Cellular interactions in variant generation, differentiation, and control of proliferation all represent points of potential therapeutic intervention. Knowledge of the rules governing "societies" of cells in tumors may answer many basic questions in cell biology, as well as provide the key to successful cancer therapeutics.

ACKNOWLEDGMENTS. The authors wish to thank Cheryl Melancon, Jessie Crowe, Sandra Trafalski, Mae Brown, and Karen Marie Schrader for secretarial assistance; Luella Kenny, Elva Winslow, Nancy Reska, Rita Ghosh, and Sarra Polanskya for technical assistance in doing the work reported in the tables and figures, and for help in locating references and proofreading; Drs. Edward Henderson, Alexander Bloch, Ron Buick, Miriam Postan, James Dvorak, Helene Smith, Gabor Markus, James Goldie, and Daniel Martin for helpful discussions; and Drs. Michael Brattain, Garth Nicolson, Helene Smith, Daniel Martin, Larry Weisenthal, and Marc Lippman for providing preprints of their work in press. We also wish to acknowledge the support of USPHS Grants CA-18420, CA-21071, and CA-24538.

REFERENCES

Abeloff, M. D., Eggleston, J. C., Mendelsohn, G., Ettinger, D. S., and Baylin, S. B., 1979a, Changes in morphologic and biochemical characteristics of small cell carcinoma of the lung—A clinicopathologic study, Am. J. Med. **66**:757–764.

Abeloff, M. D., Ettinger, D. S., Khouri, N. F., and Lenhard, R. E., 1979b, Intensive induction therapy for small cell carcinoma of the lung, Cancer Treat. Rep. **63**:519–524.

Adams, A. T., and Emerman, J. T., 1984, Quantitative analysis of heterogeneity of estrogen binding in human breast tumor specimens, Anal. Quant. Cytol. **6**:287–292.

Agrez, M. V., Kovach, J. S., and Lieber, M. M., 1982, Cell aggregates in the soft agar "human tumour stem-cell assay," Br. J. Cancer **46**:880–887.

Ajani, J. A., Shailendra, K. S., Spitzer, G., Hug, V. M., and Bodey, G. P., 1983, Cloning of human tumor stem cells in soft agar—An overview, Cancer Bull. **35**:(1):16–19.

Alabaster, O., Andreeff, M., Spooner, C., and Clagett, K., 1984, Flow cytometric measurement of intracellular pH—A dosimetric approach to metabolic heterogeneity, in: Biological Dosimetry: Cytometric Approaches to Mammalian Systems (W. G. Eisert and M. L. Mendelsohn, eds.), Springer-Verlag, Berlin, pp. 299–310.

Alberts, D. S., Chen, H.-S. G., and Salmon, S. E., 1980, In vitro drug assays: Pharmacologic considerations, in: Progress in Clinical and Biological Research, Volume 48 (S. Salmon, ed.), Liss, New York, pp. 197–207.

Albino, A. P., Lloyd, K. O., Houghton, A. N., Ottgen, H., and Old, L. J., 1981, Heterogeneity in surface antigen and glycoprotein expression of cell lines derived from different melanoma metastases of the same patient, J. Exp. Med. 154:1764–1778.

Albino, A. P., Le Strange, R., Oliff, A. I., Furth, M. E., and Old, L. J., 1984, Transforming ras genes from human melanoma: A manifestation of tumour heterogeneity?, Nature 308:69–72.

Allegra, J. C., Barlock, A., Huff, K. K., and Lipmann, M. E., 1980, Changes in multiple or sequential estrogen receptor determinations in breast cancer, Cancer 45:792–794.

Alley, M. C., Uhl, C. B., and Lieber, M. M., 1982, Improved detection of drug cytotoxicity in the soft agar colony formation assay through use of a metabolizable tetrazolium salt, Life Sci. 31:3071–3078.

American Cancer Society, 1982, Cancer Facts and Figures, American Cancer Society, New York.

Asano, S., and Mandel, T. E., 1981, Colonies formed in agar from human breast cancer and their identification as T-lymphocytes, J. Natl. Cancer Inst. 67:25–32.

Ashton, P. R., Hollingsworth, A. S., Jr., and Johnston, W. W., 1975, The cytopathology of metastastic breast cancer, Acta Cytol. 19(1):1–6.

Atkin, N. B., 1979, Premature chromosome condensation in carcinoma of the bladder: Presumptive evidence for fusion of normal and malignant cells, Cytogenet. Cell Genet. 23:217–219.

Atkin, N. B., and Kay, R., 1979, Prognostic significance of model DNA value and other factors in malignant tumours, based on 1465 cases, Br. J. Cancer 40:210–221.

Atkin, N. B., and Richards, B. M., 1956, Deoxyribonucleic acid in human tumours as measured by microspectrophotometry of Feulgen stain: A comparison of tumours arising at different sites, Br. J. Cancer 10:769–786.

Atkin, N. B., Mattinson, G., and Baker, M. C., 1966, A comparison of the DNA content and chromosome number of fifty human tumours, Br. J. Cancer 20:87–101.

Aubert, C., Rouge, F., and Galindo, J. R., 1980, Tumorigenicity of human malignant melanocytes in nude mice in relation to their differentiation in vitro, J. Natl. Cancer Inst. 64:1029–1040.

Azarnia, R., and Larsen, W. J., 1977, Intercellular communication and cancer, in: Intercellular Communication (W. C. DeMello, ed.), Plenum Press, New York, pp. 145–172.

Bahler, D. W., Lord, E. M., Kennel, S. J., and Horan, P. K., 1984, Heterogeneity and clonal variation related to cell surface expression of a mouse lung tumor-associated antigen quantified using flow cytometry, Cancer Res. 44:3317–3323.

Barlogie, B., Drewinko, B., Schumann, J., Gohde, W., Dosik, G., Latreille, J., Johnston, D. A., and Freireich, E. J., 1980, Cellular DNA content as a marker of neoplasia in man, Am. J. Med. 69:195–203.

Barlogie, B., Raber, M. N., Schumann, J., Johnson, T. S., Drewinko, B., Swartzendruber, D. E., Gohde, W., Andreeff, M. and Freireich, E. J., 1983, Flow cytometry in clinical cancer research, Cancer Res. 43:3982–3997.

Barranco, S. C., Ho, D. H. W., Drewinko, B., Romsdahl, M. M., and Humphrey, R. M., 1972, Differential sensitivity of human melanoma cell growth in vitro to arabinosylcytosine, Cancer Res. 32:2733–2736.

Barranco, S. C., Drewinko, B., and Humphrey, R. M., 1973, Differential response by human melanoma cells to 1,3-bis-(2-chloroethyl)-1-nitrosourea and bleomycin, Mutat. Res. 19:277–280.

Barrett, K. E., and Metcalfe, D. D., 1984, Mast cell heterogeneity: Evidence and implications, J. Clin. Immunol. 4(4):253–261.

Baylin, S. B., 1980, Clonal selection and heterogeneity of human solid neoplasms, in: Design of Models for Testing Cancer Therapeutic Agents (I. J. Fidler and R. J. White, eds.), Van Nostrand–Reinhold, Princeton, N. J. pp. 50–63.

Baylin, S. B., and Mendelsohn, G., 1982, Medullary thyroid carcinoma: A model for the study of human tumor progression and cell heterogeneity, in: Tumor Cell Heterogeneity: Origins and Implications (Bristol-Meyers Cancer Symposia, Volume 4) (A. H. Owens, D. S. Coffey, and S. B. Baylin, eds.), Academic Press, New York, pp. 9–27.

Baylin, S. B., Abeloff, M. D., Wieman, K. C., Tomford, J. W., and Ettinger, D. S., 1975, Elevated histaminase (diamine oxidase) activity in small-cell carcinoma of the lung, N. Engl. J. Med. 293:1286–1290.

Baylin, S. B., Weisburger, W. R., Eggleston, J. C., Mendelsohn, G., Beaven, M. A., Abeloff, M. D., and Ettinger, D. S., 1978, Variable content of histaminase, L-dopa decarboxylase and calcitonin in small-cell carcinoma of the lung, N. Engl. J. med. 299:105–110.

Baylin, S. B., Mendelsohn, G., Weisburger, W. R., Gann, D. S., and Eggleston, J. C., 1979, Levels of histaminase and L-dopa decarboxylase activity in the transition from L-cell hyperplasia to familial medullary thyroid carcinoma, Cancer 44:1315–1321.

Baylin, S. B., Abeloff, M. D., Goodwin, G., Carney, D. N., and Gazdar, A. F., 1980, Activities of L-dopa decarboxylase and diamine oxidase (histaminase) in human lung cancers and decarboxylase as a marker for small (oat) cell cancer in cell culture, Cancer Res. 40:1990–1994.

Baylin, S. B., Jackson, R. H., Lennarz, W., Jr., and Shaper, J. H., 1984, The spectrum of human lung cancer cells in culture: A potential model for studying molecular determinants of tumor progression and metastasis, in: Cancer Invasion and Metastasis: Biologic and Therapeutic Aspects (G. L. Nicolson and L. Milas, eds.), Raven Press, New York, pp. 281–291.

Beattie, G. M., Knowles, A. F., Jensen, F. C., Baird, S. M., and Kaplan, N. O., 1982, Induction of sarcomas in athymic mice, Proc. Natl. Acad. Sci. USA 79:3033–3036.

Bennett, D. C., Peachey, L. A., Durkin, H., and Rudland, P. S., 1978, A possible mammary stem cell line, Cell 15:283–298.

Benson, M. C., McDougal, D. C., and Coffey, D. S., 1984, The use of multiparameter flow cytometry to assess tumor cell heterogeneity and grade prostate cancer, Prostate 5(1):27–45.

Ber, R., Wiener, F., and Fenyo, E. M., 1978, Proof of in vivo fusion of murine tumor cells with host cells by universal fusers: Brief communication, J. Natl. Cancer Inst. 60:931–933.

Bernal, S., Thompson, R. A., Gilbert, F., and Baylin, S. B., 1983, In vitro and in vivo growth characteristics of two different cell populations in an established line of human neuroblastoma, Cancer Res. 43:1256–1260.

Berry, R. J., Laing, A. H., and Wells, J., 1975, Fresh explant culture of human tumors in vitro and the assessment of sensitivity to cytotoxic chemotherapy, Br. J. Cancer 31:218–227.

Bertelsen, C. A., Korn, E. I., Morton, D. L., and Kern, D. H., 1983, Heterogeneity of human metastatic clones in vitro chemosensitivity testing: Implications for the clinical application of the clonogenic assay, Arch. Surg. 118(12):1406–1409.

Bertelsen, C. A., Sondak, V. K., Mann, B. D., Korn, E. L., and Kern, D. H., 1984, Chemosensitivity testing to human solid tumors, Cancer 53:1240–1245.

Besch, G. J., Wolberg, W. H., Gilchrist, K. W., Voelker, J. G., and Gould, M. N., 1983, A comparison of methods for the production of monodispersed cell suspensions from human primary breast carcinomas, Breast Cancer Res. Treat. 3:15–22.

Bigner, D. D., Schold, C., Bigner, S. H., Bullard, D. E., and Wikstrand, C., 1981, How heterogeneous are gliomas?, Cancer Treat. Rep. 65(Suppl. 2):45–49.

Biorklund, A., Hakansson, L., Stenstam, B., Trope, C., and Akerman, M., 1980, On heterogeneity of non-Hodgkin's lymphomas as regards sensitivity to cytostatic drugs, Eur. J. Cancer 16:647–654.

Bissell, M. J., Hall, H. G., and Parry, G., 1982, How does extracellular matrix direct gene expression?, J. Theor. Biol. 99:31–68.

Blasberg, R. G., Gazendan, J., Patlak, C. S., Shapiro, W. R., and Fernstermacher, J. D., 1980, Changes in blood–brain transfer parameters induced by hyperosmolar intracarotid infusion and by metastatic tumor growth, Adv. Exp. Med. Biol. 131:307–319.

Bloch, A., 1984, Induced cell differentiation in cancer therapy, Cancer Treat. Rep. 68(1):199–205.

Bloemendal, H. (ed.), 1977, Cell Separation Methods, North-Holland, Amsterdam.

Bodansky, O., 1975, Biochemistry of Human Cancer, Academic Press, New York.

Bodenham, D. C., 1968, A study off 650 observed malignant melanomas in the South-West region, Ann. R. Coll. Surg. Engl. 43:218–239.

Bogden, A. E., and Von Hoff, D. D., 1984, Comparison of the human tumor cloning and subrenal capsule assays, Cancer Res. 44:1087–1090.

Bogden, A. E., Haskell, P. M., LePage, D. J., Kelton, D. E., Cobb, W. R., and Esker, H. J., 1979,

Growth of human tumor xenografts implanted under the renal capsule of normal immunocompetent mice, Exp. Cell Biol. **47**:281–293.

Bowen, J. A., Cailleau, R., Giovenella, B. C., Pathak, S., and Siciliano, M. J., 1983, A retrovirus-producing transformed mouse cell line derived from a human breast adenocarcinoma transplanted in a nude mouse, In Vitro **19**:635–641.

Brattain, M. G., Kimball, P. M., Pretlow, T. G., II, and Pitts, A. M., 1977a, Partial purification of human colonic carcinoma cells by sedimentation, Br. J. Cancer **35**:850–857.

Brattain, M. G., Pretlow, T. P., and Pretlow, T. G., II, 1977b, Cell fractionation of large bowel cancer, Cancer **40**:2479–2486.

Brattain, M. G., Fine, W. D., Khaled, F. M., Thompson, J., and Brattain, D. E., 1981, Heterogeneity of malignant cells from human colonic carcinoma, Cancer Res. **41**:1751–1756.

Brattain, M. G., Marks, M. E., McCombs, J., Finley, W., and Brattain, D. E., 1983, Characterization of human colon carcinoma cell lines isolated from a single primary tumour, Br. J. Cancer **47**:373–381.

Brattain, M. G., Levine, A. E., Chakrabarty, S., Yeoman, L. C., Willson, J. K. V., and Long, B., 1984, Heterogeneity of human colon carcinoma, Cancer Metastasis Rev. **3**(3):179–191.

Brennan, M. J., Donegan, W. L., and Appleby, D. E., 1979, The variability of estrogen receptors in metastatic breast cancer, Am. J. Surg. **137**:260–262.

Brereton, H. D., Matthews, M. M., Costa, J., Kent, H., and Johnson, R. E., 1978, Mixed anaplastic small-cell and squamous-cell carcinoma of the lung, Ann. Intern. Med. **88**:805–806.

Brinster, R. L., 1974, The effect of cells transferred into the mouse blastocyst on subsequent development, J. Exp. Med. **140**:1049–1056.

Buick, R. N., and Fry, S. E., 1980, A comparison of human tumour-cell clonogenicity in methylcellulose and agar culture, Br. J. Cancer **42**:933–936.

Buick, R. N., and Mackillop, W. J., 1981, Measurement of self-renewal in culture of clonogenic cells from human ovarian carcinoma, Br. J. Cancer **44**:349–355.

Buick, R. N., and Pollak, M. N., 1984, Perspectives on clonogenic tumor cells, stem cells, and oncogenes, Cancer Res. **44**:4909–4918.

Burchiel, S. W., Martin, J. C., Imai, K., Ferrone, S., and Warner, N. L., 1982, Heterogeneity of HLA-A, B, Ia-like, and melanoma-associated antigen expression by human melanoma cell lines analyzed with monoclonal antibodies and flow cytometry, Cancer Res. **42**:4110–4115.

Byar, P., and Mostofi, F., 1972, Carcinoma of the prostate: Prognostic evaluation of certain pathologic features in 208 radical prostatectomies, Cancer **30**:5–13.

Byers, V. S., and Johnston, J. O., 1977, Antigenic differences among osteogenic sarcoma tumor cells taken from different locations in human tumors, Cancer Res. **37**:3173–3183.

Cairns, J., 1975, Mutation selection and the natural history of cancer, Nature **255**:197–200.

Cairns, J., 1981, The origin of human cancer, Nature **289**:353–357.

Calabresi, P., and Dexter, D. L., 1982, Clinical implications of cancer cell heterogeneity, in: Tumor Cell Heterogeneity: Origins and Implications (Bristol-Meyers Cancer Symposia, Volume 4) (A. H. Owens, D. S. Coffey, and S. B. Baylin, eds.), Academic Press, New York, pp. 181–201.

Calabresi, P., Dexter, D. L., and Heppner, G. H., 1979, Clinical and pharmacological implications of cancer cell differentiation and heterogeneity, Biochem. Pharmacol. **28**:1933–1941.

Carter, J. H., Carter, H., Nussbaum, J., and Eicholz, A., 1982, Isolation of hamster intestinal epithelial cells using hypoosmotic media and PVP, J. Cell. Physiol. **111**:55–67.

Castagnetta, L., LoCasto, M., Mercadante, T., Polito, L., Cowan, S., and Leake, R. E., 1983, Intratumoural variation of oestrogen receptor status in endometrial cancer, Br. J. Cancer **47**:261–267.

Catsimpoolas, N., 1977, Methods of Cell Separation, Volume 1, Plenum Press, New York.

Cederholm-Williams, S. A., 1981, Molecular mechanism of fibrinolysis: A system involved with malignant cells, Invasion Metastasis **1**:85–98.

Chabner, B. A. (ed.), 1983, UCLA Symposium on Molecular and Cellular Biology Series, Volume 4, Liss, New York.

Chen, T. R., 1978, Evolution in vitro of stem lines with minimal karyotype deviations in a human heteroploid cell line, J. Natl. Cancer Inst. **61**:277–284.

Chen, T. R., Hay, R. J., and Macy, M. L., 1982, Karyotypic consistency in human colorectal carcinoma cell lines established in vitro, Cancer Genet. Cytogenet. **6**:93–117.

Chow, D. A., and Greenberg, A. H., 1980, The generation of tumor heterogeneity *in vivo, Int. J. Cancer* **25:**261–265.

Cifone, M., and Fidler, I. J., 1981, Increasing metastatic potential is associated with increasing genetic instability of clones isolated from murine neoplasms, *Proc. Natl. Acad. Sci. USA* **78:**6949–6952.

Cillo, C., Mach, J.-P., Schreyer, M., and Carrel, S., 1984, Antigenic heterogeneity of clones and subclones from human melanoma cell lines demonstrated by a panel of monoclonal antibodies and flow microfluorimetry analysis, *Int. J. Cancer* **34:**11–20.

Clark, J. H., Watson, C. S., Markauerich, B. M., Syne, J. S., and Panko, W. B., 1983, Heterogeneity of estrogen binding sites in mammary tumors, *Breast Cancer Res. Treat.* **3:**61–65.

Cortes, E., Holland, J. F., and Glidewell, O., 1979, Adjuvant therapy of operable primary osteosarcoma-cancer and leukemia Group B experience, *Recent Results Cancer Res.* **68:**16–24.

Courtenay, V. D., and Mills, J., 1978, An *in vitro* colony assay for human tumors grown in immune-suppressed mice and treated *in vivo* with cytotoxic agents, *Br. J. Cancer* **37:**261–268.

Courtenay, V. D., Selby, P. J., Smith, I. E., Mills, J., and Peckham, M. J., 1978, Growth of human tumour cell colonies from biopsies using two soft agar techniques, *Br. J. Cancer* **38:**77–81.

Cowan, J. D., Von Hoff, D. D., Neuenfeldt, B., Mills, G. M., and Clark, G. M., 1984, Predictive value of trypan blue exclusion viability measurements for colony formation in a human tumor cloning assay, *Cancer Drug Delivery* **1:**95–100.

Cox, K. P., Kraus, M. R., Balis, M. E., and Dancis, J., 1976, Studies on cell communication with enucleated human fibroblasts, *J. Cell Biol.* **71:**693–703.

Crickard, K., Crickard, U., and Yoonessi, M., 1983, Human ovarian cells maintained on extracellular matrix versus plastic, *Cancer Res.* **43:**2762–2767.

Curt, G. A., Clendeninn, N. J., and Chabner, B. A., 1984, Drug resistance in cancer, *Cancer Treat. Rep.* **68:**87–99.

Daar, A. S., and Fabre, J. W., 1983, The membrane antigens of human colorectal cancer cells: Demonstration with monoclonal antibodies of heterogeneity within and between tumours and of anomalous expression of HLA-DR, *Eur. J. Cancer Clin. Oncol.* **19:**209–220.

Daley, M. J., 1981, Intratumoral maturational heterogeneity within the murine myeloma MOPC-315, *Cancer Res.* **41:**187–191.

Day, D. W., 1981, Histopathology of gastric cancer, *Adv. Biosci.* **32:**95–109.

De Baetselier, P., Gorelik, E., Eshar, Z., Ron, Y., Katzav, S., Feldman, M., and Segal, S., 1981, Metastatic properties conferred on nonmetastatic tumors by hybridization of spleen B-lymphocytes with plasmacytoma cells, *J. Natl. Cancer Inst.* **67:**1079–1087.

De Baetselier, P., Roos, E., Brys, L., Remels, L., Gobert, M., Dekegel, D., Segal, S., and Feldman, M., 1984, Nonmetastatic tumor cells acquire metastatic properties following somatic hybridization with normal cells, *Cancer Metastasis Rev.* **3**(1):5–24.

Dendy, P. P. (ed.), 1976, *Human Tumors in Short Term Culture*, Academic Press, New York.

Dethlefsen, L. A., Bauer, K. D., and Riley, R. M., 1980, Analytical cytometric approaches to heterogeneous cell populations in solid tumors: A review, *Cytometry* **1:**89–97.

Deuchar, E. M. (ed.), 1975, *Cellular Interactions in Animal Development*, Wiley, New York.

DeVita, V. T., 1983, The relationship between tumor mass and resistance to chemotherapy: Implications for surgical adjuvant treatment of cancer, *Cancer* **51:**1209–1220.

DeVita, V. T., Young, R. C., and Canellos, G. P., 1975, Combination versus single agent chemotherapy: A review of the basis for selection of drug treatment of cancer, *Cancer* **35:**98–110.

Dexter, D. L., 1984, Heterogeneity in human colon cancer, in: *Cancer Invasion and Metastasis: Biologic and Therapeutic Aspects* (G. L. Nicolson and L. Milas, eds.), Raven Press, New York, pp. 265–279.

Dexter, D. L., Barbosa, J. A., and Calabresi, P., 1979, N,N-dimethylformamide-induced alteration of cell culture characteristics and loss of tumorigenity in cultures of human colon carcinoma cells, *Cancer Res.* **39:**1020–1025.

Dexter, D. L., Spremulli, E. N., Fligiel, Z., Barbosa, J. A., Vogel, R., Van Voorhees, A., and Calabresi, P., 1981, Heterogeneity of cancer cells from a single human colon carcinoma, *Am. J. Med.* **71:**949–956.

Dolnick, B. J., and Bertino, J. R., 1982, Gene amplification in human tumor systems, in: *Tumor Cell Heterogeneity: Origins and Implications (Bristol-Meyers Cancer Symposia,*

Volume 4) (A. H. Owen, D. S. Coffey, and S. B. Baylin, eds.), Academic Press, New York, pp. 169–180.

Dulbecco, R., Henahan, M., Bowman, M., Okada, S., Battifora, H., and Unger, M., 1981, Generation of fibroblast-like cells from cloned epithelial mammary cells in vitro: A possible new cell type, Proc. Natl. Acad. Sci. USA 78:2345–2349.

Dunning, W. F., 1963, Prostate cancer in the rat, Natl. Cancer Inst. Monogr. 12:351–369.

Durie, B. G. M., Persky, B., Soehnlen, B. J., Grogan, T. M., and Salmon, S. E., 1982, Amyloid production in human myeloma stem-cell culture, with morphologic evidence of amyloid secretion by associated macrophages, N. Engl. J. Med. 307:1689–1692.

Durkin, W. J., Ghanta, V. K., Balch, C. M., Davis, D. W., and Hiramoto, R. N., 1979, A methodological approach to the prediction of anticancer drug effect in humans, Cancer Res. 39:402–407.

Dvorak, J. A., 1984, The natural heterogeneity of Trypanosoma cruzi: Biological and medical implications, J. Cell. Biochem. 24(4):357–371.

Editorial, 1982, Clonogenic assays for the chemotherapeutic sensitivity of human tumours, Lancet 1:780–781.

Ejeckam, G. C., Huang, S. N., McCaughey, W. T. E., and Gold, P., 1979, Immunohistopathological study on carcinoembryonic antigen (CEA)-like material and immunoglobulin A in gastric malignancies, Cancer 44:1606–1614.

Elmore, E., Kakunaga, T., and Barett, J. C., 1983, Comparison of spontaneous mutation rates of normal and chemically transformed human skin fibroblasts, Cancer Res. 43:1650–1655.

Erickson, E., Shealy, D. J., and Erickson, R. L., 1982, The relationship of epidermal growth factor-stimulated protein phosphorylation and protein kinase activity of RSV transforming genes product, in: Expression of Differentiated Functions in Cancer Cells (R. P. Revoltella, C. Basilico, R. C. Gallo, G. M. Pontieri, G. Rovera, and J. H. Subak-Sharpe, eds.), Raven Press, New York, pp. 417–422.

Evans, R. M., Laskin, J. D., and Hakala, M. T., 1981, Effect of excess folates and deoxyinosine on the activity and site of action of 5-fluorouracil, Cancer Res. 41:3288–3296.

Everson, L. K., Plocinick, B. A., and Rogentine, G. N., 1974, HL-A expression on the G1, S, and G2 cell-cycle stages of human lymphoid cells, J. Natl. Cancer Inst. 53:913–920.

Farram, E., and Nelson, D. S., 1980, Mouse mast cells as antitumor effector cells, Cell. Immunol. 55:294–301.

Farsund, T., and Hostmark, J., 1983, Mapping of cell cycle distribution in normal human urinary bladder epithelium, Scand. J. Urol. Nephrol. 17:51–56.

Feinberg, A. P., and Coffey, D. S., 1982, The concept of DNA rearrangement in carcinogenesis and development of tumor cell heterogeneity, in: Tumor Cell Heterogeneity: Origins and Implications (Bristol-Meyers Cancer Symposia, Volume 4) (A. H. Owens, D. S. Coffey, and S. B. Baylin, eds.), Academic Press, New York, pp. 469–494.

Feinberg, A. P., and Vogelstein, B., 1983, Hypomethylation distinguishes genes of some human cancers from their normal counterparts, Nature 301:89–92.

Fialkow, P. J., 1970, Genetic marker studies in neoplasia, in: Genetic Concepts and Neoplasia, Williams & Wilkins, Baltimore, pp. 112–130.

Fialkow, P. J., 1974, The origin and development of human tumors studied with cell markers, N. Engl. J. Med. 291:26–34.

Fialkow, P. J., 1979, Clonal origin of human tumors, Annu. Rev. Med. 30:135–143.

Fidler, I. J., and Berendt, M. J., 1982, The biological diversity of malignant neoplasms, in: Biological Responses in Cancer: Progress toward Potential Applications, Volume 1 (E. Mihich, ed.), Plenum Press, New York, pp. 269–299.

Fidler, I. J., and Hart, I. R., 1982, Biological diversity in metastatic neoplasms: Origins and implications, Science 217:998–1003.

Fidler, I. J., and Kleinerman, E. S., 1984, Lymphokine-activated human blood monocytes destroy tumor cells but not normal cells under cocultivation conditions, J. Clin. Oncol. 2(8):937–943.

Fidler, I. J., and Kripke, M. L., 1977, Metastasis results from preexisting variant cells within a malignant tumor, Science 197:893–895.

Fidler, I. J., and Poste, G., 1982a, The heterogeneity of metastatic properties in malignant tumor cells and regulation of the metastatic phenotype, in: *Tumor Cell Heterogeneity: Origins and Implications* (Bristol-Meyers Cancer Symposia, Volume 4) (A. H. Owens, D. S. Coffey, and S. B. Baylin, eds.), Academic Press, New York, pp. 127–145.

Fidler, I. J., and Poste, G., 1982b, Macrophage-mediated destruction of malignant tumor cells and new strategies for the therapy of metastatic disease, *Springer Semin. Immunopathol.* **5:**161–174.

Fidler, I. J., and Raz, A., 1981, The induction of tumoricidal capacities in mouse and rat macrophages by lymphokines, in: *Lymphokines*, Volume 3 (E. Pick, ed.), Academic Press, New York, pp. 345–363.

Fidler, I. J., and White, R. J. (eds.), 1980, *Design of Models for Testing Cancer Therapeutic Agents*, Van Nostrand–Reinhold, Princeton, N. J.

Fisher, B., 1984, Keynote address: The interdependence of laboratory and clinical research in the study of metastases, in: *Cancer Invasion and Metastasis: Biological and Therapeutic Aspects* (G. L. Nicolson and L. Milas, eds.), Raven Press, New York, pp. 27–46.

Fisher, E. R., Gregorio, R., Redmond, C., Vellios, F., Sommers, S. C., and Fisher, B., 1975, Pathologic findings from the National Surgical Adjuvant Breast Project (Protocol No. 4). I. Observations concerning the multicentricity of mammary cancer, *Cancer* **35:**247–254.

Foulds, L., 1954, Tumor progression: A review, *Cancer Res.* **14:**327–339.

Foulds, L., 1969, *Neoplastic Development*, Volume 1, Academic Press, New York.

Foulds, L., 1975, *Neoplastic Development*, Volume 2, Academic Press, New York.

Frank, J. P., and Williams, J. R., 1982, X-ray induction of persistent hypersensitivity to mutation, *Science* **216:**307–308.

Frankfurt, O., 1980, Flow cytometric analysis of double-stranded RNA content distribution, *J. Histochem. Cytochem.* **28:**663–669.

Frankfurt, O. S., 1983, Increased uptake of vital dye Hoechst 33342 during S phase in synchronized HeLa S3 cells, *Cytometry* **4:**216;–221.

Frankfurt, O. S., Slocum, H. K., Rustum, Y. M., Arbuck, S. G., Pavelic, Z. P., Petrelli, N., Huben, R. P., Pontes, E. J., and Greco, W. R., 1984a, Flow cytometric analysis of DNA aneuploidy in primary and metastatic human solid tumors, *Cytometry* **5:**71–80.

Frankfurt, O. S., Greco, W. R., Slocum, H. K., Arbuck, S. G., Gamarra, M., Pavelic, Z. P., and Rustum, Y. M., 1984b, Proliferative characteristics of primary and metastatic human solid tumors by DNA flow cytometry, *Cytometry* **5:**629–635.

Freedman, V. H., and Shin, S., 1974, Cellular tumorigenicity in nude mice: Correlation with cell growth in semi-solid medium, *Cell* **3:**355–359.

Frei, E., III, 1980, Models and the clinical dilemma, in: *Design of Models for Testing Cancer Therapeutic Agents* (I. J. Fidler and R. J. White, eds.), Van Nostrand–Rheinhold, Princeton, N. J., pp. 248–259.

Frei, E., III, and Canellos, G. P., 1980, Dose: A critical factor in cancer chemotherapy, *Am. J. Med.* **69:**585–594.

Frentz, G., and Moller, U., 1983, Clonal heterogeneity in curretted human epidermal cancers and precancers analysed by flow cytometry and compared with histology, *Br. J. Dermatol.* **109**(2):173–181.

Friedlander, M. C., Taylor, I. W., Russell, P., and Tattersall, M. H. N., 1984, Cellular DNA content—A stable feature in epithelial ovarian cancer, *Br. J. Cancer* **49:**173–179.

Friend, J. H., and Guralnik, D. B. (eds.), 1960, *Webster's New World Dictionary of the American Language*, Colleege ed., World Publishing Company, New York, p. 682.

Frost, P., and Kerbel, R. S., 1983, On a possible epigenetic mechanism(s) of tumor cell heterogeneity: The role of DNA methylation, *Cancer Metastasis Rev.* **2:**375–378.

Gazdar, A. F., Carney, D. N., and Minna, J. D., 1981a, *In vitro* study of the biology of small cell carcinoma of the lung, *Yale J. Biol. Med.* **54:**187–193.

Gazdar, A. F., Zweig, M. H., Carney, D. N., Van Steirteghen, A. C., Baylin, S. B., and Minna, J. D., 1981b, Levels of creatine kinase and its BB isoenzyme in lung cancer specimens and cultures, *Cancer Res.* **41:**2773–2777.

Geier, G. R., Schwarz, J. A., and Schlag, P., 1979, Cytologic uniformity of breast cancer from different locations: A pattern analysis study, *Exp. Cell Biol.* **47:**241–249.

Gilula, N. B., 1974, Junctions between cells, in: *Cell Communication* (R. P. Cox, ed.), Wiley–Interscience, New York, pp. 1–29.

Gioanni, J., and Lalanne, C. M., 1982, An improved method for preparing cell suspensions used for the cloning of human tumors, *Clin. Chem. Acta* **122**:289–291.

Gleason, D. F., 1977, Histologic grading and clinical staging of prostatic carcinoma, in: *Urologic Pathology: The Prostate* (M. Tannenbaum, ed.), Lea & Febiger, Philadelphia, pp. 171–197.

Gleason, D. F., Mellinger, G. T., and the Veterans Administration Cooperative Urological Research Group, 1974, Prediction of prognosis for prostatic adenocarcinoma by combined histological grading and clinical staging, *J. Urol.* **111**:58–64.

Goldenberg, D. M., and Pavia, R. A., 1981, Malignant potential of murine stromal cells after transplantation of human tumors into nude mice, *Science* **212**:65–67.

Goldenberg, D. M., Pavia, R. A., and Tsao, M. C., 1974, *In vivo* hybridisation of human tumour and normal hamster cells, *Nature* **250**:649–651.

Goldie, J. H., 1982, Drug resistance and chemotherapeutic strategy, in: *Tumor Cell Heterogeneity: Origins and Implications* (*Bristol-Meyers Cancer Symposia*, Volume 4) (A. H. Owens, D. S. Coffey, and S. B. Baylin, eds.), Academic Press, New York, pp. 115–125.

Goldie, J. H., 1983, Drug resistance and cancer chemotherapy strategy in breast cancer, *Breast Cancer Res. Treat.* **3**:129–136.

Goldie, J. H., and Coldman, A. J., 1979, A mathematic model for relating the drug sensitivity of tumors to their spontaneous mutation rate, *Cancer Treat. Rep.* **63**:1727–1733.

Goldie, J. H., and Coldman, A. J., 1983, Quantitative model for multiple levels of drug resistance in clinical tumors, *Cancer Treat. Rep.* **67**:923–931.

Goldie, J. H., and Coldman, A. J., 1984, The genetic origin of drug resistance in neoplasms: Implications for systemic therapy, *Cancer Res.* **44**:3643–3653.

Goodwin, G., Shaper, J. H., Abeloff, M. D., Mendelsohn, G., and Baylin, S. B., 1983, Analysis of cell surface proteins delineates a differentiation pathway linking endocrine and nonendocrine human lung cancers, *Proc. Natl. Acad. Sci. USA* **80**:3807–3811.

Greco, F. A., and Oldham, R. K., 1981, Clinical management of patients with small cell lung cancer, in: *Small Cell Lung Cancer* (F. A. Greco, R. K. Oldham, and P. A. Bunn, Jr., eds.), Grune & Stratton, New York, pp. 353–379.

Green, M. M., 1980, Transposable elements in Drosophila and other Diptera, *Annu. Rev. Genet.* **14**:109–120.

Griffen, J. E., Allman, D. R., Durrant, J. L., and Wilson, J. D., 1981, Variation in steroid 5 α-reductase activity in cloned human skin fibroblasts: Shift in phenotypic expression from high to low activity upon subcloning, *J. Biol. Chem.* **256**:3662–3666.

Grill, S. P., Wells, R. J., and Cheng, Y. C., 1984, Utilization of an immunostaining technique to demonstrate heterogeneity in the content of dihydrofolate reductase in peripheral blast cells from a patient with acute lymphocytic leukemia, *Cancer Res.* **44**:1252–1256.

Grossman, H. B., Wedemeyer, G., Ren, L., and Carey, T. E., 1984, UM-SCP-1, a new human cell line derived from a prostatic squamous cell carcinoma, *Cancer Res.* **44**:4111–4117.

Hager, J., Fligiel, S., Stanley, W., Richardson, A. M., and Heppner, G. H., 1981, Characterization of a variant producing tumor cell line from a heterogeneous strain BALB/cf C_3H mouse mammary tumor, *Cancer Res.* **41**:1293–1300.

Haigler, H. T., 1983, Epidermal growth factor: Cellular binding and consequences, in: *Growth and Maturation Factors*, Volume 1 (G. Guroff, ed.), Wiley, New York.

Hakala, M. T., 1973, Enzyme changes in resistant tissues, in: *Drug Resistance and Selectivity: Biochemical and Cellular Basis* (E. Mihich, ed.), Academic Press, New York, pp. 263–298.

Hall, T. C., 1971, Prediction of response in cancer therapy, *Natl. Cancer Inst. Monogr.* **34**.

Hall, T. C., 1974, Predictive tests in cancer, *Br. J. Cancer* **30**:191–198.

Hamburger, A. W., 1981, Use of *in vitro* tests in predictive cancer chemotherapy, *J. Natl. Cancer Inst.* **66**:981–988.

Hamburger, A. W., and Salmon, S. E., 1977, Primary bioassay of human tumor stem cells, *Science* **197**:461–463.

Hamburger, A. W., Salmon, S. E., Kim, M. B., Trent, J. M., Soehnlein, B. J., Alberts, D. C., and

Schmidt, H. J., 1978, Direct cloning of human ovarian carcinoma cells in agar, *Cancer Res.* **38**:3438–3444.

Hamburger, A. W., White, C. P., and Brown, R. W., 1981, Effect of epidermal growth factor on proliferation of human tumor cells in soft agar, *J. Natl. Cancer Inst.* **67**:825–830.

Hand, P. H., Nuti, M., Colcher, D., and Schlom, J., 1983, Definition of antigenic heterogeneity and modulation among human mammary carcinoma cell populations using monoclonal antibodies to tumor-associated antigens, *Cancer Res.* **43**:728–735.

Hanna, N., 1980, Expression of metastatic potential of tumor cells in young nude mice is correlated with low levels of natural killer cell-mediated cytotoxicity, *Int. J. Cancer* **26**:675–680.

Harland, R. N. L., Barnes, D. M., Howell, A., Ribeiro, G. G., Taylor, J., and Sellwood, R. A., 1983, Variation of receptor status in cancer of the breast, *Br. J. Cancer* **47**:511–515.

Hart, J. S., 1983, Chromosome abnormalities in human neoplasia, *Cancer Treat. Rev.* **10**:173–183.

Haskill, S., Kivinan, S., Nelson, K., and Fowler, W. C., Jr., 1983, Detection of intratumoral heterogeneity by simultaneous multiparameter flow cytometric analysis with enzyme and DNA markers, *Cancer Res.* **43**:1003–1009.

Hastings, R. J., and Franks, L. M., 1983, Cellular heterogeneity in a tissue culture cell line derived from a human bladder carcinoma, *Br. J. Cancer* **47**:233–244.

Hawkins, R. A., Hill, A., Freedman, B., Gore, S. M., Roberts, M. M., and Forrest, A. P. M., 1977, Reproducibility of measurements of oestrogen receptor concentration in breast cancer, *Br. J. Cancer* **36**:355–361.

Helms, S. R., Brazeal, F. I., Bueschen, A. J., and Pretlow, T. G., II, 1975, Separation of cells with histochemically demonstrable acid phosphatase activity from suspensions of human prostatic cells in an isokinetic gradient of Ficoll in tissue culture medium, *Am. J. Pathol.* **80**:79–90.

Hemstreet, G. P., III, Enoch, P. G., and Pretlow, T. G., II, 1980, Tissue disaggregation of human renal cell carcinoma with further isopycnic and isokinetic gradient purification, *Cancer Res.* **40**:1043–1049.

Henson, D. E., 1982, Heterogeneity in tumors, *Arch. Pathol. Lab. Med.* **106**:(12):597–598.

Heppner, G., 1982, Tumor subpopulation interactions, in: *Tumor Cell Heterogeneity: Origins and Implications* (*Bristol-Meyers Cancer Symposia*, Volume 4) (A. H. Owens, D. S. Coffey, and S. B. Baylin, eds.), Academic Press, New York, pp. 225–235.

Heppner, G. H., 1984, Tumor heterogeneity, *Cancer Res.* **44**:2259–2265.

Heppner, G. H., and Miller, B. E., 1983, Tumor heterogeneity: Biological implications and therapeutic consequences, *Cancer Metastasis Rev.* **2**:5–23.

Heppner, G. H., Miller, B. E., Cooper, D. N., and Miller, F. R., 1980, Growth interactions between mammary tumor cells, in: *Cell Biology of Breast Cancer* (C. M. McGrath, M. J. Brennan, and M. A. Rich, eds.), Academic Press, New York, pp. 161–172.

Heppner, G. H., Miller, B. E., and Miller, F. R., 1983, Tumor subpopulation interactions in neoplasms, *Biochim. Biophys. Acta* **695**:215–226.

Heppner, G. H., Loveless, S. E., Miller, F. R., Mahoney, K. H., and Fulton, A. M., 1984, Mammary tumor heterogeneity, in: *Cancer Invasion and Metastasis: Biologic and Therapeutic Aspects* (G. L. Nicolson and L. Milas, eds.), Raven Press, New York, pp. 209–221.

Hercend, T., Reinherz, E. L., Meuer, S., Schlossman, S. F., and Ritz, J., 1983, Phenotypic and functional heterogeneity of human cloned natural killer cell lines, *Nature* **301**:158–160.

Hirohashi, S., Ino, Y., Kodama, T., and Shimosato, Y., 1984, Distribution of blood group antigens A, B, H and I (Ma) in mucus-producing adenocarcinoma of human lung, *J. Natl. Cancer Inst.* **72**:1299–1305.

Hirsch, F. R., Ottesen, G., Podenphant, J., and Olsen, J., 1983, Tumor heterogeneity in lung cancer based on light microscopic features: A retrospective study of a consecutive series of 200 patients, treated surgically, *Virchows Arch. A* **402**:147–153.

Hockey, M. S., Stokes, H. J., Thompson, H., Woodhouse, C. S., Macdonald, F., Fielding, J. W. L., and Ford, C. H. J., 1984, Carcinoembryonic antigen (CEA) expression and heterogeneity in primary and autologous metastatic gastric tumors demonstrated by monoclonal antibody, *Br. J. Cancer* **49**:129–133.

Hoehn, W., Schroeder, F. H., Riemann, J. F., Joebsis, A. C., and Hermanek, P., 1980, Human prostatic adenocarcinoma: Some characteristics of a serially transplantable line in nude mice (PC82), *Prostate* **1**:95–104.

Hoffman, V., Berens, M., and Martz, G. (eds.), 1984, *Predictive Drug Testing on Human Tumor Cells*, Springer-Verlag, Berlin.

Hogstedt, B., and Mitelman, F., 1981, The interrelations of micronuclei, chromosomal instability, and mutational activity in acute non-lymphocytic leukemia—A hypothesis, *Hereditas* **95**:165–167.

Horoszewicz, J. S., Leong, S. S., Chu, T. M., Wajsman, Z. L., Friedman, M., Papsidero, L., Kim, U., Chai, L. S., Kakati, S., Arya, S. K., and Sandberg, A. A., 1980, The LNCaP cell line: A new model for studies on human prostatic carcinoma, in: *Models for Prostate Cancer* (G. P. Murphy, ed.), Liss, New York, pp. 115–132.

Houghton, P. J., and Houghton, J. A., 1983, Chemotherapeutic response in xenografts: Inter- and intratumor heterogeneity, in: *UCLA Symposium on Molecular and Cellular Biology Series*, Volume 4 (B. A. Chabner, ed.), Liss, New York, pp. 61–69.

Hu, F., and Pasztor, L. M., 1975, *In vivo* hybridization of cultured melanoma cells and isogeneic normal mouse cells, *Differentiation* **4**:92–97.

Hurwitz, C., and Tolmach, L. J., 1969, Time lapse cinemicrographic studies of X-irradiated Hela S3 cells. I. Cell progression and cell disintegration, *Biophys. J.* **9**:607–633.

Illmensee, K., 1978, Reversion of malignancy and normalized differentiation of teratocarcinoma cells in chimeric mice, *Basic Life Sci.* **12**:3–25.

Imada, M., and Sueoka, N., 1978, Clonal sublines of rat neurotumor RT4 and cell differentiation. I. Isolation and characterization of cell lines and cell type conversion, *Dev. Biol.* **66**:97–108.

Isaacs, J., 1982, Mechanisms for and implications of the development of heterogeneity of androgen sensitivity in prostatic cancer, in: *Tumor Cell Heterogeneity: Origins and Implications (Bristol-Meyers Cancer Symposia*, Volume 4) (A. H. Owens, D. S. Coffey, and S. B. Baylin, eds.), Academic Press, New York, pp.99–111.

Isaacs, J. T., Wake, N., Coffey, D. S., and Sandberg, A. A., 1982, Genetic instability coupled to clonal selection as a mechanism for tumor progression in the Dunning R-3327 rat prostatic adenocarcinoma system, *Cancer Res.* **42**:2353–2361.

Johnson, L. K., Baxter, J. D., Vlodavsky, I., and Gospodarowitz, D., 1980, Epidermal growth factor and expression of specific genes: Effects on cultured rat pituitary cells are dissociable from the mitogenic response, *Proc. Natl. Acad. Sci. USA* **77**:394–398.

Johnson, P. A., and Rossof, A. H., 1983, The role of the human tumor stem cell assay in medical oncology, *Arch. Intern. Med.* **143**:111–114.

Johnson, R. G., and Sheridan, J. D., 1971, Junctions between cancer cells in culture: Ultrastructure and permeability, *Science* **174**:717–719.

Kaighn, M. E., Narayan, K. S., Ohnuki, Y., Lechner, J. F., and Jones, L. W., 1979, Establishment and characterization of a human prostatic carcinoma line (PC-3), *Invest. Urol.* **17**:16–23.

Kallman, R. F., 1984, Automated autoradiographic analysis of tumor cell colonies *in vitro*, in: *Biological Dositometry: Cytometric Approaches to Mammalian Systems* (W. G. Eisert and M. L. Mendelsohn, eds.), Springer-Verlag, Berlin, pp. 255–263.

Karp, J. E., Burke, P. J., Saylor, P. L., and Humphrey, R. L., 1984, Correlation of proliferative and clonogenic tumor cells in multiple myeloma, *Cancer Res.* **44**:4197–4200.

Kaufmann, M., 1980, Clinical applications of *in vitro* chemosensitivity testing, *Adv. Biosci.* **26**:189–210.

Keng, P. C., Li, C. K. N., and Wheeler, K. T., 1981a, Characterization of the separation properties of the Beckman elutriator system, *Cell Biophys.* **3**:41–56.

Keng, P. C., Wheeler, K. T., Sieman, D. W., and Lord, E. M., 1981b, Direct synchronization of cells from solid tumors by centrifugal elutriation, *Exp. Cell Res.* **134**:15–22.

Kennedy, K. A., Teicher, B. A., Rockwell, S., and Sartorelli, A. C., 1981, Chemotherapeutic approaches to cell populations of tumors, in: *Bristol-Meyers Cancer Symposia*, Volume 2 (A. C. Sartorelli, J. S. Lazo, and J. R. Bertino, eds.), Academic Press, New York, pp. 85–101.

Kerbel, R. S., and Davies, A. J., 1982, Facilitation of tumour progression by cancer therapy, *Lancet* **2**:977–978.

Kerbel, R. S., Lagarde, A. E., Dennis, J. W., and Donaghue, T. P., 1983, Spontaneous fusion *in vivo* between normal host and tumor cells: Possible contribution to tumor progression and metastasis studied with a lectin-resistant mutant tumor, *Mol. Cell. Biol.* **3**:523–538.

Kern, D. H., Bertelsen, C. A., Mann, B. D., Campbell, M. A., Morton, D. L., and Cochran, A. J., 1983, Clinical application of the clonogenic assay, *Ann. Clin. Lab. Sci.* **13**:10–15.

Kiang, D. T., King, M., Zhang, H. J., Kennedy, B. J., and Wang, N., 1982, Cyclic biological expression in mouse mammary tumors, *Science* **216**:68–70.

King, W. J., and Greene, G. L., 1984, Monoclonal antibodies localize oestrogen receptor in the nuclei of target cells, *Nature* **307**:745–747.

Klebe, R. J., 1984, Rapid cloning of mammalian cells with honeycomb cloning plates and nonlethal vital stains, *In Vitro* **20**:127–132.

Kozlowski, J. M., Fidler, I. J., Campbell, D., Xu, Z.-L., Kaighn, M. E., and Hart, I. R., 1984, Metastatic behavior of human tumor cell lines grown in the nude mouse, *Cancer Res.* **44**:3522–3529.

Kramer, S. A., Farnham, R., Glenn, J. F., and Paulson, D. F., 1981, Comparative morphology of primary and secondary deposits of prostatic adenocarcinoma, *Cancer* **48**:271–273.

Kuo, M. T., Sen, S., Teeter, L., Cailleau, R. M., Kuesek, J. E., and Bowen, J., 1984, Expression of endogenous murine leukemia virus in transplantable tumor cells and DNA methylation of viral sequences, *Cancer Res.* **44**:3518–3521.

Kusyk, C., Edwards, C. L., Arrighi, F. E., and Romsdahl, M. M., 1979, Improved method for cytogenetic studies of solid tumors, *J. Natl. Cancer Inst.* **63**:1199–1203.

Lagarde, A. E., Donaghue, T. P., Dennis, J. W., and Kerbel, R. S., 1983, Genotypic and phenotypic evolution of a murine tumor during its progression *in vivo* toward metastasis, *J. Natl. Cancer Inst.* **71**:183–191.

Lala, P. K., Santer, V., and Rahil, K. S., 1980, Spontaneous fusion between Ehrlich ascites tumor cells and host cells *in vivo*: Kinetics of hybridization and concurrent changes in the histocompatibility profile of the tumor after propagation in different host strains, *Eur. J. Cancer Clin. Oncol.* **16**:487–510.

Lalande, M. E., Ling, V., and Miller, R. G., 1981, Hoechst 33342 dye uptake as a probe of membrane permeability changes in mammalian cells, *Proc. Natl. Acad. Sci. USA* **78**:363–367.

Larizza, L., and Schirrmacher, V., 1984, Somatic cell fusion as a source of genetic rearrangement leading to metastatic variants, *Cancer Metastasis Rev.* **3**(3):193–222.

Larner, E. H., and Rutherford, C. L., 1982, Implementation of micromethods to resolve problems of human breast tumor heterogeneity in analysis of cyclic 3':5'-nucleotide phosphodiesterase, *Cancer Res.* **42**:1661–1668.

Lasfargues, E. Y., 1973, Human mammary tumors, in: *Tissue Culture: Methods and Applications* (P. F. Kruse, Jr., and M. K. Patterson, eds.), Academic Press, New York, pp. 45–49.

Leibovitz, A., 1975, Development of media for isolation and cultivation of human cancer cells, in: *Human Tumor Cells in Vitro* (J. Fogh, ed.), Plenum Press, New York, pp. 23–44.

Leibovitz, A., Liu, R., Hayes, C., and Salmon, S. E., 1983, A hypoosmotic medium to disaggregate tumor cell clumps into viable and clonogenic single cells for the human tumor stem cell clonogenic assay, *Int. J. Cell Cloning* **1**(6):478–485.

Leith, J. T., Brenner, H. J., DeWyngaert, J. K., Dexter, D. L., Calabresi, P., and Glicksman, A. S., 1981, Selective modification of the X-ray response of two mouse mammary adenocarcinoma sublines by N,N-dimethylformamide, *Int. J. Radiat. Oncol. Biol. Phys.* **7**:943–947.

Leith, J. T., Bliven, S. F., Lee, E. S., Glicksman, A. S., and Dexter, D. L., 1984, Intrinsic and extrinsic heterogeneity in the responses of parent and clonal human colon carcinoma xenografts to photon irradiation, *Cancer Res.* **44**:3757–3762.

Levine, A. E., Hamilton, D. A., Yeoman, L. C., Busch, H., and Brattain, M. G., 1984, Identification of a tumor inhibitory factor in rat ascites fluid, *Biochem. Biophys. Res. Commun.* **119**:76–82.

Lewis, R. A., and Austen, K. F., 1981, Mediation of local homeostasis and inflammation by leukotrienes and other mast cell-dependent compounds, *Nature* **293**:103–108.

Lieber, M. M., and Kovach, J. S., 1982, Soft agar colony formation assay for chemotherapy sensitivity testing of human solid tumors, *Mayo Clin. Proc.* **57**:527–528.

Linder, D., and Gartler, S. M., 1965, Glucose-6-phosphate dehydrogenase mosaicism: Utilization as a cell marker in the study of leiomyomas, *Science* **150**:67–69.

Ling, V., Gerlach, J., and Kartner, 1984, Multidrug resistance, *Breast Cancer Res. Treat.* **4**:89–94.

Lippman, S. M., Mendelsohn, G., Trump, D. L., Wells, S. A., and Baylin, S. B., 1982, The prognostic and biological significance of cellular heterogeneity in medullary thyroid carcinoma: A study of calcitonin, L-dopa decarboxylase, and histaminase, *J. Clin. Endocrinol. Metab.* **5**:233–240.

Livingston, R. B., 1978, Treatment of small cell carcinoma: Evolution and future directions, *Semin. Oncol.* **5**:299–308.

Loewenstein, W. R., 1979, Junctional intercellular communication and the control of growth, *Biochim. Biophys. Acta* **560**:1–65.

Loveless, S. E., and Heppner, G. H., 1983, Tumor associated macrophages of mouse mammary tumors. I. Differential cytotoxicity of macrophages from metastatic and non-metastatic tumors, *J. Immunol.* **131**:2074–2078.

Lowe, F. C., and Isaacs, J. T., 1984, Biochemical methods for predicting metastatic ability of prostatic cancer utilizing the Dunning R-3327 rat prostatic adenocarcinoma system, *Cancer Res.* **44**:744–752.

McCulloch, E. A., Buick, R. N., and Till, J. E., 1978, Cellular differentiation in the myeloblastic leukemias of man, in: *Cell Differentiation and Neoplasia* (G. F. Saunders, ed.), Raven Press, New York, pp. 211–221.

McDowell, E. M., Sorokin, S. P., Hoyt, R. F., and Trump, B. F., 1981, An unusual bronchial carcinoid tumor: Light and electron microscopy, *Hum. Pathol.* **12**:338–348.

Mackillop, W. J., Stewart, S. S., and Buick, R. N., 1982, Density/volume analysis in the study of cellular heterogeneity in human ovarian carcinoma, *Br. J. Cancer* **45**:812–820.

Mackillop, W. J., Ciampi, A., Till, J. E., and Buick, R. N., 1983, A stem cell model of humam tumor growth: Implications for tumor cell clonogenic assays, *J. Natl. Cancer Inst.* **70**:-9–16.

Macpherson, I. A., 1973, Soft agar techniques, in: *Tissue Culture Methods and Applications* (P. F. Kruse and M. K. Patterson, Jr., eds.), Academic Press, New York, pp. 267–273.

Madajewicz, S., Petrelli, N., Rustum, Y. M., Campbell, J., Herrera, L., Mittelman, A., Perry, A., and Creaven, P. J., 1984, Phase I-II trial of high-dose calcium leucovorin and 5-fluorouracil in advanced colorectal cancer, *Cancer Res.* **44**:4667–4669.

Maeda, M., and Ichikawa, Y., 1980, Production of a colony-stimulating factor following differentiation of leukemic myeloblasts to macrophages, *J. Cell. Physiol.* **102**:323–331.

Makino, S., 1957, The chromosome cytology of the ascites tumors of rats, with special reference to the concept of the stemline cell, *Int. Rev. Cytol.* **6**:25–84.

Marangos, P. J., Gazdar, A. F., and Carney, D. N., 1982, Neuron-specific enolase in human small cell carcinoma cultures, *Cancer Lett.* **15**:67–71.

Markert, C. L., 1982, Cell differentiation in neoplasia, in: *Tumor Cell Heterogeneity: Origins and Implications* (*Bristol-Meyers Cancer Symposia*, Volume 4) (A. H. Owens, D. S. Coffey, and S. B. Baylin, eds.), Academic Press, New York, pp. 237–247.

Markert, C. L., 1984, Genetic control of cell interaction in chimeras, *Dev. Genet.* **4**(4):267–280.

Markus, G., 1983, Plasminogen activators in malignant growth, in: *Progress in Fibrinolysis, Volume 6* (J. F. Davidson, ed.), Churchill–Livingstone, Edinburgh, pp. 587–604.

Markus, G., 1984, The role of hemostasis and fibrinolysis in the metastatic spread of cancer, *Semin. Thromb. Hemost.* **10**(1):61–70.

Markus, G., Camiolo, S. M., Kohga, S., Madeja, J. M., and Mittelman, A., 1983, Plasminogen activator secretion of human tumors in short term organ culture, including a comparison of primary and metastatic colon tumors, *Cancer Res.* **43**:5517–5525.

Marshall, M. J., Shone, D. G., Windle, J. M., and Worsfold, M., 1982, Spontaneous fusion of malignant and host mouse cells in culture detected by phosphoglucose isomerase (PGI) isoenzymes, *Br. J. Cancer* **46**:811–816.

Martin, D. S., 1958, Discussion of experimental drugs in combination chemotherapy, *Ann. N. Y. Acad. Sci.* **76**:926–929.

Martin, D. S., Stolfi, R. L., Sawyer, R. C., Spiegelman, S., Casper, E. S., and Young, C. W., 1983a, Therapeutic utility of utilizing low doses of N-(phosphonacetyl)-L-aspartic acid in combination with 5-fluorouracil: A murine study with clinical relevance, *Cancer Res.* **43**:2317–2321.

Martin, D. S., Stolfi, R. L., Sawyer, R. C., Spiegelman, S., and Young, C. W., 1983b, Improved therapeutic index with sequential N-phosphonacetyl-L-aspartate plus high-dose methotrexate plus high-dose 5-fluorouracil and appropriate rescue, Cancer Res. **43**:4653–4661.

Martin, D. S., Stolfi, R. L., Sawyer, R. C., and Young, C. W., 1985, The application of biochemical modulation with a therapeutically inactive modulating agent in clinical trials of cancer, Cancer Treat. Rep. **69**:421–423.

Mattern, J., and Volm, M., 1982, Clinical relevance of predictive tests for cancer chemotherapy, Cancer Treat. Rev. **9**:267–298.

Matthews, M. J., 1979, Effects of therapy on the morphology and behavior of small cell carcinoma of the lung—A clinicopathologic study, Prog. Cancer Res. Ther. **11**:155–165.

Melamed, M. R., Darzynkiewicz, Z., Trazonos, F., and Sharpless, T., 1977, Cytology automation by flow cytometry, Cancer Res. **37**:2806–2812.

Mendelsohn, G., Eggleston, J. C., Weisburger, W. R., Gann, D. S., and Baylin, S. B., 1978, Calcitonin and histaminase in C cell hyperplasia and medullary thyroid carcinoma: A light microscopic and immunohistochemical study, Am. J. Pathol. **92**:35–52.

Meyer, J. S., McDivitt, R. W., Stone, K. R., Prey, M. U., and Bauer, W. C., 1984, Practical breast carcinoma cell kinetics: Review and update, Breast Cancer Res. Treat. **4**:79–88.

Meyskens, F. L., Thomson, S. P., and Moon, T. E., 1984, Quantitation of the number of cells within tumor colonies in semisolid media and their growth as oblate spheroids, Cancer Res. **44**:271–277.

Mihich, E. (ed.), 1973, Drug Resistance and Selectivity: Biochemical and Cellular Basis, Academic Press, New York.

Milas, L., 1984, Tumor metastasis: Achievements, dilemmas and future, a summary of the conference, in: Cancer Invasion Metastasis: Biologic and Therapeutic Aspects (G. L. Nicolson and L. Milas, eds.), Raven Press, New York, pp. 457–467.

Miller, B. E., Miller, F. R., Leith, J., and Heppner, G. H., 1980, Growth interaction in vivo between tumor subpopulations derived from a single mouse mammary tumor, Cancer Res. **40**:3977–3981.

Miller, B. E., Miller, F. R., and Heppner, G. H., 1981, Interactions between tumor subpopulations affecting their sensitivity to the antineoplastic agents cyclophosphamide and methotrexate, Cancer Res. **41**:4378–4381.

Miller, B. E., Miller, F. R., and Heppner, G. H., 1983, Development of a drug-sensitivity assay for heterogeneous tumors based on growth in 3-dimensional collagen gels, in: UCLA Symposium on Molecular and Cellular Biology Series, Volume 4 (B. A. Chabner, ed.), Liss, New York, pp. 107–118.

Miller, F. R., 1983, Tumor subpopulation interactions in metastasis, Invasion Metastasis **3**:234–242.

Milstein, C., Frangione, B., and Pink, J. R. L., 1967, Studies on the variability of immunoglobulin sequence, Cold Spring Harbor Symp. Quant. Biol. **32**:31–36.

Miner, K. M., and Nicolson, G. L., 1983, Differences in the sensitivities of murine metastatic lymphoma/lymphosarcoma variants to macrophage-mediated cytolysis and/or cytostasis, Cancer Res. **43**:2063–2071.

Miner, K. M., Kawaguchi, T., Uba, G. W., and Nicolson, G. L., 1982, Clonal drift of cell surface, melanogenic, and experimental metastatic properties of in vivo-selected, brain meninges-colonizing murine B16 melanoma, Cancer Res. **42**:4631–4638.

Miner, K. M., Klostergaard, J., Granger, G. A., and Nicolson, G. L., 1983, Differences in the cytotoxic effects of activated murine peritoneal macrophages and J774 monocytic cells on metastatic variants of B16 melanoma, J. Natl. Cancer Inst. **70**:717–724.

Minna, J. D., Gazdar, A. F., Carney, D. N., Radice, P. A., and Simms, E., 1980, In vitro and in vivo models for the study of small cell carcinoma of the lung, in: Design of Models for Testing Cancer Therapeutic Agents (I. J. Fidler and R. J. White, eds.), Van Nostrand–Reinhold, Princeton, N. J., pp. 148–157.

Minna, J. D., Carney, D. N., Alvarez, R., Bunn, P. A., Jr., Cuttitta, F., Ihde, D. C., Matthews, M. J., Oie, H., Rosen, S., Whang-Peng, J., and Gazdar, A. F., 1982, Heterogeneity and homogeneity of human small cell lung cancer, in: Tumor Cell Heterogeneity: Origins and Implications (Bristol-Meyers Cancer Symposia, Volume 4) (A. H. Owens, D. S. Coffey, and S. B. Baylin, eds.), Academic Press, New York, pp. 29–52.

Mintz, B., and Illmensee, K., 1975, Normal genetically mosaic mice produced from malignant teratocarcinoma cells, Proc. Natl. Acad. Sci. USA 72:3585–3589.

Molenaar, W. M., van den Berg, M., Halie, M. R., and Poppema, S., 1983, The heterogeneity of follicular center cell lymphomas. I. Cytohistologic, immunologic, and enzymehistochemical aspects, Cancer 52:2269–2276.

Moody, T. W., Pert, C. B., Gazdar, A. F., Carney, D. N., and Minna, J. D., 1981, High levels of intracellular bombesin characterize human small-cell lung carcinoma, Science 214:1246–1248.

Moon, J. E., Salmon, S. E., White, C. S., Chen, H.-S. G., Meyskens, F. L., Durie, B. G. M., and Alberts, D. S., 1981, Quantitative association between the in vitro human tumor stem cell assay and clinical response to cancer chemotherapy, Cancer Chemother. Pharmacol. 6:211–218.

Moore, M. A. S., 1984, Proliferation and differentiation control mechanisms in myeloid leukemia, in: Biological Responses in Cancer: Progress toward Potential Applications, Volume 2 (E. Mihich, ed.), Plenum Press, New York, pp. 94–119.

Morasca, L., 1979, In vitro testing for tumor sensitivity to anticancer agents, in: Chemotherapy of Solid Tumors (F. Pannuti and P. J. Creaven, eds.), Casa Editrice Patron, Bologna, pp. 63–68.

Natali, P. G., Giacomini, P., Bigotti, A., Imai, K., Nicotra, M. R., Ng, A. K., and Ferrone, S., 1983a, Heterogeneity in the expression of HLA and tumor-associated antigens by surgically removed and cultured breast carcinoma cells, Cancer Res. 43:660–668.

Natali, P. G., Viora, M., Nicotra, M. R., Giacomini, P., Bigotti, A., and Ferrone, S., 1983b, Antigenic heterogeneity of skin tumors of nonmelanocyte origin: Analysis with monoclonal antibodies to tumor-associated antigens and to histocompatibility antigens, J. Natl. Cancer Inst. 71:439–447.

Nelson, K. G., Siegfried, J. M., Siegal, G. P., Becker, R., Walton, L. A., and Kaufman, D. G., 1984, The heterogeneity of LDH isozyme patterns of human uterine sarcomas and cultured sarcoma cell lines, Am. J. Pathol. 116:85–93.

Neri, A., Welch, D., Kawaguchi, T., and Nicolson, G. L., 1982, The development and biologic properties of malignant cell sublines and clones of a spontaneously metastasizing rat mammary adenocarcinoma, J. Natl. Cancer Inst. 68:507–517.

Nervi, C., Badaracco, G., Maisto, A., Mauro, F., Tirindella-Danesi, D., and Starace, G., 1982, Cytometric evidence of cytogenetic and proliferative heterogeneity of human solid tumors, Cytometry 2:303–308.

Neugut, A. I., and Weinstein, I. B., 1979, The use of agarose in the determination of anchorage independent growth, In Vitro 15:351–356.

Nicolson, G. L., 1984a, Tumor progression, oncogenes and the evolution of metastatic phenotypic diversity, Clin. Exp. Metastasis 2(2):85–106.

Nicolson, G. L., 1984b, Generation of phenotypic diversity and progression in metastatic tumor cells, Cancer Metastasis Rev. 3(1):25–42.

Nicolson, G. L., and Custead, S. E., 1982, Tumor metastasis is not due to adaptation of cells to a new organ environment, Science 215:176–178.

Nicolson, G. L., and Milas, L. (eds.), 1984, Cancer Invasion and Metastasis: Biologic and Therapeutic Aspects, Raven Press, New York.

Nicolson, G. L., Steck, P. A., Welch, D. R., and Lembo, T., 1983, Heterogeneity and instability of phenotypic and metastatic properties of local tumor- and metastasis-derived clones of a mammary adenocarcinoma, in: Understanding Breast Cancer: Clinical and Laboratory Concepts (M. Rich, J. Hager, and P. Furmanski, eds.), Dekker, New York, pp. 145–166.

Niell, H. B., Neely, C. L., Wood, C. A., Soloway, M. S., Maxwell, T. A., Buxton, B. H., Dilawari, R. A., and Kim, W. S., 1983, Use of tumor colony assay in clinical oncology, South. Med. J. 76:1376–1379.

Nowell, P. C., 1976, The clonal evolution of cell populations, Science 194:23–28.

Nowell, P. C., 1982, Genetic instability in cancer cells: Relationship to tumor cell heterogeneity, in: Tumor Cell Heterogeneity: Origins and Implications (Bristol-Meyers Cancer Symposia, Volume 4) (A. H. Owens, D. S. Coffey, and S. B. Baylin, eds.), Academic Press, New York, pp. 351–365.

Nowell, P. C., 1983, Tumor progression and clonal evolution: The role of genetic instability, in: *Chromosome Mutation and Neoplasia* (J. German, ed.), Liss, New York, pp. 413–432.

Nowell, P. C., and Hungerford, D. A., 1960, A minute chromosome in human chronic granulocytic leukemia, *Science* **132**:1497.

Ochi, H., Wake, N., Rao, U., Takeuchi, J., Slocum, H. K., Rustum, Y. M., Karakousis, C., and Sandberg, A. A., 1984, Serial cytogenetic analysis of a recurrent malignant melanoma, *Cancer Genet. Cytogenet.* **11**:175–183.

Ohno, S., 1971, Genetic implication of karyological instability of malignant somatic cells, *Physiol. Rev.* **51**:496–526.

Okabe, T., Suzuki, A., Hirono, M., Tamaoki, N., Oshimura, M., and Takaku, F., 1983, Establishment of different clonal strains from a human sarcoma of the stomach: Tumorigenic heterogeneity in athymic nude mice, *Cancer Res.* **43**:5456–5461.

Okamura, S., Chechik, B. E., Lee, C., Gelfand, E. W., and Mak, T. W., 1981, Heterogeneity of human thymocytes and a malignant T-lymphoblast cell line, MOLT-3, *Cancer Res.* **41**:1664–1668.

Oksala, T., and Therman, E., 1974, Mitotic abnormalities and cancer, in: *Chromosomes and Cancer* (J. German, ed.), Wiley, New York, pp. 239–263.

Osieka, R., Seeber, S., and Schmidt, C. G., 1984, Predictive tests in cancer chemotherapy: A reappraisal, *Klin. Wochenschr.* **62**:203–212.

Owens, A. H., Coffey, D. S., and Baylin, S. B. (eds.), 1982, *Tumor Cell Heterogeneity: Origins and Implications* (Bristol-Meyers Cancer Symposia, Volume 4) Academic Press, New York.

Papaioannou, V. E., McBurney, M. W., Gardner, R. L., and Evans, R. L., 1975, Fate of teratocarcinoma cells injected into early mouse embryos, *Nature* **258**:70–73.

Papaioannou, V. E., Evans, E. P., Gardner, R. L., and Graham, C. F., 1979, Growth and differentiation of an embryonal carcinoma cell line (C145b), *J. Embryol. Exp. Morphol.* **54**:277–295.

Parbhoo, S. P., 1981, Heterogeneity in human mammary cancer, in: *New Aspects of Breast Cancer*, Volume 4 (B. A. Stoll, ed.), Heinemann, London, pp. 55–77.

Pavelic, Z. P., Nowak, N. J., Slocum, H. K., and Rustum, Y. M., 1983, Correlation of tumor-cell growth in four semisolid systems, *J. Cancer Res. Clin. Oncol.* **105**:94–97.

Pavlik, E. J., Kenady, D. E., Van Nagell, J. R., Keaton, K., Donaldson, E. S., Hanson, M. B., and Flanigan, R. C., 1983, The proliferation of human tumor cell lines in the presence of different agars, agaroses, and methyl cellulose, *In Vitro* **19**:538–550.

Pearse, A. G. E., 1969, The cytochemistry and ultrastructure of polypeptide hormone-producing cells of the APUD series and the embryologic, physiologic, and pathologic implications of the concept, *J. Histochem. Cytochem.* **17**:303–313.

Perez, D. J., Taylor, I. W., Milthorpe, B. K., McGovern, V. J., and Tattersall, M. H. N., 1981, Identification and quantitation of tumor cells in cell suspensions: A comparison of cytology and flow cytometry, *Br. J. Cancer* **43**:526–531.

Perloff, M., Holland, J. F., and Frei, E., III, 1982, Adjuvant chemotherapy, in: *Cancer Medicine*, 2nd ed. (J. F. Holland and E. Frei, III, eds.), Lea & Febiger, Philadelphia, pp. 515–526.

Pertoff, H., Robin, K., and Kjellen, L., 1977, The viability of cells grown or centrifuged in a new density gradient medium Percoll (TM), *Exp. Cell Res.* **110**:449–457.

Pertschuk, L. P., Tobin, E. H., Brigat, D. J., Kim, D. S., Bloom, N. D., Gaetjens, E., Berman, P. J., Carter, A. C., and Degenshein, G. A., 1978, Immunofluorescent detection of estrogen receptors in breast cancer, *Cancer* **41**:907–911.

Petersen, S. E., Lorentzen, M., and Bichel, P., 1981, A mosaic subpopulation structure of human colorectal carcinomas demonstrated by flow cytometry, *Acta Pathol. Microbiol. Scand. Suppl.* **274**:412–416.

Peterson, J. A., Ceriani, R. L., Blank, E. W., and Osvaldo, L., 1983, Comparison of rates of phenotypic variability in surface antigen expression in normal and cancerous human breast epithelial cells, *Cancer Res.* **43**:4291–4296.

Petricciani, J. C., 1980, On the origin of human tumors, *In Vitro* **16**:361–364.

Pierce, G. B., 1974, Cellular heterogeneity of cancers, in: *Chemical Carcinogenesis*, Part B (P. O. P. Ts'o and J. A. DiPaolo, eds.), Dekker, New York, pp. 463–472.

Pierce, G. B., and Dixon, F. J., Jr., 1959, Testicular teratomas. I. Demonstration of teratogenesis by metamorphosis of multipotential cells, *Cancer* **12**:573–583.

Pierce, G. B., and Wallace, C., 1971, Differentiation of malignant to benign cells, *Cancer Res.* **31**:127–134.

Pierce, G. G., and Wells, R. S., 1982, Embryologic microenvironment in the regulation of cancer cells, in: *Tumor Cell Heterogeneity: Origins and Implications (Bristol-Meyers Cancer Symposia,* Volume 4) (A. H. Owens, D. S. Coffey, and S. B. Baylin, eds.), Academic Press, New York, pp. 249–258.

Pierce, G. B., Lewis, S. H., Miller, G. J., Moritz, E., and Miller, P., 1979, Tumorigenicity of embryonal carcinoma as an assay to study control of malignancy by the murine blastocyst, *Proc. Natl. Acad. Sci. USA* **76**:6649–6651.

Pizzolo, G., Semenzato, G., Chilosi, M., Morittu, L., Ambrosetti, A., Warner, N., Bofill, M., and Janossy, G., 1984, Distribution and heterogeneity of cells detected by HNK-1 monoclonal antibody in blood and tissues in normal, reactive, and neoplastic conditions, *Clin. Exp. Immunol.* **57**:195–206.

Pollister, A. W., and Ris, H., 1947, Nucleoprotein determinations in cytological preparations, *Cold Spring Harbor Symp. Quant. Biol.* **12**:147–157.

Poste, G., 1984, *Oncology Overview: Selected Abstracts on Tumor Heterogeneity,* National Cancer Institute, International Research Data Bank Program, Bethesda.

Poste, G., and Fidler, I. J., 1980, Therapeutic application of macrophage-mediated destruction of tumor cells: An approach to cancer therapy that addresses the problem of tumor cell heterogeneity, in: *Design of Models for Testing Cancer Therapeutic Agents* (I. J. Fidler and R. J. White, eds.), Van Nostrand–Reinhold, Princeton, N. J., pp. 225–238.

Poste, G., and Greig, R., 1982, On the genesis and regulation of cellular heterogeneity in malignant tumors, *Invasion Metastasis* **2**:137–176.

Poste, G., Doll, J., and Fidler, I. J., 1981, Interactions among clonal subpopulations affect stability of the metastatic phenotype in polyclonal populations of B16 melanoma cells, *Proc. Natl. Acad. Sci. USA* **78**:6226–6230.

Poste, G., Doll, J., Brown, A. E., Tzeng, J., and Zeidman, I., 1982, A comparison of the metastatic properties of B16 melanoma clones isolated from cultured cell lines, subcutaneous tumors, and individual lung metastases, *Cancer Res.* **42**:2770–2778.

Poste, G., Greig, R., Tzeng, J., Koestler, T., and Corwin, S., 1984, Interactions between tumor cell subpopulations in malignant tumors, in: *Cancer Invasion and Metastasis: Biologic and Therapeutic Aspects* (G. L. Nicolson and L. Milas, eds.), Raven Press, New York, pp. 224–243.

Prehn, R. T., 1982, Antigenic heterogeneity: A possible basis for progression, in: *Tumor Cell Heterogeneity: Origins and Implications (Bristol-Meyers Cancer Symposia,* Volume 4) (A. H. Owens, D. S. Coffey, and S. B. Baylin, eds.), Academic Press, New York, pp. 73–80.

Preisler, H. D., 1980, Prediction of response to chemotherapy in acute myelocytic leukemia, *Blood* **56**:361–367.

Preisler, H. D., Rustum, Y. M., and Priore, R. L., 1985, Relationship between leukemic cell retention of cytosine arabinoside triphosphate and the duration of remission in patients with acute nonlymphocytic leukemia, *Eur. J. Cancer Clin. Oncol.* **21**:23–30.

Pretlow, T. G., and Pretlow, T. P. (eds.), 1984, *Cell Separation,* Volume 3, Academic Press, New York.

Pretlow, T. G., II, Weir, E. E., and Zettergren, J. G., 1975, Problems connected with the separation of different kinds of cells, *Int. Rev. Exp. Pathol.* **14**:91–204.

Pretlow, T. G., Jones, C. M., and Pretlow, T. P., 1976, Separation of tumor cells by density gradient centrifugation: Recent work with human tumors and a discussion of the kind of quantitation needed in cell separation experiments, *Biophys. Chem.* **5**:99–106.

Pretlow, T. P., Boohaker, E. A., Pitts, A. M., Macfadyin, A. J., Bradley, E. L., Jr., and Pretlow, T. G., II, 1984, Heterogeneity and subcompartmentalization in the distribution of eosinophils in human colonic carcinoma, *Am. J. Pathol.* **116**(2):207–213.

Prockop, D. J., 1984, Osteogenesis imperfecta, phenotypic heterogeneity, protein suicide, short and long collagen, *Am. J. Hum. Genet.* **36**:(3):499–505.

Ranadive, K. J., and Bhide, S. V., 1962, Tissue interactions between normal and malignant cells, in: *Biological Interactions in Normal and Neoplastic Growth* (M. J. Brennan and W. L. Simpson, eds.), Little, Brown, Boston, pp. 337–354.

Raza, A., and Preisler, H. D., 1984, Use of BrdU and ^{3}H-TdR for the double-labeling of human leukemic cells, *BioTechniques* **2**(4):262–266.

Raza, A., Preisler, H. D., Mayers, G. L., and Bankert, R., 1984, Rapid enumeration of S-phase cells by means of monoclonal antibodies, *N. Engl. J. Med.* **310**:991.

Reddy, A. L., and Fialkow, P. J., 1979, Multicellular origin of fibrosarcomas in mice induced by the chemical carcinogen 3-methylcholanthrene, *J. Exp. Med.* **150**:878–887.

Reinhold, H. S., 1965, A cell dispension technique for use in quantitative transplantation studies with solid tumours, *Eur. J. Cancer* **1**:67–71.

Rheinwald, J. G., and Beckett, M. A., 1980, Defective terminal differentiation in culture as a consistent and selectable character of malignant human keratinocytes, *Cell* **22**:629–632.

Rigby, P. W. J., 1982, The oncogenic circle closes, *Nature* **297**:451–453.

Rogan, A. M., Hamilton, T. C., Young, R. C., Klecker, R. W., Jr., and Ozols, R. F., 1984, Reversal of adriamycin resistance by verapamil in human ovarian cancer, *Science* **224**:994–996.

Rognum, T. O., Brandtzaeg, P., and Thorud, E., 1983, Is heterogeneous expression of HLA-dr antigens and CEA along with DNA-profile variations evidence of phenotypic instability and clonal proliferation in human large bowel carcinomas?, *Br. J. Cancer* **48**:543–551.

Roper, P. R., and Drewinko, B., 1976, Comparison of *in vitro* methods to determine drug-induced cell lethality, *Cancer Res.* **36**:2182–2188.

Rosen, S. T., Mulshine, J. L., Cuttitta, F., Fedorko, J., Carney, D. N., Gazdar, A. F., and Minna, J. D., 1984, Analysis of human small cell lung cancer differentiation antigens using a panel of rat monoclonal antibodies, *Cancer Res.* **44**:2052–2061.

Rosenblum, M. L., Dougherty, D. V., Deen, D. F., and Wilson, C. B., 1981, Potentials and limitations of a clonogenic cell assay for human brain tumors, *Cancer Treat. Rep.* **65**(Suppl. 2):61–66.

Rowley, J. D., 1973, A new consistent chromosomal abnormality in chronic myelogenous leukemia identified by quinacrin fluorescence and Giemsa staining, *Nature* **243**:290–293.

Rubin, H., and Chu, B. M., 1982, Self-normalization of highly transformed 3T3 cells through maximized contact interaction, *Proc. Natl. Acad. Sci. USA* **79**:1903–1907.

Rubin, H., and Chu, B. M., 1984, Solute concentration effects on the expression of cellular heterogeneity of anchorage-independent growth among spontaneously transformed BALB/c 3T3 cells, *In Vitro* **20**:585–596.

Rupniak, H. T., and Hill, B. T., 1980, The poor cloning ability in agar of human tumour cells from biopsies of primary tumors, *Cell Biol. Int. Rep.* **4**:479–486.

Rustum, Y. M., and Preisler, H. D., 1979, Correlation between leukemic cell retention of 1-beta-D-arabinofuranosylcytosine-5′-triphosphate and response to therapy, *Cancer Res.* **39**:42–49.

Sachs, L., 1980, Constitutive uncoupling of pathways of gene expression that control growth and differentiation in myeloid leukemia: A model for the origin and progression of malignancy, *Proc. Natl. Acad. Sci. USA* **77**:6152–6156.

Sager, R., 1982, The role of genomic rearrangements in tumor cell heterogeneity. in: *Tumor Cell Heterogeneity: Origins and Implications* (Bristol-Meyers Cancer Symposia, Volume 4) (A. H. Owens, D. S. Coffey, and S. B. Baylin, eds.), Academic Press, New York, pp. 411–423.

Salmon, S. E. (ed.), 1980, *Cloning of Human Tumor Stem Cells*, Liss, New York.

Salmon, S. E., and Trent, J. M., 1984, *Human Tumor Cloning*, Grune & Stratton, New York.

Salmon, S. E., Alberts, D. S., Meyskens, F. L., Jr., and Moon, T. E., 1983, Human tumor stem-cell assay, *N. Engl. J. Med.* **308**:1478.

Salomon, D. S., Zwiebel, J. A., Bano, M., Losonczy, I., Fehnel, P., and Kidwell, W. R., 1984, Presence of transforming growth factors in human breast cancer cells, *Cancer Res.* **44**:4069–4077.

Sandberg, A. A., 1982, Chromosomal changes in human cancers: Specificity and heterogeneity, in: *Tumor Cell Heterogeneity: Origins and Implications* (Bristol-Meyers Cancer Symposia,

Volume 4) (A. H. Owens, D. S. Coffey, and S. B. Baylin, eds.), Academic Press, New York, pp. 367–397.

Saxen, L., Kankinen-Jaaskelainen, M., Lehtonen, E., Nordling, S., and Wartionvaara, J., 1976, Inducive tissue interactions, in: Cell Surface Reviews, Volume 1 (G. Poste and G. L. Nicolson, eds.), North-Holland, Amsterdam, pp. 331–407.

Scheen, S. R., III, Banks, P. M., and Winkelmann, R. K., 1984, Morphologic heterogeneity of malignant lymphomas developing in mycosis fungoides, Mayo Clin. Proc. 59:(2):95–106.

Schirrmacher, V., 1980, Shifts in tumor cell phenotypes induced by signals from the microenvironment: Relevance for the immunobiology of cancer metastasis, Immunobiology 157:89–98.

Schlag, P., and Schreml, W., 1982, Heterogeneity in growth pattern and drug sensitivity of primary tumor and metastases in the human tumor colony-forming assays, Cancer Res. 42:4086–4089.

Schmid, F. A., Hutchison, D. J., Otter, G. M., and Stock, C. C., 1976, Development of resistance to combinations of six antimetabolites in mice with L1210 leukemia, Cancer Treat. Rep. 60:23–27.

Seabright, M., 1976, Patterns of induced aberrations in humans with abnormal autosome complement, in: Chromosomes Today, Volume 5 (P. L. Pearson and K. R. Lewis, eds.), Kieger, Melbourne, Fla., pp. 293–297.

Segre, G., 1979, Pharmacokinetics and antineoplastic drug therapy, in: Chemotherapy of Solid Tumors (F. Pannuti and P. J. Creaven, eds.), Casa Editrice Patron, Bologna, pp. 45–62.

Selby, P., Buick, R. N., and Tannock, I., 1983, A critical appraisal of the "human tumor stem-cell assay," N. Engl. J. Med. 308:129–134.

Selby, P. J., Thomas, J. M., and Peckham, M. J., 1979, A comparison of the chemosensitivity of a primary tumor and its metastases using a human tumor xenograft, Eur. J. Cancer Clin. Oncol. 15:1425–1429.

Shanahan, F., Denburg, J. A., Bienenstock, J., and Befus, A. D., 1984, Mast cell heterogeneity, Can. J. Physiol. Pharmacol. 62:734–737.

Shapiro, J. R., Yung, W.-K. A., and Shapiro, W. R., 1981, Isolation, karyotype, and clonal growth of heterogeneous subpopulations of human malignant gliomas, Cancer Res. 41:2349–2359.

Shapiro, J. R., Pu, P.-Y., Mohamed, S. L., Nielsen, N., Sundaresan, N., and Shapiro, W. R., 1984, Regional heterogeneity in high grade human gliomas, Proc. Am. Assoc. Cancer Res. 25:375a.

Shapiro, W. R., Yung, W.-K. A., Basler, G. A., and Shapiro, J. R., 1981, Heterogeneous response to chemotherapy of human gliomas grown in nude mice and as clones in vitro, Cancer Treat. Res. 65(Suppl. 2):55–59.

Sharkey, F. E., 1983, Morphometric analysis of differentiation of human breast carcinoma: Tumor heterogeneity, Arch. Pathol. Lab. Med. 107:411–414.

Sherwin, S. A., Twardzik, D. R., Bohn, W. H., Cockley, K. D., and Todaro, G. J., 1983, High molecular-weight transforming growth factor activity in the urine of patients with disseminated cancer, Cancer Res. 43:403–407.

Shoemaker, R., Wolpert-Defilippes, M., Kern, D., Lieber, M., Melnick, N., Miller, W., Salmon, S., Simon, R., Venditti, J., and Von Hoff, D., 1984, Antitumor drug screening with a human tumor colony forming assay (HTCFA), Proc. Am. Assoc. Cancer Res. 25:326a.

Shortman, K., 1972, Physical procedures for the separation of animal cells, Annu. Rev. Biophys. Bioeng. 1:93–130.

Siegal, G. P., Barsky, S. H., Terranova, V. P., and Liotta, L. A., 1981, Stages of neoplastic transformation of human breast tissue as monitored by dissolution of basement membrane components, Invasion Metastasis 1:54–70.

Sinkovics, J. G., 1979, Medical Oncology: An Advanced Course, Dekker, New York.

Siracky, J., 1979, An approach to the problem of heterogeneity of human tumor cell population, Br. J. Cancer 39:570–577.

Slack, N. H., and Bross, I. D. J., 1975, The influence of site of metastasis on tumor growth and response to chemotherapy, Br. J. Cancer 32:78–86.

Slocum, H. K., Pavelic, Z. P., and Rustum, Y. M., 1980, An enzymatic method for the disaggregation of human solid tumors for studies of clonogenicity and biochemical determinants of drug action, in: *Progress in Clinical and Biological Research*, Volume 48 (S. Salmon, ed.), Liss, New York, pp. 339–343.

Slocum, H. K., Pavelic, Z. P., Rustum, Y. M., Creaven, P. J., Karakousis, C., Takita, H., and Greco, W. R., 1981a, Characterization of cells obtained by mechanical and enzymatic means from human melanoma, sarcoma, and lung tumors, *Cancer Res.* **41:**1428–1434.

Slocum, H. K., Pavelic, Z. P., Kanter, P. M., Nowak, N.J., and Rustum, Y. M., 1981b, The soft agar clonogenicity and characterization of cells obtained from human solid tumors by mechanical and enzymatic means, *Cancer Chemother. Pharmacol.* **6:**219–225.

Slocum, H. K., Frankfurt, O. S., Pavelic, Z. P., Arbuck, S., and Rustum, Y. M., 1983, Populations of cells from human solid tumors obtained by centrifugal elutriation and characterized by Coulter volume analysis, flow cytometry, and colony formation in soft agar, *Proc. Am. Assoc. Cancer Res.* 24:126a.

Slocum, H. K., Pavelic, Z. P., Greco, W. R., and Rustum, Y. M., 1984, The roles of aggregates in soft agar colony formation assays, *Proc. Am. Assoc. Cancer Res.* 25:377a.

Smith, H. S., Lan, S., Ceriani, R., Hackett, A. J., and Stampfer, M. R., 1981, Clonal proliferation of cultured nonmalignant and malignant human breast epithelia, *Cancer Res.* **41:**4637–4643.

Smith, H. S., Wolman, S. R., and Hackett, A. J., 1984, The biology of breast cancer at the cellular level, *Biochim. Biophys. Acta* **738:**103–123.

Sorg, C., Bruggen, J. Seibert, E., and Macher, E., 1978, Membrane-associated antigens of human malignant melanoma. IV. Changes in expression of antigens on cultured melanoma cells, *Cancer Immunol. Immunother.* **3:**259–271.

Spears, C. P., Gustavsson, B. G., Mitchell, M. S., Spicer, D., Berne, M., Bernstein, L., and Danenberg, P. V., 1984, Thymidylate synthetase inhibition in malignant tumors and normal liver of patients given intravenous 5-fluorouracil, *Cancer Res.* **44:**4144–4150.

Spremulli, E. N., and Dexter, D. I.., 1983, Human tumor cell herogeneity and metastasis, *J. Clin. Oncol.* **1**(8):496–509.

Steel, G. G., Courtenary, V. D., and Peckham, M. J., 1983, The response to chemotherapy of a variety of human tumor xenografts, *Br. J. Cancer* **47:**1–13.

Stephen, J., and Ambrose, E. J., 1983, Application of *in vitro* autoradiography for monitoring drug response in cancer chemotherapy, *Acta Cytol.* **27**(3):362–364.

Stephens, T. C., Peacock, J. H., and Steel, G. G., 1977, Cell survival in B16 melanoma after treatment with combinations of cytotoxic agents: Lack of potentiation, *Br. J. Cancer* **36:**84–93.

Stitch, H. F., and Steele, H. D., 1962, DNA content of tumor cells. III. Mosaic composition of sarcomas and carcinomas in man, *J. Natl. Cancer Inst.* **28:**1207–1218.

Stone, K. R., Mickey, D. D., Wunderli, H., Mickey, G. H., and Paulson, D. F., 1978, Isolation of a human prostate carcinoma cell line (DU145), *Int. J. Cancer* **21:**273–281.

Strauli, P., and Haemmerli, G., 1984, The role of cancer cell motility in invasion, *Cancer Metastasis Rev.* **3**(2):127–141.

Sturani, E., Toschi, L., Zippel, R., Mategani, E., and Alberghina, L., 1984, G1 phase heterogeneity in exponentially growing Swiss 3T3 mouse fibroblasts, *Exp. Cell Res.* **153:**135–144.

Subak-Sharpe, H., Burk, R. R., and Pitts, J. D., 1969, Metabolic cooperation between biochemically marked mammalian cells in tissue culture, *J. Cell Sci.* **4:**353–367.

Sugarbaker, E. V., Cohen, A. M., and Ketcham, A. S., 1971, Do metastases metastasize?, *Ann. Surg.* **174:**161–166.

Talmadge, J. E., Benedict, K., Madsen, J., and Fidler, I. J., 1984, Development of biological diversity and susceptibility to chemotherapy in murine cancer metastases, *Cancer Res.* **44:**3801–3805.

Tan, M. N., Shimano, T., and Chu, T. M., 1981, Differential localization of human pancreas cancer-associated antigen and carcinoembryonic antigen in homologous pancreatic tumoral xenograft, *J. Natl. Cancer Inst.* **67:**563–569.

Tanke, H. J., Van Driel-Kulker, A. M. J., Cornelisse, C. J., and Ploem, J. S., 1983, Combined flow cytometry and image cytometry of the same cytological sample, *J. Microsc.* **130:**11–22.

Tanneberger, S., 1979, Individual cell biology: Bases and prospects for rational cancer chemotherapy, in: *Chemotherapy of Solid Tumors* (F. Pannuti, and P. J. Creaven, eds.), Casa Editrice Patron, Bologna, pp. 27–44.

Tanneberger, S., and Nissen, E., 1983, Predicting response of human solid tumors to chemotherapy, *Cancer Treat. Rev.* **10**:203–219.

Tannock, I. F., 1968, The relation between cell proliferation and the vascular system in a transplanted mouse mammary tumor, *Br. J. Cancer* **22**:258–273.

Teicher, B. A., and Sartorelli, A. C., 1982, Selective attack of hypoxic tumor cells, in: *Design of Models for Testing Cancer Therapeutic Agents* (I. J. Fidler and R. J. White, eds.), Van Nostrand–Reinhold, Princeton, N. J., pp. 19–36.

Teodori, L., Tirindelli-Danesi, D., Mauro, F., DeVita, R., Ucelli, R., Botti, C., Mondini, C., Nervi, C., and Stipa, S., 1983, Non-small-cell lung carcinoma: Tumor characterization on the basis of flow cytometrically determined cellular heterogeneity, *Cytometry* **4**:174–183.

Thompson, L. H., and Suit, H. D., 1969, Proliferation kinetics of X-irradiated mouse cells studied with time-lapse photography. II, *Int. J. Radiat. Biol.* **15**:347–362.

Thomson, S. P., and Meyskens, F. L., 1982, Method for measurement of self-renewal capacity of clonogenic cells from biopsies of metastatic malignant melanoma, *Cancer Res.* **42**:4606–4613.

Till, J. E., and McCulloch, E. A., 1980, Hemopoietic stem cell differentiation, *Biochim. Biophys. Acta* **605**:431–459.

Tisman, G., Hsu, M. Y. K., and Neuman, D., 1982, Human tumor stromal cell assay (HTSCA), *Clin. Res.* **30**:748A.

Todaro, G. J., Marquardt, H., Twardzik, D. R., Johnson, P. A., Fryling, C. M., and De Larco, J. E., 1982, Transforming growth factors produced by tumor cells, in: *Tumor Cell Heterogeneity: Origins and Implications (Bristol-Meyers Cancer Symposia*, Volume 4) (A. H. Owens, D. S. Coffey, and S. B. Baylin, eds.), Academic Press, New York, pp. 205–224.

Torosian, M. H., Tsou, K. C., Daly, J. M., Muller, J. L., Stein, T. P., Miller, E. E., and Buzby, G. P., 1984, Alteration of tumor cell kinetics by pulse total parenteral nutrition, *Cancer* **53**:1409–1415.

Trope, C., 1980, Different susceptibilities of tumor cell subpopulations to cytotoxic agents, in: *Design of Models for Testing Cancer Therapeutic Agents* (I. J. Fidler and R. J. White, eds.), Van Nostrand–Reinhold, Princeton, N. J., pp. 64–79.

Trope, C., 1982, Different susceptibilities of tumor cell subpopulations to cytotoxic agents and therapeutic consequences, in: *Tumor Cell Heterogeneity: Origins and Implications (Bristol-Meyers Cancer Symposia*, Volume 4) (A. H. Owens, D. S. Coffey, and S. B. Baylin, eds.), Academic Press, New York, pp. 147–168.

Trope, C., Hakansson, L., and Dencker, H., 1975, Heterogeneity of human adenocarcinoma of the colon and the stomach as regards sensitivity to cytostatic drugs, *Neoplasma* **22**(4):423–430.

Trope, C., Aspeyran, K., Kullander, S., and Astedt, B., 1979, Heterogeneous response of disseminated human ovarian cancers to cytostatis *in vitro*, *Acta Obstet. Gynecol. Scand.* **58**:543–546.

Vaage, J., 1980, Inherent changes in the *in vivo* growth characteristics of C3H/He mammary carcinomas, *Cancer Res.* **40**:3495–3501.

van den Berg, H. M., Molenaar, W. M., Poppema, S., and Halie, M. R., 1983, The heterogeneity of follicular follicle center cell tumors. II. Clinical follow-up of 30 patients, *Cancer* **52**:2264–2268.

van Zeeland, A. A., van Diggelen, M. C. E., and Simons, T. W. I. M., 1972, The role of metabolic cooperation in selection of hypoxanthine-guanine-phosphoribosyl-transferase (HG-PRT)-deficient mutants from diploid mammalian cell strains, *Mutat. Res.* **14**:355–363.

Vaupel, P. W., Frinak, S., and Bicher, H. I., 1981, Heterogeneous oxygen partial pressure and pH distribution in C3H mouse mammary adenocarcinoma, *Cancer Res.* **41**:2008–2013.

Vindelov, L. L., Hansen, H. H., Christensen, I. J., Sprang-Thomsen, M., Hirsch, F. R., Hansen, M., and Nissen, N. I., 1980, Clonal heterogeneity of small-cell anaplastic carcinoma of the lung demonstrated by flow-cytometric DNA analysis, *Cancer Res.* **40**:4295–4300.

Vlodavsky, I., Lui, M., and Gospodarowicz, D., 1980, Morphological appearance, growth behavior, and migratory activity of human tumor cells maintained on extracellular matrix versus plastic, *Cell* **19**:607–616.

Von Hoff, D. D., 1983, "Send this patient's tumor for culture and sensitivity," N. Engl. J. Med. **308**:154–155.

Von Hoff, D. D., and Weisenthal, L., 1980, In vitro methods to predict for patient response to chemotherapy, Adv. Pharmacol. Chemother. **17**:133–156.

Von Hoff, D. D., Casper, J., Bradley, E., Sanbach, J., Jones, D., and Makuch, R., 1981a, Association between human tumor colony-forming assay results and response of an individual patient's tumor to chemotherapy, Am. J. Med. **70**:1027–1032.

Von Hoff, D. D., Sandbach, J., Osborne, C. K., Metelmann, C., Clark, G. M., O'Brien, M., and the South Central Taxas Human Tumor Cloning Group, 1981b, Potential and problems with growth of breast cancer in a human tumor cloning system, Breast Cancer Res. Treat. **1**:141–148.

Wake, N., Slocum, H. K., Rustum, Y. M., Matsui, S., and Sandberg, A. A., 1981, Chromosomes and causation of human cancer and leukemia. LXIV. A method for chromosome analysis of solid tumors, Cancer Genet. Cytogenet. **3**:1–10.

Wake, N., Isaacs, J. T., and Sandberg, A. A., 1982, Chromosomal changes associated with progression of the Dunning R-3327 rat prostatic adenocarcinoma system, Cancer Res. **42**:4131–4142.

Walle, A., and Niedermayer, W., 1984, Separation of diploid from aneuploid cells in acute lymphoblastic leukaemia, Br. J. Haematol. **57**:571–576.

Warr, D., McKinney, S., and Tannock, I., 1984, Influence of measurement error on assessment of response to anticancer chemotherapy: Proposal for new criteria of tumor response, J. Clin. Oncol. **2**(9):1040–1046.

Waymouth, C., 1974, To disaggregate or not to disaggregate, injury and cell disaggregation, transient or permanent?, In Vitro **10**:97–111.

Weinberg, R. A., 1980, Integrated genomes of animal viruses, Annu. Rev. Biochem. **49**:197–226.

Weiner, F., Fenyo, E. M., Klein, G., and Harris, H., 1972, Fusion of tumour cells with host cells, Nature New Biol. **238**:155–159.

Weisenthal, L. M., 1981, In vitro assays in preclinical antineoplastic drug screening, Semin. Oncol. **8**:362–376.

Weisenthal, L. M., and Lippman, M. E., 1985, Clonogenic and nonclonogenic in vitro chemosensitivity assays, Cancer Treat. Rep. (in press).

Weisenthal, L. M., Marsden, J. A., Dill, P. L., and Macaluso, C. K., 1983, A novel dye exclusion method for testing in vitro chemosensitivity of human tumors, Cancer Res. **43**:749–757.

Weiss, L., 1980, Metastasis: Differences between cancer cells in primary and secondary tumors, Pathobiol. Annu. **10**:51–80.

Weiss, L., 1983, Random and nonrandom processes in metastasis, and metastatic inefficiency, Invasion Metastasis **3**:193–207.

Weiss, L., Holmes, J. C., and Ward, P. M., 1983, Do metastases arise from preexisting subpopulations of cancer cells?, Br. J. Cancer **47**:81–89.

Weiss, M. A., Michael, P. G., Pesce, A. J., and DiPersio, L., 1981, Heterogeneity of B_2-microglobulin in human breast carcinoma, Lab. Invest. **45**:46–57.

Welander, C. E., Homesley, H. D., and Jobson, V. W., 1983, In vitro chemotherapy testing of gynecologic tumors: Basis for planning therapy, Am. J. Obstet. Gynecol. **147**(12):188–195.

Welch, D. R., and Nicolson, G. L., 1983, Phenotypic drift and heterogeneity in response of metastatic mammary adenocarcinoma cell clones to adriamycin, 5-fluoro-2'-deoxyuridine, and methotrexate treatment in vitro, Clin. Exp. Metastasis **1**:317–325.

Welch, D. R., Milas, L., Tomasovic, S. P., and Nicolson, G. L., 1983, Heterogeneous response and clonal drift of sensitivities of metastatic 13762NF mammary adenocarcinoma clones to gamma-radiation in vitro, Cancer Res. **43**:6–10.

Werrlein, R. J., and Glinos, A. D., 1974, Oxygen microenvironment and respiratory oscillations in cultured mammalian cells, Nature **251**:317–319.

Wheeler, K. T., Wallen, C. A., Wolf, K. L., and Siemann, D. W., 1984, Hypoxic cells and in situ chemopotentiation of the nitrosoureas by misonidazole, Br. J. Cancer **49**:787–793.

Wilson, R. E., Antman, K. H., Brodsky, G., and Greenberger, J. S., 1984, Tumor-cell heterogeneity in soft tissue sarcomas as defined by chemoradiotherapy, Cancer **53**:1420–1425.

Wolf, M. K., and Aronson, S. B., 1961, Growth, Fluorescence and metachromasy of cells cultured in the presence of acridine orange, *J. Histochem. Cytochem.* **9**:22–29.

Wolman, S. R., 1983, Karyotypic progression in human tumors, *Cancer Metastasis Rev.* **2**:257–293.

Woodruff, M. F. A., 1983, Cellular heterogeneity in tumours, *Br. J. Cancer* **47**:589–594.

Wright, S., 1982, The shifting balance theory and macroevolution, Annu. Rev. Genet. **16**:1–19.

Yang, J., Guzman, R., Richards, J., and Nandi, S., 1980, Primary culture of mouse mammary tumor epithelial cells embedded in collagen gels, *In Vitro* **16**:502–506.

Yang, K.-P., and Samaan, N. A., 1983, Reduction of estrogen receptor concentration in MCF-7 human breast carcinoma cells following exposure to chemotherapeutic drugs, *Cancer Res.* **43**:3534–3538.

Yung, W.-K. A., Shapiro, J. R., and Shapiro, W. R., 1982, Heterogeneous chemosensitivity of subpopulations of human glioma cells in culture, *Cancer Res.* **42**:992–998.

INDEX